1992
YEAR BOOK OF
TRANSPLANTATION

The 1992 Year Book® Series

Year Book of Anesthesia and Pain Management: Drs. Miller, Abram, Kirby, Ostheimer, Roizen, and Stoelting

Year Book of Cardiology®: Drs. Schlant, Collins, Engle, Frye, Kaplan, and O'Rourke

Year Book of Critical Care Medicine®: Drs. Rogers and Parrillo

Year Book of Dentistry®: Drs. Meskin, Currier, Kennedy, Leinfelder, Matukas, and Rovin

Year Book of Dermatologic Surgery: Drs. Swanson, Salasche, and Glogau

Year Book of Dermatology®: Drs. Sober and Fitzpatrick

Year Book of Diagnostic Radiology®: Drs. Federle, Clark, Gross, Madewell, Maynard, Sackett, and Young

Year Book of Digestive Diseases®: Drs. Greenberger and Moody

Year Book of Drug Therapy®: Drs. Lasagna and Weintraub

Year Book of Emergency Medicine®: Drs. Wagner, Burdick, Davidson, Roberts, and Spivey

Year Book of Endocrinology®: Drs. Bagdade, Braverman, Horton, Kannan, Landsberg, Molitch, Morley, Odell, Rogol, Ryan, and Sherwin

Year Book of Family Practice®: Drs. Berg, Bowman, Davidson, Dietrich, and Scherger

Year Book of Geriatrics and Gerontology®: Drs. Beck, Abrass, Burton, Cummings, Makinodan, and Small

Year Book of Hand Surgery®: Drs. Amadio and Hentz

Year Book of Health Care Management: Drs. Heyssel, Brock, King, and Steinberg, Ms. Avakian, and Messrs. Berman, Kues, and Rosenberg

Year Book of Hematology®: Drs. Spivak, Bell, Ness, Quesenberry, and Wiernik

Year Book of Infectious Diseases®: Drs. Wolff, Barza, Keusch, Klempner, and Snydman

Year Book of Infertility: Drs. Mishell, Paulsen, and Lobo

Year Book of Medicine®: Drs. Rogers, Bone, Cline, Braunwald, Greenberger, Utiger, Epstein, and Malawista

Year Book of Neonatal and Perinatal Medicine®: Drs. Klaus and Fanaroff

Year Book of Nephrology: Drs. Coe, Favus, Henderson, Kashgarian, Luke, Myers, and Strom

Year Book of Neurology and Neurosurgery®: Drs. Currier and Crowell

Year Book of Neuroradiology: Drs. Osborn, Harnsberger, Halbach, and Grossman

Year Book of Nuclear Medicine®: Drs. Hoffer, Gore, Gottschalk, Sostman, Zaret, and Zubal

Year Book of Obstetrics and Gynecology®: Drs. Mishell, Kirschbaum, and Morrow

Year Book of Occupational and Environmental Medicine: Drs. Emmett, Brooks, Harris, and Schenker

Year Book of Oncology®: Drs. Young, Longo, Ozols, Simone, Steele, and Weichselbaum

Year Book of Ophthalmology®: Drs. Laibson, Adams, Augsburger, Benson, Cohen, Eagle, Flanagan, Nelson, Reinecke, Sergott, and Wilson

Year Book of Orthopedics®: Drs. Sledge, Poss, Cofield, Frymoyer, Griffin, Hansen, Johnson, Simmons, and Springfield

Year Book of Otolaryngology–Head and Neck Surgery®: Drs. Bailey and Paparella

Year Book of Pathology and Clinical Pathology®: Drs. Gardner, Bennett, Cousar, Garvin, and Worsham

Year Book of Pediatrics®: Dr. Stockman

Year Book of Plastic, Reconstructive, and Aesthetic Surgery: Drs. Miller, Cohen, McKinney, Robson, Ruberg, and Whitaker

Year Book of Podiatric Medicine and Surgery®: Dr. Kominsky

Year Book of Psychiatry and Applied Mental Health®: Drs. Talbott, Frances, Freedman, Meltzer, Perry, Schowalter, and Yudofsky

Year Book of Pulmonary Disease®: Drs. Bone and Petty

Year Book of Sports Medicine®: Drs. Shephard, Eichner, Sutton, and Torg, Col. Anderson, and Mr. George

Year Book of Surgery®: Drs. Schwartz, Jonasson, Robson, Shires, Spencer, and Thompson

Year Book of Transplantation: Drs. Ascher, Hansen, and Strom

Year Book of Ultrasound: Drs. Merritt, Mittelstaedt, Carroll, and Nyberg

Year Book of Urology®: Drs. Gillenwater and Howards

Year Book of Vascular Surgery®: Dr. Bergan

Roundsmanship®: '92–'93: A Student's Survival Guide to Clinical Medicine Using Current Literature: Drs. Dan, Feigin, Quilligan, Schrock, Stein, and Talbott

1992

The Year Book of TRANSPLANTATION

Editor-in-Chief

Nancy L. Ascher, M.D., Ph.D.
Chief, Liver Transplant Division, Professor of Surgery, University of California, San Francisco

Editors

John A. Hansen, M.D.
Senior Vice President and Director, Clinical Research Division, Professor of Medicine, University of Washington, Seattle

Terry Strom, M.D.
Professor of Medicine, Harvard Medical School; Director, Division of Clinical Immunology, Beth Israel Hospital

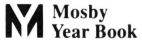
Mosby Year Book

St. Louis   Baltimore   Boston   Chicago   London   Philadelphia   Sydney   Toronto

Editor-in-Chief, Year Book Publishing: Kenneth H. Killion
Sponsoring Editor: Kelly Blossfeld
Manager, Literature Services: Edith M. Podrazik
Senior Information Specialist: Terri Santo
Senior Medical Writer: David A. Cramer, M.D.
Assistant Director, Manuscript Services: Frances M. Perveiler
Associate Managing Editor, Year Book Editing Services: Connie Murray
Senior Production/Desktop Publishing Manager: Max F. Perez
Proofroom Manager: Barbara M. Kelly

Editorial Office:
Mosby–Year Book, Inc.
200 North LaSalle St.
Chicago, IL 60601

International Standard Serial Number: 1060-2968
International Standard Book Number: 0-8151-0251-8

Table of Contents

Journals Represented

Mosby–Year Book subscribes to and surveys nearly 900 U.S. and foreign medical and allied health journals. From these journals, the Editors select the articles to be abstracted. Journals represented in this YEAR BOOK are listed below.

American Journal of Cardiology
American Journal of Diseases of Children
American Journal of Gastroenterology
American Journal of Kidney Diseases
American Journal of Medicine
American Journal of Roentgenology
American Journal of Surgical Pathology
Annals of Internal Medicine
Annals of Surgery
Blood
Bone Marrow Transplantation
British Journal of Surgery
British Medical Journal
Canadian Journal of Surgery
Chest
Clinical Genetics
Clinical Nephrology
Clinical Transplantation
Clinical and Experimental Immunology
Diabetes
Diabetologia
European Heart Journal
European Journal of Surgery
Gastroenterology
Hepatology
Journal of Clinical Microbiology
Journal of Clinical Pathology
Journal of Experimental Medicine
Journal of Heart Transplantation
Journal of Heart and Lung Transplantation
Journal of Immunology
Journal of Pediatric Surgery
Journal of Pediatrics
Journal of Thoracic and Cardiovascular Surgery
Journal of Urology
Journal of the American Medical Association
Journal of the American Society of Nephrology
Kidney International
Lancet
Lung
Medical Journal of Australia
Medicine
Metabolism
Microsurgery
Nephrology, Dialysis, Transplantation
Nephron
New England Journal of Medicine
New York State Journal of Medicine

Proceedings of the National Academy of Sciences
Quarterly Journal of Medicine
Radiology
Reviews of Infectious Diseases
Scandinavian Journal of Immunology
Science
Seminars in Hematology
Surgery
Surgery, Gynecology and Obstetrics
Therapeutic Drug Monitoring
Transplantation
Transplantation Proceedings
Virchows Archiv A: Pathological Anatomy and Histopathology

STANDARD ABBREVIATIONS

The following terms are abbreviated in this edition: acquired immunodeficiency syndrome (AIDS), central nervous system (CNS), cerebrospinal fluid (CSF), computed tomography (CT), electrocardiography (ECG), human immunodeficiency virus (HIV), and magnetic resonance (MR) imaging (MRI).

Publisher's Preface

We are pleased to present the premier volume of the YEAR BOOK OF TRANSPLANTATION. We are grateful to Dr. Nancy Ascher and her editorial colleagues Dr. John Hansen and Dr. Terry Strom for their belief in the need for this new series; for the hard conceptual work that went into defining the scope, structure, and limits of the content; and of course for the week-to-week work of developing the content for our readers.

Mosby-Year Book, Inc., started this series because organ transplantation has become a large, diverse clinical reality supported by an extraordinary range of scientific disciplines. We believe that all who are engaged in organ transplantation can benefit from "the YEAR BOOK service" — *surveillance* of the world medical literature, *selection* by experts of the most significant articles, *condensation* of those articles by skilled medical writers, and *commentary* from the experts who selected the articles.

We sincerely hope that this new publication will be of real value to its intended audience, and we invite your comments.

As Publishers, we feel challenged to seek ways of presenting complex information in a clear and readable manner. To this end, the 1992 YEAR BOOK OF TRANSPLANTATION provides structured abstracts in which the various components of a study can easily be identified through headings. These headings are not the same in all abstracts, but, rather are those that most accurately designate the content of each particular journal article. We are confident that our readers will find the information contained in our abstracts to be clear, concise, and easily accessible.

1 Kidney Transplantation

Role of HLA Matching in Renal Transplantation

▶ ↓ As the transplant community moves sluggishly to expand the role of HLA matching in kidney grafts, the evidence continues to mount that the rate of engraftment—especially long-term—improves with the quality of the match. It has been long known that the quality of serologic matching for HLA class II molecules (DR, etc.) is inferior to the accuracy of matching for HLA class I molecules (A,B,C). Molecular genetic techniques are now shown to be more accurate than serologic analysis (1) for class II typing. Can these techniques be used within the time restraints imposed by current organ preservation techniques? Probably!—Terry Strom, M.D.

Reference

1. Mytilineous J, et al: *Transplantation* 50:870, 1990.

National Allocation of Cadaveric Kidneys by HLA Matching: Projected Effect on Outcome and Costs
Gjertson DW, Terasaki PI, Takemoto S, Mickey MR (UCLA Tissue Typing Laboratory, Los Angeles)
N Engl J Med 324:1032–1036, 1991
1–1

Introduction.—Transplantation of a cadaveric kidney matched at the HLA-A, B, and DR loci enhances graft survival in cyclosporine-treated patients. The value of a national system of kidney allocation based on HLA matching remains controversial. The costs of such a system may be unjustified. The effect of HLA matching on graft survival for all allocations of cadaveric kidneys in the United States was estimated.

Methods.—Data on 22,190 first-time cadaveric kidney recipients were partitioned to estimate the graft-survival rates in 5 mutually exclusive groups of transplants with increasing numbers of HLA mismatches. Overall graft survival was projected as a weighted average, using percentages of transplants in the hierarchical groups in recipient waiting pools of various sizes. The costs and benefits of HLA matching in a national system were compared with those of cyclosporine introduction, which was estimated to enhance graft survival by 7% of 10 years.

Results.—Sharing kidneys nationally based on hierarchical HLA matching enhanced graft survival by an estimated 5% at 10 years. The anticipated 5-year cost of this national system for 7,000 recipients would be $6.5 million less than the cost of using cyclosporine alone. This estimated cost included costs of graft removal and dialysis after transplant rejection (Fig 1–1).

Conclusions.—A national HLA allocation system will not add to the

1

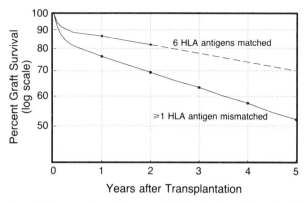

Fig 1–1.—Actuarial 5-year graft-survival curves *(solid lines)* and projections *(dashed line)* for 365 first-time recipients of cadaver kidneys matched for 6 HLA antigens and 21,621 recipients of transplants with at least 1 HLA-antigen mismatch. The differences between groups after 3, 6, 12, and 24 months were all significant ($P < .001$). (Courtesy of Gjertson DW, Terasaki PI, Takemoto S, et al: *N Engl J Med* 324:1032–1036, 1991.)

cost of renal transplantation. It will improve the long-term results by 5%, similar to that of cyclosporine. The initiation of a national kidney-sharing system based on hierarchical levels of HLA matches is proposed.

▶ What increases long-term kidney transplant engraftment, does not have serious side effects, is cost efficient and is hardly ever used in practice? You got it! The correct answer is HLA typing. I still don't understand why we don't use this powerful tool more effectively.—T. Strom, M.D.

A Report of 504 Six Antigen-Matched Transplants
Takemoto S, Carnahan E, Terasaki PI (UCLA Tissue Typing Laboratory, Los Angeles)
Transplant Proc 23:1318–1320, 1991   1–2

Background.—Since 1987, more than 500 transplants have been performed in recipients matched for 6 antigens (6Ag). Two-year survival rates were calculated using data from those cases.

Methods and Results.—The results in 6Ag, homozygous, and non-shipped kidneys from the University of California, Los Angeles Transplant Registry having more than zero mismatches transplanted in the same period were compared. The 6Ag results were significant from 3 months to 2 years for first cadavers. Second graft results were significantly better for up to 1 year. The matching effect disappeared for subsequent transplants. The poor results in 6Ag-matched recipients with multiple regrafts may have been a result of mismatches at other histocompatibility loci. Sixty-three percent of the first 6Ag grafts had a cold ischemia time (CIT) of less than 24 hours, whereas longer CITs did not adversely

Effect of High Plasma Renin Activity Percent in 6-Antigen
Transplants

	No. of Cases	3 mos	6 mos	1 yr	2 yr
First Graft					
0%-10%	194	93.1	88.7	88.7	85.3
11%-50%	51	93.8	87.3	87.3	81.7
51%-80%	23	90.9	90.9	90.0	
>80%	46	88.9	88.9	83.3	83.3
>First Graft					
0%-10%	28	96.2	88.2	74.9	74.9
11%-50%	29	86.0	75.0	70.2	70.2
51%-80%	18	88.2	75.6	62.1	62.1
>80%	49	93.7	79.9	74.5	

(Courtesy of Takemoto S, Carnahan E, Terasaki PI: *Transplant Proc* 23:1318–1320, 1991.)

affect graft survival. No detrimental effect for high plasma renin activity was found for first or regraft 6Ag transplants (table). Forty percent of the regrafts had a plasma renin activity greater than 80%.

Conclusions.—The Six-Antigen Match Program, started in 1987, has been successful. One-year graft survival was 87%, compared with 79% for transplant Registry controls and 76% for contralateral controls. Hospital stays were shorter and serum creatinine levels were lower for 6Hg-matched recipients. Despite the fact that a higher than expected number of patients with 6Hg-matched transplants had diabetes, their 1-year graft survival rate was 89%.

▶ The reports from Teraski and Opelz' laboratories consistently demonstrate a salutary effect of HLA typing upon renal engraftment. This report joins a list of publications making this important point (see Table 1 in the original article). Perhaps the most profound impact of matching is noted in highly presensitized patients (table). This group fares miserably with HLA mismatched transplants but excellent engraftment can be achieved with HLA matched grafts. This study, which uses conventional serologic DR typing methods almost certainly underestimates the benefits of HLA typing because DNA-based methodologies will provide additional benefits because of their heightened accuracy.—T. Strom, M.D.

HLA Matching Enhances Long-Term Renal Graft Survival But Does Not Relate to Acute Rejection

Baltzan MA, Baltzan RB, Baltzan BL, Cunningham TC, Pylypchuk GB, Dyck RF, West ML (University of Saskatchewan, Saskatoon, Canada)
Medicine 69:227–231, 1990

Background.—The HLA system's effect on graft survival would be manifested in the rejection process. Forty living donor kidney grafts of patients with more than 1 but less than 2 haplotype matches were examined.

Patients.—The patients, average age 32 years, were treated during a 25-year period. The most common cause of renal failure was chronic glomerulonephritis. Thirty-one patients had 2 haplotype matches, and 9 had more than 1 but less than 2. There were 33 primary oper-ations. Prophylactic corticosteroids were used in all patients. Azathioprine was used in 34 patients and cyclosporine was used in 6.

Findings.—Among patients who were not treated with cyclosporine and who had 5 or fewer units of blood preoperatively, 65% had acute rejection. However, in those who had more than 5 units, only 18% had acute rejection. All such patients had successful reversal with high-dose steroids. There were 2 patients with chronic rejection, but no patient undergoing a second graft had irreversible rejection. One patient had chronic glomerulonephritis, perhaps because of recurrent disease. Technical and immunosuppressive complications resulted in the loss of 1 graft each, whereas 3 more patients died incidentally. As a whole, the group had a 1-year actuarial graft survival rate of 95% and a 10-year survival rate of 84%. Survivors were leading normal lives with no significant restrictions and minimal medications.

Conclusions.—In kidney transplantation, chronic rejection appears to be dependent on HLA factors and is largely preventable by close HLA matching. Acute cellular rejection appears to be independent of HLA. There may be a relationship between hyperacute and chronic rejection that represents parts of a spectrum of humoral immunity.

▶ OK, I picked this article because I believe the conclusions are correct (even if the sample size is too small to draw any firm conclusions). The large registries headed by Opelz and Terasaki show that the salubrious influence of HLA matching on successful engraftment grow with time. Whereas differences are modest at 1–2 years posttransplantation between well and poorly matched transplants, the typing effect is quite powerful at 5–10 years posttransplant. Shouldn't we aim for more transplant "keepers?" So what if surgeons hate the notion of allocating kidneys on the basis of histocompatibility.—T. Strom, M.D.

The Effect of Individual HLA-A and -B Mismatches on the Generation of Cytotoxic T Lymphocyte Precursors
Zhang L, van Bree S, van Rood JJ, Claas FHJ (University Hospital, Leiden, The Netherlands)
Transplantation 50:1008–1010, 1990   1–4

Background.—Both the HLA system and cytotoxic T cells are known to play important roles in graft rejection, but there has been little study of the interrelationship between these factors. A limiting dilution analysis was used to study the correlation between HLA mismatching and cytotoxic T lymphocyte (CTL) precursor frequency.

Methods.—The subjects were 21 highly sensitized patients waiting for renal transplantation. The limiting dilution culture technique was used to ascertain CTL precursor frequencies against the patients' individual mismatched HLA-A and HLA-B alloantigens. A total of 33 HLA-A alloantigens and 55 HLA-B antigens was tested.

Results.—Cytotoxic T lymphocyte precursor frequencies against HLA-A antigens were significantly lower on the average than those against HLA-B antigens (Fig 1–2). High CTL precursor frequencies were induced by 44% of HLA-B antigens compared with only 15% of the HLA-A antigens. Frequencies were unaffected by the number of DR mismatches or the age and sex of the patients.

Conclusions.—Cytotoxic T lymphocyte precursor frequencies are higher

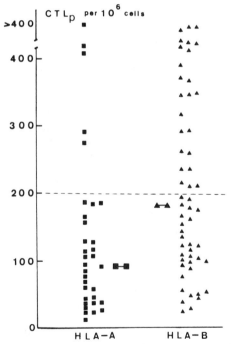

Fig 1–2.—Cytotoxic T lymphocyte precursor (CTLp) frequencies against individually mismatched HLA-A *(filled square)* and HLA-B *(filled triangle)* antigens in 21 patients. *Filled squares connected by a line* and *filled triangles connected by a line* represent the medians of CTLp frequencies against 33 HLA-A antigens and 55 HLA-B antigens, respectively. Mismatched HLA-B antigens showed significantly higher CTLp frequencies compared with those generated by mismatches of HLA-A locus antigens. ($P <$ .002). (Courtesy of Zhang L, van Bree S, van Rood JJ, et al: *Transplantation* 50:1008–1010, 1990.)

in response to mismatched HLA-B than HLA-A antigens. The differential effect of these antigens on the generation of donor-specific CTL precursors may explain the greater importance of matching HLA-B antigens.

▶ The number of potential killer cells (cytotoxic T lymphocytes or CTLs) that can be activated by a given antigenic stimulus can be quantitated by limiting dilution techniques. The precursor frequency of CTLs activated by a stimulus can be determined. This article offers an interesting vignette. Mismatches for HLA-B locus antigen result in activation of a higher number of activated CTLs than mismatches for HLA-A locus antigens (Fig 1–2). This is especially interesting if you buy the notion that HLA-B locus matching is more important than HLA-A locus matching. I'm an agnostic on this topic. I'd like to see DNA typing used to assess the relative importance of HLA-A and HLA-B locus matching before I subscribe to this view.—T. Strom, M.D.

Comparison of RFLP-DR Beta and Serological HLA-DR Typing in 1500 Individuals
Mytilineos J, Scherer S, Opelz G (University of Heidelberg, West Germany)
Transplantation 50:870–873, 1990   1–5

Background.—For technical reasons, serologic typing of HLA-DR antigens is often problematic. Typing of HLA-DR by analysis of DNA restriction fragment-length polymorphism (RFLP), introduced recently, permits an exact definition of HLA-DR alleles. The reliability of RFLP typing was tested in a clinical laboratory setting.
Methods and Findings.—The standard serologic technique and the RFLP method were both used to type 1,522 people. Although 11% of the serologic typings were unsuccessful or doubtful technically, all RFLP typings were successful. An error rate of 25% was noted in the results of the remaining 1,358 serologic typings. In 16%, a serologic "blank" was found to be a definable allele by RFLP. In 9%, an allele was incorrectly interpreted serologically. Eleven percent of individuals tested were HLA-DR homozygous by RFLP.
Conclusions.—Although the RFLP method for HLA-DR typing is time-consuming and involves the use of radioactivity, it has an impressive qualitative advantage over serology. All serologic typing failures in this study could be typed successfully by RFLP. Nearly all "blanks" were resolved. Another important advantage of this method is that it can recognize homozygous individuals without family typing. The RFLP typing is especially useful for typing bone marrow transplant recipients in whom serology often fails and for kidney transplant candidates with "blanks."

▶ Given the remarkably high error rate of serologic typing for DR, it is amazing that HLA typing exerts a strong influence for long-term renal engraftment. Of course, the technically, less demanding procedures for HLA class I typing are far more accurate. There is simply no doubt that RFLP or other molecular genetic techniques must be quickly developed for cadaver donor kidney transplantation. The effect of accurate DNA-based typing may prove almost revolutionary in its impact on long-term engraftment.—T. Strom, M.D.

Immune Status in Renal Transplant Recipients

▶ ↓ Patients who harbor high titer anti-HLA antibodies are at high risk for immunologic graft loss. As a consequence, efforts in several quarters proceed to remove HLA antibodies from circulation. The specific and nonspecific immune status of transplant recipients is important in predicting outcome.—Terry Strom, M.D.

Extracorporeal Removal of Anti-HLA Antibodies in Transplant Candidates
Hakim RM, Milford E, Himmelfarb J, Wingard R, Lazarus JM, Watt RM
(Vanderbilt Univ, Nashville; Brigham and Women's Hosp, Harvard Med School, Boston; El Du Pont de Nemours & Company, Glenolden, Penn)
Am J Kidney Dis 16:423–431, 1990   1–6

Background.—When antibodies play an important part in an underlying disease process, they are usually of the immunoglobulin G class. However, current methods of immunoglobulin removal, such as plasma exchange, are not specific, lowering all plasma proteins indiscriminately. The safety and efficacy of an extracorporeal system for removing immunoglobulin and its effect on HLA antibody activity were studied in highly sensitized hemodialysis patients awaiting cadaveric transplantation.

Methods.—Fourteen transplant candidates were enrolled in the clinical trial. Treatment consisted of an extracorporeal immunoadsorption system using Protein A that selectively removes immunoglobulin from plasma. The dynamics of anti-HLA antibody as a model of IgG removal and reequilibration were also assessed.

Results.—At the end of a course of treatment, plasmas IgG levels had dropped by a mean 90% compared with control values. Albumin levels were decreased by only 15%. Specific cytotoxic anti-HLA antibody titers were decreased about 18-fold. Nine patients had a significant reduction in panel reactivity, measured as the proportion of a 40-member cell donor panel killed by patients' serum in the presence of complement. Anti-HLA antibody titers returned to baseline values during the 4-week follow-up. Blood chemistry evaluation showed no remarkable changes. There were no unanticipated adverse reactions.

Conclusions.—Transient, significant reduction of IgG and HLA antibodies in patients awaiting cadaveric transplantation is a safe and effective procedure. The device used improves the selectivity of plasmapheresis used in many treatment protocols of active immunologic disease. The cost and efficacy of plasmapheresis were also improved. This procedure may become useful in managing highly sensitized transplant candidates, and in other diseases in which antibody plays a pathogenetic role.

▶ Staphylococcal protein A avidly binds to IgG and binds IgA and IgM with lesser affinity. Hence, immobilized protein A can be used to deplete IgG from a given fluid. This principle has been tested in clinical practice as a means to deplete anti-HLA antibodies from the circulation of highly presensitized transplant candidates by extracorporeal immunoadsorption. This is a far more selective means of depleting anti-HLA antibodies than plasmapheresis, which depletes bulk plasma. Using this approach, the titer of anti-HLA antibodies was reduced in most, but not all, subjects. The IgG3, which is known to bind to protein A with lower affinity than the other IgG isotypes, was only partially depleted. This manipulation proved safe. Other workers have shown that at least some highly presensitized patients can be successfully transplanted following this form of pretreatment. Should this treatment be regularly instituted in highly presensitized individuals? It is expensive. It is dubious that the success rate will rival that achieved in primary, unsensitized graft recipients. Because the organ supply cannot satisfy the need to supply organs to patients with a better prognosis for long-term graft function, I do not favor routine use of this treatment. Isn't the goal in clinical transplantation to rehabilitate as many patients as possible? This technique, while suitable for preparing patients for emergency or urgent transplants, does not support these Millsian goals. As a consequence, I agree wholeheartedly with the trend to preferentially transplant blue ribbon unsensitized candidates because they are more likely to gain long-term engraftment. Moreover, Terasaki and his colleagues maintain that a superb rate of engraftment in highly presensitized patients can be achieved by use of 6 antigen matched donors. I'd think matching, rather than expensive treatment, is the way to go.—T. Strom, M.D.

Adsorption of Cytotoxic Anti-HLA Antibodies With HLA Class I Immunosorbant Beads

DeVito LD, Sollinger HW, Burlingham WJ (Univ of Wisconsin Hosp and Clinics, Madison)
Transplantation 49:925–931, 1990   1–7

Background.—The growing number of highly sensitized patients is a major problem in clinical transplantation today. For such patients, the provision of a negatively crossmatched donor kidney is unlikely or impossible. Treatment must include removing the cytotoxic anti-HLA class I antibodies and preventing their resynthesis.

Methods.—In an effort to generate HLA immunosorbants to specifically remove anti-HLA antibodies from sera of highly sensitized patients, HLA proteins were purified and coupled covalently onto Sepharose. Antisera was adsorbed from 5 patients with narrowly reactive cytotoxic anti-HLA antibodies and from 1 patient with broadly reactive antibodies.

Findings.—An HLA-A2 immunosorbant depleted anti-HLA-A2 cytotoxic antibodies but not anti-HLA-B7 or anti-HLA-B44 cytotoxic antibodies from the narrowly reactive sera. In 1 patient high panel-reactive antibody developed with strong cytotoxicity against HLA-A1 and HLA-A2 after an HLA-A1, HLA-B57 mismatched kidney was rejected. His sera was adsorbed with 5 HLA immunosorbants, including HLA-A2 and HLA-A1, 28. The HLA-A2 immunosorbant depleted antibodies to

HLA-A2$^+$ and HLA-B57$^+$ cells but not to HLA-A1$^+$ cells. The HLA-A1, A28 immunosorbant depleted antibodies to both HLA-A1$^+$ and HLA-A28 cross-reactive HLA-A2$^+$ cells. Adsorption was specific for HLA-A alleles to which the patient was sensitized.

Conclusions.—The HLA immunosorbants are stable to sequential cycles of adsorption and elution. Therefore, they may be of future value in the treatment of sensitized patients.

Decreased Lymphokine-Activated Killer Cells in Kidney Transplant Recipients: Correlation With a Diminished Number of CD3$^-$/NKH1$^+$ Cells

Alard P, Lantz O, Ramirez A, Perrot JY, Chavanel G, Fries D, Charpentier B, Senik A (Institut de Recherches Scientifiques sur le Cancer, Villejuif, France; Hôpital de Bicdêtre, Kremlin-Bicêtre, France; Université Paris VI, Paris, France)
Transplantation 50:250–257, 1990   1–8

Background.—There is a high incidence of malignancies in patients who have had kidney transplantation. Natural killer cell activity is known to be impaired, but there have been no studies of lymphokine-activated killer (LAK) cell activity in these patients. Lymphokine-activated killer activity in kidney transplant recipients was compared to that of hemodialysis patients with chronic renal insufficiency and normal controls.

Methods.—Subjects were 30 kidney transplant recipients, mean follow-up 42 months since operation. These randomly selected patients had normal renal function and had received various immunosuppressive regimens depending on the date of their transplant. Thirteen hemodialysis patients who were on a waiting list for transplantation or had some contraindication to it were also studied. Eighteen normal controls were studied. All subjects had measurement of LAK cell activity by a clonal or polyclonal technique.

Results.—Lymphokine-activated killer cell activity was decreased to a highly significant degree in the renal transplant recipients compared to the other 2 groups. The transplant group also had a lower percentage of CD3$^-$/NKH1$^+$ cells. There was a strong correlation between LAK activity and percentage of CD3$^-$ cells, but not between LAK activity and percentage of double-positive CD3$^+$/NKH1$^+$ cells. Percentage of CD3$^-$/NKH1$^+$ cells was the only significant variable in determining LAK activity; even pathologic status was insignificant. The T cell-specific functions of interleukin-2 secretion and specific cytotoxic activity were preserved in the kidney transplant recipients.

Conclusions.—Kidney transplant recipients appear to have deficient LAK cell activity mainly because of a decreased number of CD3$^-$/NKH1$^+$ cells. T cell function is normal in these patients, suggesting that their high rate of malignancies is related to their LAK deficiency. In vivo, CD3$^+$ cells do not appear to make a significant contribution to LAK precursors.

▶ This analysis was undertaken because natural killer (NK) cells can lyse certain, but not all, tumor cells in vitro without an obvious need for pre-immunization. Lymphokine-activated killer (LAK) cells are derived from NK cells. As the term LAK cells suggests, NK cells are cytokine (IL-2) activated NK cells. Because transplant patients are subject to an increased incidence of tumors, NK cells have been studied extensively posttransplantation. Cells expressing NK function are a heterogenous lot. I don't believe NK cells express a single surface phenotype, but I do agree that the majority of NK cells have the CD3⁻ CD16⁺, NK⁺ phenotype.

A comparative analysis of LAK activity, LAK precursor cell frequency and alloreactive T cell functions was undertaken in a dialysis population and in patients 6 months to 12 years posttransplantation. In keeping with observations made in many laboratories, it was found that T cell functions were essentially normal in transplant recipients no longer taking early posttransplant high dose regimens. It is interesting—maybe even curious—that LAK activity selectivity deteriorated posttransplantation. Moreover, this defect was associated with a decreased circulating number of CD3⁻NK⁺ cells. The authors go on to postulate that this defect contributes to the increased number of malignancies noted in posttransplant patients. This postulate may be correct, but the support—other than guilt by association—is weak. Are there data to indicate that NK/LAK cells are of special importance in protecting the host from the curious types of cancers that occur most commonly in posttransplant patients—skin cancer, EBV transformed lymphomas, etc.? Nonetheless, this interesting study cannot be dismissed ex cathedra.—T. Strom, M.D.

Recovery of Decreased Ability of Peripheral-Blood Mononuclear Cells From Chronic Renal Failure to Produce Interleukin-1α and β After Renal Transplantation
Kang X-X, Hirano T, Oka K, Tamaki T, Sakurai E, Kaji N, Yoshida M, Kozaki M (Hachioji Medical Center Tokyo, Tokyo College of Pharmacy, Tokyo)
Nephron 58:450–455, 1991   1–9

Background.—Defective immune function has been implicated in nephrotic syndrome, and recent studies have found suppressive plasma factors that counter blood lymphocyte responses to mitogens in this disorder. Because release of interleukin-1 (IL-1) by monocytes is involved in many immune and inflammatory processes, monocyte-macrophage function may be altered in nephrotic syndrome.

Study.—The ability of cultured peripheral-blood mononuclear cells to release interleukin in response to concanavalin A was estimated in 42 patients with chronic renal failure (CRF) and in 69 renal transplant recipients with functioning grafts. Forty-two healthy age-matched subjects also were studied.

Findings.—Blood cells from patients with CRF released less IL-1α than cells from the renal transplant patients or control subjects. A similar difference was found in levels of IL-1β release. Interleukin release declined for 2–3 weeks after renal transplantation and then gradually increased. The transient decline in IL-1 release did not correlate with acute allograft rejection.

Conclusions.—Monitoring the ability of stimulated blood mononuclear cells to release IL-1 may help predict the course of CRF. Interleukin release is only temporarily suppressed after uncomplicated renal transplantation.

▶ This study calls attention, once again, to the immunodeficiency state that is associated with chronic renal failure. Numerous studies have documented this immunodeficiency using different end points. Many years ago, my mentor, John Merrill, and his colleagues demonstrated that hosts with renal failure mounted impaired delayed-type hypersensitivity reactions. In this study, peripheral-blood mononuclear cells were stimulated with Con A and IL-1 production into supernatants was measured (see Figure 1 in the original article). As expected, patients with chronic failure produced only meager quantities of IL-1. After transplantation, IL-1 production plummeted even further. This further decrease in IL-1 production is undoubtedly due to the effects of corticosteroid therapy since steroids have been shown to block production of IL-1 and IL-6 at the transcriptional or pretranscriptional level. Corticosteroids also block production of TNF, IL-2, gamma interferon. Cyclosporine also blocks production of IL-2 and gamma IFN but not IL-1. Only IL-1 production was measured in this study. Production of IL-2 is also deficient in patients with chronic renal failure.

Following dose reduction in steroid therapy, IL-1 production increased in transplant recipients. Indeed, in these patients, IL-1 production exceeded levels noted in CRF patients and was equivalent to production in normal subjects. It has been noted in many other studies that low-dose maintenance immunosuppression has little effect on de novo immune responses. In clinical practice, opportunistic infection is almost exclusive to heavily immunosuppressed patients in the early posttransplant period. Following dose reductions, this phenomenon disappears. This study catalogues the aspect of this scenario. Early posttransplantation, the hefty maintenance doses usually used cause a marked immunodeficiency, but later immune function is remarkably normal.—T. Strom, M.D.

T Cell Subsets Mediating Rejection of Established Fetal Pancreas Grafts and Failure to Observe Graft Adaptation
Rees MA, Rosenberg AS, Singer A (Natl Cancer Inst, Natl Insts of Health: Food and Drug Administration, Bethesda, Md)
*Transplantation*49:1130–1133, 1990   1–10

Background.—Research has shown a difference in the immunogenicity of freshly transplanted fetal pancreas grafts compared with isolated adult pancreatic islet grafts. Although CD4$^+$ cell depletion in vivo does not interfere with the ability of animals to reject fresh fetal pancreas grafts, it does abrogate their ability to reject pancreatic islet allografts. Also, as the fetal pancreatic graft matures, the exocrine part of the fetal pancreas dies away, leaving mostly intact islets of Langerhans and a few contaminating ductal elements. The rejection response directed against long-term established fetal pancreatic grafts was studied, because these grafts should represent an intermediary between fresh fetal pancreas and isolated islet grafts.

Methods.—In the experimental model used, H-2^b nude mice were made hyperglycemic by streptozotocin treatment, then engrafted with allogeneic fetal pancreas grafts. Engrafted animals returned to near normoglycemia, and the unengrafted animals subsequently died. Fetal pancreas grafts were left to reside in the immunoincompetent nude host for 6 to 9 months before T cell reconstitution. At this time, animals were reconstituted with either negatively selected CD4$^+$ or CD8$^+$ H-2^b T cell subpopulations.

Results.—A 6- to 9-month residence in an immunoincompetent host did not result in a change in the immunogenicity of fetal pancreatic grafts. Both CD4$^+$ and CD8$^+$ T cell subsets were able to reject the long-term established fetal pancreas grafts.

Conclusions.—There is a difference in the ability of isolated CD8$^+$ T cells to effect rejection of long-term established fetal pancreas allografts and their ability to effect islet allograft rejection. This difference is probably attributable to the absence of donor-derived APC in the islet allografts able to activate class I allospecific CD8$^+$ T$_h$ cells. This means that the purified islet allografts contain donor-derived APC able to activate only CD4$^+$ and not CD8$^+$ T$_h$ cells or are wholly devoid of donor-derived APC. In the latter case, antigen presentation would be accomplished only by reprocessing of exogenous donor-derived alloantigens by host APC and presentation of these reprocessed antigens to major histocompatibility complex (MHC) class II-restricted CD4$^+$ T$_h$ cells, as exogenous antigens do not activate MHC class I-restricted CD8$^+$ T$_h$ cells.

Differential Effects of Interleukin 2 Receptor-Targeted Therapy on Heart and Kidney Allografts in Rats: Depression of Effectiveness of ART-18 Monoclonal Antibody Treatment by Uremia
Ueda H, Hancock WW, Cheung Y-C, Tanaka K, Kupiec-Weglinski JW, Tilney NL (Harvard Med School; Brigham and Women's Hosp, Boston)
Transplantation 49:1124–1129, 1990   1–11

Background.—There is an impression that organs and tissues may differ substantially in immunogenicity and may also influence host immune responses differentially. Expression of major histocompatibility complex (MHC) antigens may be a dynamic, organ-dependent process in allograft rejection. The route of host immunization may also be a factor in differential tissue and organ effects, especially for skin and islet allografts.

Objective.—The differences in host immunity between cardiac and renal allografts were examined using established rat models. Treatment targeted against interleukin-2 receptors (IL-2R) on activated cells served as a probe. Immunosuppression was done with ART-18, a mouse IgG1 antibody that recognizes the IL-2-binding domain of the rat p55 subunit IL-2R molecule. It inhibits both IL-2 binding and IL-2-dependent T cell growth.

Observations.—Both kidney and heart allografts survived about 3 weeks in ART-18-treated rats, but the host responses varied. Although the splenic ratio of CD4+ to CD8+ cells was similar in treated and un-

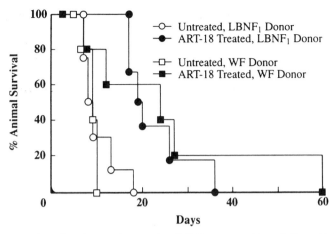

Fig 1–3.—Kidney allograft survival in rats after ART-18 treatment (300 μg/kg/day x 10 days intravenously). The death of animals from uremia was used as the time of graft injection ($n = 5-8$). (Courtesy of Ueda H, Hancock WW, Cheung Y-C, et al: *Transplantation* 49:1124–1129, 1990.)

treated animals given cardiac allografts, it decreased significantly in kidney recipients conditioned with ART-18. Both CD4+ and CD8+ cells from kidney-grafted hosts suppressed the mixed lymphocyte reaction (MLR) in vivo, but only the CD8$^+$ cells were effective in the cardiac allograft model. A significant proportion of the renal cell infiltrate remained IL-2R$^+$ despite continued monoclonal antibody treatment, but IL-2R$^+$ cells were absent from the cardiac grafts of treated hosts. Although ART-18 prolonged renal graft survival significantly (Fig 1–3), prolonged graft function was poor and the animals remained uremic. If a native kidney was retained and renal function remained normal, the Il-2R$^+$ cells were absent from the graft infiltrate.

Implications.—Treatment with ART-18 affects host responses differently in animals with renal and cardiac allografts, despite comparable prolongation of survival. Uremia prevents the elimination of infiltrating IL-2R$^+$ mononuclear cells by monoclonal antibody, possibly explaining why such treatment has been less effective than expected.

▶ All antigen-activated T cells express, at least transiently, high affinity IL-2 receptors. Indeed, the alpha chain of the receptor complex is expressed exclusively on activated T cells. As a consequence, we originally hypothesized that targeting the IL-2R with cytocidal agents should produce effective and highly selective immunosuppression. We first tested this hypothesis in a mouse model of heart transplantation and produced tolerance (1). The powerful effect of anti-IL-2R mAbs was extended to a rat model of cardiac transplantation in collaboration with the group undertaking the present study (2). In a DTH model, we demonstrated that cytocidal, not receptor blockade effects were crucial to achieve full immunosuppression (3).

In the present study, the authors exploit the differing effects of anti-IL-2R mAb treatment on rat cardiac and renal transplantation. The immunosuppressive effects of anti-IL-2R mAb treatment were far more profound in recipients of cardiac allografts than in nephrectomized recipients of kidney allografts (Fig 1–3). When this paradox was analyzed, the uremic state accounted for the differential effect since mAb treatment was quite potent in kidney graft recipients who were spared pretransplant nephrectomy. The pathologic correlate to this situation was revealed when it was discovered that anti-IL-2R mAb treatment failed to lyse infiltrating leukocytes in uremic hosts. This failure probably results from a defective ADCC mechanism in uremic hosts. In any event, these results validate the concept that IL-2 receptor-targeted therapy requires cytocidal agents. First generation murine mAbs are not potent in this regard. Humanized mAbs and/or chimeric toxins may provide useful cytocidal agents for clinical use.—T. Strom, M.D.

References

1. Kirkman RL, et al: *J Exp Med* 162:358, 1985.
2. Kupiec-Weglinski J, et al: *Proc Natl Acad Sci USA* 83:2624, 1986.
3. Kelley VE, et al: *J Immunol* 138:2771, 1987.

Donor-Specific Cytotoxic T Lymphocyte Hyporesponsiveness Following Renal Transplantation in Patients Pretreated With Donor-Specific Transfusions
Grailer AP, Sollinger HW, Kawamura T, Burlingham WJ (Univ of Wisconsin Hosp and Clinics, Madison)
Transplantation 51:320–324, 1991   1–12

Background.—Research on donor-specific transfusion (DST) has shown numerous effects on donor-specific T lymphocyte responses. Although the effects of DST on the mixed leukocyte culture response are generally suppressive, there are a variety of effects on cytotoxic T lymphocyte (CTL) responses. Posttransplant CTL hyporesponsiveness to donor alloantigens has been described in prednisone/azathioprine-immunosuppressed renal transplant recipients with cadaveric organs. Whether the development of antidonor CTL hyporesponsiveness correlates with decreased rejection incidence was investigated in DST-treated patients in the first year after transplantation.

Methods and Findings.—Donor-specific CTL hyporesponsiveness developed in peripheral blood lymphocytes up to 2 years after transplantation in patients preconditioned with 3 donor-specific transfusions plus azathioprine. In 12 patients, the hyporesponsiveness developed gradually. It became detectable in some patients as soon as 1 month after transplantation. It was statistically significant for the whole group at 9 to 12 months after the transplant. Some patients had a complete specificity for donor alloantigens, and others had partial suppression of the response to a third party HLA-mismatched control. In 1 patient, the mechanism of donor-specific CTL hyporesponsiveness was explored 2 years after transplantation. This patient had received a 2-HLA haplotype-mismatched kidney transplant from her husband. Bulk culture CTL analysis demonstrated specific nonresponsiveness to donor stimulators. However, the antidonor response was restored to pretransplant peripheral blood lymphocyte levels in the presence of exogenous recombinant IL-2. Limiting dilution analysis showed equivalent precursor frequency of antidonor CTL in pretransplant and posttransplant peripheral blood lymphocytes.

Conclusions.—Posttransplant CTL hyporesponsiveness to donor develops gradually in peripheral blood of kidney transplant recipients after DST treatment. Although clonal deletion of antidonor CTL precursors may contribute to the protective effect of DST in some cases, defective lymphokine production may be a more important mechanism in other cases.

Multivariate Analysis of Donor-Specific Versus Random Transfusion Protocols in Haploidentical Living-Related Transplants
Reed A, Pirsch J, Armbrust MJ, Burlingham WJ, Knechtle SJ, D'Alessandro AM, Sollinger HW, Lorentzen D, Kalayoglu M, Belzer FO (Univ of Wisconsin Hosp and Clinics, Madison)
Transplantation 51:382–384, 1991   1–13

Background.—The role of blood transfusions in the preconditioning of renal allograft recipients continues to be debated. The use of preoperative donor-specific transfusion (DST) was compared with random transfusion (RT) in one-haplotype-matched living-related transplants.

Methods.—One hundred twenty-seven haploidentical living-related transplants were studied retrospectively. Seventy-four patients had a DST plus azathioprine, and 53 had RT. All patients were given cyclosporine beginning 1 week before transplantation. In both groups, immunosuppression consisted of triple induction treatment with prednisone, cyclosporine, and thioprine. Seven patients were sensitized in the first group and 1 in the second group, leaving 67 and 52 patients, respectively, for analysis.

Findings.—Actuarial graft survival was comparable in the 2 groups. Two-year graft survival was 95% in the DST group and 91% in the RT group. Patients with RT had significantly more rejection episodes and had them sooner than the DST group. At 1 year, 50% of those in the DST group had at least 1 episode, compared with 75% in the RT group. According to a multivariate analysis of 10 variables, only DST and pregnancy significantly predicted rejection episodes; both were protective.

Conclusions.—Although the difference in rejection episodes and their timing between the DST and RT groups was significant, this difference has not yet translated into a significant difference in graft survival between the groups. The potential benefit of DST may lie in its capacity to allow early steroid withdrawal. Further research is needed to establish the effect of transfusion group on long-term graft survival and to test this hypothesis.

The Flow Cytometric Crossmatch and Early Renal Transplant Loss

Mahoney RJ, Ault KA, Given SR, Adams RJ, Breggia AC, Paris PA, Palomaki GE, Hitchcox SA, White BW, Himmelfarb J, Leeber DA (Found for Blood Research, Scarborough, Me; Maine Cytometry Research Inst, Portland, Me)
Transplantation 49:527–535, 1990   1–14

Background.—T and B cell-bound class-specific antibody can be very sensitively detected by the flow cytometric crossmatch test (FCXM). A positive FCXM has been found to be associated with episodes of rejection and graft failure. Flow cytometric crossmatch test results, HLA antibody levels, rejection episodes, and graft survival were studied in 90 cadaveric renal allograft recipients.

Findings.—There were 67 primary and 23 regraft procedures. Eight of the primary grafts and 6 of the regrafts were lost within 2 months; 10 of these were HLA sensitized and FCXM positive. Of the remaining 76 allografts, 12 were FCXM positive. The FCXM tests, therefore, had a sensitivity of 71% and specificity of 84% in detecting early graft loss. At 2 months, the primary grafts had a 33% loss rate and FCXM-positive regrafts had a 60% loss rate. These figures contrasted with the 7% rate for primary and 0% rate for FCXM-negative regrafts. Among FCXM-positive graft recipients, a previous early graft loss appeared to be a contraindication for transplantation of a FCXM-positive regraft. There was no association between panel reactive antibody of 10% or less at crossmatch and early graft loss. At 1 year, there was no difference in graft survival between primary and regrafts, regardless of FCXM status. Of the 12 FCXM-positive grafts that survived 2 months, all continued to function at 2 years. The FCXM was shown to be the best predictor of early graft loss, and an FCXM channel shift of 29 or greater on a 1,024-channel log scale increased the risk of early graft failure 7 times compared with the first and second tertiles.

Conclusions.—The FCXM test may represent a useful supplementary approach to identifying sensitized patients at risk of early kidney allograft loss. There are associations between positive FCXM, high rates of irreversible rejection, and level of sensitization and early graft failure. Early failure is not related to the number of HLA mismatched antigens or the donor's age, gender, or cause of death.

▶ Conventional crossmatches detect preformed antidonor antibodies in many, but not all, patients bearing such antibodies. The incidence of accelerated rejection and immunologic graft failure remains higher in crossmatch-negative highly presensitized than in nonsensitized patients. Hence, pre-existant antidonor immunity must be missed in patients destined to experience accelerated rejection. Although it is uncertain whether this immunity is cellular, humoral, or a mix, it is certainly reasonable to determine whether more sensitive screening methods for detecting antidonor antibodies provide clinically useful data. Detection of antibody binding to donor cells by flow cytometric detection is clearly more sensitive than tests that use target cell lysis as an end point. It has been a matter of controversy whether flow cytometric testing is too sensitive and picks up clinically irrelevant antibodies. This study indicates that flow cytometric detection can identify patients at very high risk to reject their graft (see Figure 3 in the original article). Should this analysis be verified, we may have taken an important step toward improved donor selection.—T. Strom, M.D.

Local Events in Renal Allograft Rejection

▶ ↓ As Yogi Berra once pointed out, you can see a lot just by looking. Pathologic investigation of transplant continues to yield important clinical and scientific data. Fine needle aspiration cytology and conventional histologic analysis have been used to evaluate long-term transplants. The possible participation of hyurolan has been invesigated and use of in situ hybridization to detect intergraft transcripts has now been exploited. New molecular genetic techniques are almost certain to add a new layer of sophistication to our understanding of the events of graft rejection.—Terry Strom, M.D.

Fine-Needle Aspiration Cytology and Conventional Histology in 200 Renal Allografts
Reinholt FP, Bohman S-O, Wilczek H, von Willebrand E, Häyry P (Karolinska Institutet, Stockholm; Huddinge University Hospital, Huddinge; University of Helsinki)
Transplantation 49:910–912, 1990   1–15

Background.—Fine-needle aspiration biopsy (FNAB) is used as an adjunct or alternative to conventional core biopsy in monitoring renal allografts in many centers. The FNAB findings have been compared to those of conventional core biopsies, but the number of studies is limited. A systematic comparison of 200 parallel fine- and core-needle biopsies from human renal allografts was assessed.

Methods.—Parallel fine-needle and core biopsies were obtained from 200 patients. Of these, 162 had reduced kidney function and 38 had biopsies performed as protocol follow-up during phases of stable kidney function. The diagnoses in parallel fine-needle and core biopsies were compared.

Results.—Fine-needle aspiration biopsy was a reliable diagnostic tool. Its sensitivity and specificity in acute cellular rejection was 81% and 92%, respectively. In normal kidney grafts, its sensitivity and specificity was 78% and 82%, respectively. However, it was less valuable in diagnosing vascular rejection or interstitial fibrosis.

Conclusions.—Although FNAB is an excellent tool for the diagnosis of acute cellular rejection, further study is needed of the diagnostic implications of isometric vacuolization of tubular cells in FNAB specimens as a marker for acute cyclosporine nephrotoxicity.

▶ Fine-needle aspiration biopsy appears to be a reliable means to monitor intragraft events in the first several weeks following engraftment. During this period, it is often critical to establish or discard the diagnosis of cellular rejection during periods of graft dysfunction. The FNAB technique is well suited to aid in this enterprise (see Table 1 in the original article). As time elapses, however, it becomes crucial to monitor for vascular rejection and severe CsA toxicity. Immunologic endothelial damage and intense interstitial fibrosis are not detected by this means. Hence, I would not be comfortable relying on FNAB after the first month after transplantation.—T. Strom, M.D.

Immunopathological Patterns in Long-Term Renal Allografts
Bohman S-O, Wilczek HE, Reinholt FP, von Willebrand E, Häyry P (Karolinska Institutet, Stockholm; Huddinge Hospital, Huddinge; University of Helsinki)
Transplantation 51:610–613, 1991   1–16

Background.—The factors that determine the long-term outcome of renal allografts are not well defined. In many cases, the reasons for late failure of a graft remain unknown. The occurrence and pattern of various immunologic markers were studied in renal allograft biopsy specimens obtained after transplantation.

Methods.—Forty-eight consecutive core-needle biopsy specimens were obtained 12 to 158 months after transplantation. Assessments included a conventional histologic investigation, an immunohistochemical analysis of various immune system markers, and cytologic analyses of simultaneously obtained fine-needle aspiration biopsy specimens. Findings in grafts with excellent and reduced function were compared, as well as those in patients who were immunosuppressed with azathioprine or cyclosporine.

Results.—All those with excellent renal graft function had normal cytologic immunohistologic patterns, regardless of the type of immunosuppression they received. The presence of inflammatory cell infiltration in a long-term renal graft therefore suggests a pathologic process that may be clinically significant. Biopsy specimens from cyclosporine-treated patients with reduced renal function that showed a normal picture or focal interstitial fibrosis histologically were also usually normal in cytologic and immunohistologic patterns. Five of 36 specimens from grafts with reduced function had immunohistochemical patterns with signs of immune activation that could not be distinguished from those seen in early acute rejection. The immunopathologic pattern varied in cases with histologic signs of chronic rejection, suggesting that different pathogenetic mechanisms were involved.

Conclusions.—The finding of cellular infiltration in a long-term renal allograft indicates the presence of a pathologic process of clinical importance. This study also confirms the nonimmunologic nature of chronic cyclosporine nephrotoxicity. Clear signs of immune activation may sometimes be found in long-term allografts with deteriorating function.

▶ Conventional immunohistology and FNAB specimens obtained from long-term renal allograft recipients were examined. The biopsies were categorized as normal, immune activation (interstitial diffuse mononuclear leukocytic infiltrate with IL-2 receptor positive cells), focal lymphocytic infiltrate, diffuse lymphocytic infiltration (infiltrating cells lack expression of the IL-2 receptor), and thrombocytic aggregation (see Table 4 in the original article). The grafts with "normal" pathology had excellent function. The presence of any pattern of lymphocytic infiltration was associated with reduced function. Many biopsies of grafts with impaired function in CsA-treated but not azathioprine-treated patients lacked meaningful lymphocytic infiltration, thereby indicating that CsA toxicity, a nonimmunologic mechanism, is likely to have caused graft dysfunction.—T. Strom, M.D.

The Localization of Hyaluronan in Normal and Rejected Human Kidneys
Wells AF, Larsson E, Tengblad A, Fellström B, Tufveson G, Klareskog L, Laurent TC (Uppsala University, Sweden)
Transplantation 50:240–243, 1990   1–17

Background.—Hyaluronan (HYA) is a large glycosaminoglycan with a considerable capacity to immobilize water. Increased levels of HYA have been found in plasma and in tissues associated with various inflammatory disorders.

Objective.—A biotin-labeled HYA binding protein was used as a probe to determine the distribution of HYA in normal and rejected human kidneys. Six biopsies of normal kidney tissue and 6 irreversibly rejected renal grafts were studied.

Observations.—In the normal kidneys, HYA was found exclusively in the connective tissue and in the medulla. The tubular cells themselves were negative. Increased HYA staining, especially in the cortex, was observed in the rejected kidneys. The sclerotic glomeruli were also stained. The amount of HYA was also increased interstitially, especially in areas of prominent tubular atrophy.

Summary.—In the normal renal medulla, HYA is present in a peritubular distribution. It is increased in both the medulla and the cortex of rejected kidneys, and it also appears in the sclerotic vessels. Increased amounts of HYA may contribute to local edema formation in a rejecting kidney allograft. Monitoring HYA in renal grafts may help to predict rejection.

▶ The substance HYA (aka, hyaluranon or hyaluronic acid) accumulates in the medulla and cortex and in sclerotic vessels of rejected kidneys (see Figures 1 and 2 of the original article). This substance joins an enormous number of molecules that can be localized to rejected organs. It is certain that HYA accumulation results from a complicated chain reaction of events that are proximal to generation of HYA. It is hard to believe that this fascinating phenomena is central to graft rejection. While this is an interesting report, I'm not about to make anti-HYA mAbs to block rejection.—T. Strom, M.D.

Differential In Situ Expression of Cytokines in Renal Allograft Rejection
Vandenbroecke C, Caillat-Zucman S, Legendre C, Noel L-H, Kreis H, Woodrow D, Bach J-F, Tovey MG (INSERM U25, Hôpital Necker, Paris; Charing Cross and Westminster Medical School, London)
Transplantation 51:602–609, 1991   1–18

Background.—Although renal transplantation has become an established practice in clinical medicine, the mechanisms underlying allograft rejection remain largely unknown. The hallmark of acute graft rejection is damage to endothelial and parenchymal cells, resulting in impaired renal function. The expression of interleukin 6 (IL-6), tumor necrosis factor α (TNFα), and interferon γ (IFN-γ) genes was examined in renal biopsy specimens from persons without evidence of kidney disease and from patients undergoing acute renal allograft rejection.

Methods.—A method of in situ hybridization capable of detecting 1 to 5 copies of a specific cellular messenger RNA in individual cells was used. None of the sections of normal human kidneys showed IL-6, TNF-α, or IFN-γ RNA transcripts. However, sections of the renal biopsies from 6 of 8 patients showing acute rejection showed increased levels of IL-6 mRNA. There was a uniform level of IL-6 mRNA expression in all cells examined, including glomerular cells, tubular epithelia, smooth muscle cells, vascular endothelia, and the interstitial mononuclear infiltrate. In 1 patient with acute rejection, juxtatubular clusters of TNF-α mRNA were detected in the absence of IL-6 mRNA. Only a small number of grains in the urinary space or in tubular or vascular lumen was noted after hybridization with the IL-6 or TNF-α probes. By contrast, transplant recipients with stable renal function had no significant labeling with the IL-6, TNF-α, or IFN-γ probes. All the sections of normal and transplanted kidneys studied had a similar level of expression of actin mRNA, suggesting that the overall level of RNA synthesis was comparable in the 2 groups.

Conclusions.—Through the use of a highly sensitive, specific method of in situ hybridization, it was shown that the expression of IL-6 but not IFN-γ mRNA is substantially increased during acute cellular rejection of human kidney allografts compared with normal kidney and grafted kidney with normal function. This is the first report of the use of a direct means for detecting cytokine gene expression within human allografts undergoing rejection.

▶ The techniques of molecular immunology are now being applied to clinical and preclinical transplant specimens. Because of the great importance of cytokines in immunologic and inflammatory reactions, several groups are probing the expression of various cytokines in such specimens. Some workers are using labeled anticytokine antibodies for this purpose. Each tissue section can be tested for expression of cytokines if the cytokine is exuberantly expressed. Most laboratories, including mine, have attempted to detect specific cytokine mRNAs. Northern blot analysis, the simplest means of detecting a specific mRNA, has proven too insensitive to detect intralesional mRNAs. My laboratory has used a polymerase chain reaction (PCR) assisted reverse transcription analysis. This powerful technique can detect the proverbial needle in a haystack. Sensitivity is not a problem. On the other hand, we and others have found that it is imperative to use quantitative methods for PCR analysis because many transplant specimens contain at least a few activated inflammatory cells. Even small scale expression of cytokine mRNAs can be detected. Hence, it becomes important to determine how much of a given mRNA is present. Is abundant, but not meager, expression of a given cytokine gene associated with rejection? This PCR-based method uses mRNA extracted from the biopsy so that the nature of the cell transcribing a given gene and not the influence of local gene transcription on neighboring cells can be established.

In situ labeling of specific mRNAs can be accomplished on biopsy specimens. The sensitivity of this method can be higher than that of Northern blot analysis if a minority of the cells within a given sample are transcribing the gene. This is the circumstance with transplant tissues. While the in situ hybridization technique is not as sensitive as PCR, the cell actively transcribing the test gene can be identified. As the field of molecular diagnostics evolves, the reader will need to understand the strengths and weaknesses of these alternative techniques, because perfect concordance between these techniques will occur only when a specimen is laden with a specific transcript or it lacks the transcript entirely. In the circumstance where a modest number of transcripts are present, PCR is more likely to detect, but not to localize, the transcript. This report indicates that IL-6 encoding mRNA is present in acute rejection specimens as detected by in situ hybridization (see Figure 1 in the original article). In keeping with the foregoing commentary, we detect IL-6 mRNA in both rejecting and nonrejecting samples by PCR. Hence, we are now evaluating the quantity of IL-6 transcripts in these samples.—T. Strom, M.D.

Cardiac Evaluation in the Renal Transplant Recipient

▶ ↓ Transplantation is a zero sum game. To allocate a transplant to 1 patient on the waiting list automatically deprives another individual of a transplant. Obviously it is of the utmost importance to allocate a transplant—this precious resource—in a utilitarian manner. Clearly, the stress of transplant surgical procedure should not be used as a vehicle to determine whether a recipient has life-endangering cardiovascular disease. Renal failure patients are plagued by a high incidence of cardiovascular disease. The consequences of hypertension, hyperlipidemia, and perhaps altered mineral metabolism lay the ground work for cardiovascular disease. Diabetics are especially prone to the development of coronary artery disease. The following 4 articles deal with evaluation of cardiac function and coronary artery potency in patients being considered for transplant.

The report from Van den Broek et al. emphasizes the potential reversible nature of left ventricular dysfunction in uremic patients. The remaining 3 articles deal with pretransplant evaluation of coronary artery disease. It is important to note that while exercise radionucleotide angiocardiography (Cottier et al.) accurately identifies the presence or absence of coronary artery disease in most uremic patients, this technique is not effective in diabetic patients with ESRD (Holley et al.). In diabetic patients, intravenous dipyridamole thallium imaging is a more accurate means of identifying patients with coronary artery disease (Camp et al.).—Terry Strom, M.D.

Improved Left Ventricular Function After Renal Transplantation
Van Den Broek JH, Boxall JA, Thomson NM (Prince Henry's Hospital, Melbourne)
Med J Aust 154:279–280, 1991   1–19

Background.—Even in patients with normal renal function, left ventricular impairment is considered a poor prognostic sign. When this condition occurs in a patient with concomitant renal failure, kidney transplantation is sometimes not offered as an option. A patient in whom left ventricular function improved dramatically after kidney transplantation was studied.

Case Report.—Man, 20, who was seen with a headache was found to have IgA nephropathy with advanced renal damage. The next year, he became uremic and began hemodialysis; he tolerated this treatment poorly and was admitted for continuous ambulatory peritoneal dialysis. At this time, he was found to have a murmur of mitral incompetence, raised jugular venous pressure, and radiologic cardiomegaly. He had a left ventricular end-diastolic diameter of 5.8 cm and fractional shortening of 7%. His condition deteriorated to left ventricular failure, severe peripheral neuropathy, and reactive depression. The next year, he complained of symptoms of weakness; he had ECG signs of left ventricular hypertrophy and strain, a left ventricular end-diastolic diameter of 6.7 cm, and fractional shortening of 4%. Renal transplantation was done as the only real chance for recovery in this patient, almost 2 years from the initial presentation. His postoperative course was mostly uneventful; his cardiac function improved; and his mitral regurgitation murmur disappeared. At 6 months after transplantation, he had a left ventricular end-diastolic diameter of 5.6 cm and a fractional shortening of 30%.

Conclusions.—Hemodialysis patients with severe left ventricular impairment may show dramatic improvement in their heart condition with kidney transplantation. It cannot be predicted which patients will show this response, but kidney transplant may resolve the problem alone in some patients, making cardiac transplant unnecessary. The probable cause of left ventricular disease in the study patient was "uremic cardiomyopathy."

▶ We have recently begun to study our middle-older age transplant candidates by echocardiography. To our surprise, left ventricular function can improve markedly after transplantation. This fascinating case report dramatizes this point. "Uremic cardiomyopathy" is not a contraindication to transplantation. Indeed, the development of severe uremic cardiomyopathy may be an indication for emergency transplantation.—T. Strom, M.D.

Cardiac Evaluation of Candidates for Kidney Transplantation: Value of Exercise Radionuclide Angiocardiography
Cottier C, Pfisterer M, Müller-Brand J, Thiel G, Burkart F (University Hospital Basel, Switzerland)
Eur Heart J 11:832–838, 1990   1–20

Background.—Renal transplant recipients have a high incidence of and mortality from coronary artery disease (CAD). It is important therefore, to identify patients with significant CAD before kidney transplantation.

Methods.—A protocol for systematic cardiac assessment was set up and prospectively followed from 1984 to 1987. One hundred three patients with uremia who were eligible for transplantation were studied. After clinical assessment, 28 patients with symptoms of CAD or diabetes mellitus were directly referred for coronary angiography. The remaining 75 had rest and exercise radionuclide angiocardiography for assessment of possible asymptomatic CAD.

Findings.—Left ventricular ejection fraction (EF) was below 40% at rest or fell during exercise by at least 5 EF% in 12 cases. Coronary angiography was clone in 9 patients and showed CAD in 4 and hypertensive heart disease in 5. A mean 28-month follow-up of the remaining 63 without severe resting left ventricular dysfunction or exercise ischemia showed no clinical manifestations of CAD. The overall incidence of CAD in symptomatic and asymptomatic patients during the 27-month follow-up after cardiac assessment was 20% and 25% in those without diabetes and those with diabetes, respectively.

Conclusions.—Clinical assessment combined with exercise radionuclide angiocardiography in patients without signs or symptoms of heart disease had a high predictive accuracy for the presence or absence of late manifestations of CAD. Thus, exercise radionuclide angiography is a useful way to screen candidates for kidney transplantation for asymptomatic CAD.

▶ As demonstrated in this and other analyses, many patients with end-stage renal disease have coronary artery disease. In a group of nondiabetic patients with end-stage renal disease, exercise radionuclide angiocardiograms proved to be a valuable method—even in asymptomatic subjects—of screening for coronary artery disease.—T. Strom, M.D.

Thallium Stress Testing Does Not Predict Cardiovascular Risk in Diabetic Patients With End-Stage Renal Disease Undergoing Cadaveric Renal Transplantation
Holley JL, Fenton RA, Arthur RS (Univ of Pittsburgh)
Am J Med 90:563–570, 1991   1–21

Background.—The appropriate cardiovascular assessment for diabetic patients before cadaveric kidney transplantation is controversial. The use of thallium stress testing was evaluated as a predictor of perioperative cardiovascular risk in such patients with end-stage renal disease.

Methods.—The records were reviewed of 189 consecutive patients with diabetic nephropathy assessed for cadaveric renal transplantation. In 141 patients the initial examination of cardiovascular status was thallium stress testing, and in 44 it was cardiac catheterization. In 4 patients no formal cardiovascular assessment was done before transplantation.

Results.—Sixty-four patients who had thallium stress testing had adequate and normal findings. In this group the incidence of perioperative

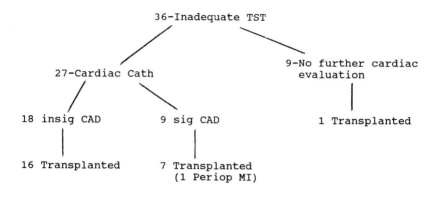

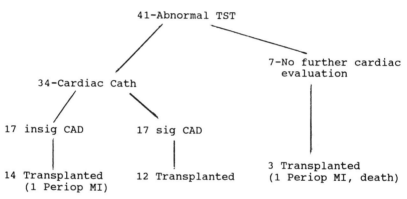

Fig 1–4.—Evaluation outcomes of patients with abnormal or inadequate thallium stress tests. *TST*, thallium stress test; *cath*, catheterization; *CAD*, coronary artery disease; *Periop*, perioperative; *MI*, myocardial infarction. (Courtesy of Holley JL, Fenton RA, Arthur RS: *Am J Med* 90:563–570, 1991.)

cardiac events was 2%. Forty-one others had abnormal findings on the thallium stress test, and in 36 the test was inadequate. Sixty-one of these 77 patients then had coronary angiography. The only factor predicting an abnormal or inadequate test was the use of β-blockers. Of the patients with an inadequate or abnormal thallium stress test, 43% had significant coronary artery disease according to cardiac catheterization. The perioperative risk of cardiac events was similar in those who had a normal and adequate thallium stress test and in the other patient groups combined. Patients with normal and adequate tests had a survival similar to that of patients with an abnormal or inadequate test. This survival was significantly longer than that in patients undergoing cardiac catheterization as the initial test. Thallium stress testing was less expensive than cardiac catheterization (Fig 1–4).

Conclusions.—Thallium stress testing allowed 45% of the patients in this series to avoid cardiac catheterization. Discontinuing β-blockers before stress testing may increase exercise performance. The relatively low predictive value of thallium stress testing for significant coronary artery disease and perioperative cardiac events in this patient population suggests the need for a more cost-effective, noninvasive screening tool.

▶ Patients who have diabetes mellitus, especially those with end-stage renal disease, are exceptionally prone to develop atherosclerosis. Given the propensity of patients with diabetes mellitus to sustain bouts of painless myocardial ischemia, it seems reasonable that the transplant operation should not serve as a trial by fire procedure to determine the identify of patients stricken with covert coronary artery disease. Do all diabetics require preoperative coronary arteriograms? First the good news. A previous study by this group indicated that diabetics who achieved at least 70% of this maximal predicted heart rate during a thallium stress test rarely had significant coronary artery disease; however, only 45% of patients reached the described heart rate.

In this follow-up study, treatment of diabetic end-stage renal disease patients with β-blockers was identified as an important impediment to reaching the desired heart rate. More worrisome was the poor predictability of noninvasive testing in the analysis that includes data from multiple centers and included 30 observers.

Because of the failure of many diabetics to achieve an adequate heart rate, we use dipyrimadole-thallium scans as a screening test. Nonetheless, several groups have maintained that the pattern of reperfusion is different in patients with end-stage renal disease than in other patient populations.

Organ transplantation is a zero sum game. Allocation of an organ to 1 patient deprives another potential recipient of that organ. An effective means of assessing coronary artery disease in diabetics before transplantation is an urgent need. We may not be able to accomplish this goal by means other than coronary arteriography.—T. Strom, M.D.

Prognostic Value of Intravenous Dipyridamole Thallium Imaging in Patients With Diabetes Mellitus Considered for Renal Transplantation
Camp AD, Garvin PJ, Hoff J, Marsh J, Byers SL, Chaitman BR (St Louis Univ, St Louis, Mo)
Am J Cardiol 65:1459–1463, 1990   1–22

Background.—Diabetic patients with end-stage renal failure are at high risk for cardiac morbidity and mortality associated with renal transplantation. The best way to establish preoperative cardiac risk has not been determined. The efficacy of intravenous dipyridamole thallium imaging was assessed in predicting cardiac events.

Methods.—A total of 40 diabetic renal transplant candidates were enrolled in the prospective trial. The patients were aged 27 to 64 years, with a mean of 42 years; 88% were hypertensive and 53% smoked cigarettes. Whereas 6 of the patients had chest pain, 3 had prior myocardial infarction. Dipyridamole thallium imaging was done using .56 mg/kg of dipyridamole infused intravenously for 4 minutes.

Findings.—Dipyridamole thallium imaging showed that 9 patients had reversible defects, 8 had fixed defects, and 23 had normal findings. Cardiac events occurred only in the 6 patients with reversible thallium defects. Of these 6 patients, 3 had cardiac events before transplantation and 3 had them in the early postoperative period (within 6 weeks of surgery). Of the 21 patients who underwent renal transplantation, 3 had cardiac events within 6 weeks of surgery.

Conclusions.—Dipyridamole thallium imaging is an effective way to identify those renal transplant candidates who are likely to develop cardiac complications. Routine coronary angiography may not be needed to screen all renal transplant candidates preoperatively.

▶ It is crucial to screen for the presence of coronary artery disease in diabetic candidates for organ transplantation. These patients are notorious for experiencing silent bouts of myocardial ischemia, and yet the incidence of coronary artery disease is very high among diabetics with end-stage renal disease. Routine stress electrocardiograms or stress thallium scans do not get the job done. Most of these patients cannot exercise vigorously enough to reach the target heart rate. In other patient populations, thallium imaging combined with the use of dipyridamole to induce maximal vasodilation has proven useful. These benefits can apparently be extended to this target patient population (see Figure 1 in the original article). Should this report be verified, many patients will be spared the necessity for coronary arteriograms—obviously a far more invasive procedure.—T. Strom, M.D.

Role of Ultrasonography in Kidney Transplantation

▶ ↓ I have long believed that sonography provides a lovely means to delineate the anatomical attributes of the graft and surrounding tissues. I have also believed that the individuals who claimed they could distinguish rejection from acute tubular necrosis were either using different and better instrumentation than I had available or were also great tea leaf readers. The following cluster of articles reinforces my own prejudice that over-reliance on the sonogram can unnecessarily delay obtaining a biopsy—a procedure that can provide real answers about the presence or absence of rejection.—Terry Strom, M.D.

Ultrasonography of Renal Allografts: Collecting System Dilatation and Its Clinical Significance
Kashi SH, Lodge JPA, Giles GR, Irving HC (St James's University Hospital, Leeds, England)
Nephrol Dial Transplant 6:358–362, 1991   1–23

Objective—Ultrasound is used routinely to assess the complications of renal transplantation and to diagnose pelvicalyceal dilatation. The degrees of pelvicalyceal dilatation in patients with good or poor renal function and the long-term outcome and problems associated with early dilatation were assessed. The impact of ureteral blockage on graft survival and function was also investigated.

Study Plan.—The results of ultrasound procedures were reviewed for 135 patients (49 females, 86 males) with a median age of 38.5 years (range, 5–71 years) undergoing renal transplantation between January 1987 and December 1988. Ultrasound examinations occurred on day 3 after transplantation, then weekly, providing 658 ultrasound scans for analysis. Long-term follow-up of at least 18 months was recorded for each subject.

Findings.—Of the 658 ultrasound scans from the 135 patients who received kidney transplants, 522 were categorized as normal, whereas 112 and 24 showed mild and moderate-to-severe dilatation of the pelvicalyceal area, respectively. Fifty-eight patients had some evidence of dilatation at least once. Eleven individuals with mild dilatation had moderate-to-severe dilatation during the follow-up. Four of the 42 patients (9.5%) with mild dilatations eventually had a ureteral obstruction; 10 of 16 patients with moderate-to-severe dilatation eventually had such an obstruction. Cyclosporine nephrotoxicity occurred in 40 (33%) of the 121 nonobstructed and in 5 (36%) of the 14 blocked kidney grafts. In 5 of 26 grafts with acute tubular necrosis a blockage developed. Twenty patients either had rejection of the allograft or died, for a 1-year survival rate of 85%. Renal function was significantly worse in patients with ureteral obstruction.

Conclusion.—A patient with moderate-to-severe dilatation of the allograft should undergo aggressive and persistent follow-up immediately to reduce potential renal damage.

▶ A simple message. Ultrasonographic detection of progressive collecting system dilatation or severe dilatation accurately detects ureteric obstruction. Detection of ureteric obstruction prevents early graft failure but does not prevent modest graft dysfunction.—T. Strom, M.D.

Evaluation of Renal Transplant Dysfunction by Duplex Doppler Sonography: A Prospective Study and Review of the Literature
Perrella RR, Duerinckx AJ, Tessler FN, Danovitch GM, Wilkinson A, Gonzalez S, Cohen AH, Grant EG (Univ of California, Los Angeles)
Am J Kidney Dis 15:544–550, 1990   1–24

Background.—How effective duplex Doppler sonography is in detecting acute renal transplant rejection was examined. Widely varying sensitivities have been reported, depending on the diagnostic criteria used. This double-blind prospective study was comprised of 157 duplex Doppler sonograms acquired from 49 consecutive renal transplant recipients because of suspected acute rejection. Most patients had received cadaver kidney transplants.

Findings.—The sensitivity of sonography for detecting acute rejection declined markedly at a high detection threshold. The test had a positive predictive value of 67% using a high threshold and 73% using a low threshold value. A resistive index exceeding .85 consistently correlated with cellular rejection, whereas a lesser value usually also was associated with cellular rejection.

Conclusion.—Duplex Doppler sonography does not avoid biopsy in the setting of suspected acute rejection, but duplex and color Doppler studies do have value in monitoring the response to treatment and assessing allografts for other vascular abnormalities.

Duplex Doppler Sonography in Renal Allografts: The Significance of Reversed Flow in Diastole
Kaveggia LP, Perrella RR, Grant EG, Tessler FN, Rosenthal JT, Wilkinson A, Danovitch GM (Univ of California, Los Angeles)
AJR 155:295–298, 1990   1–25

Introduction.—In imaging renal transplants by Doppler sonography, a poor outcome has been associated with very high vascular resistance as evidenced by reversal of flow in diastole.

Methods.—To evaluate the significance of diastolic flow reversal seen on duplex Doppler sonograms of patients with renal transplant dysfunction, 533 studies were performed in 270 patients after renal transplantation. Most of the scans were acquired within 6 weeks after surgery. A 3- or 5-MHz mechanical sector or phased-array transducer was used for color and/or variable-gate pulsed Doppler imaging.

Results.—In 9 patients, diastolic flow reversal was seen in all Doppler samples. All of them had cadaver kidney transplants. In all patients, flow reversal was evident less than 6 weeks after transplantation. Serum creatinine levels ranged from 5 to 14 mg/dL. There was acute rejection in 4 patients, acute tubular necrosis in 4, vascular thrombosis in 2, and acute interstitial nephritis in 1.

Conclusion.—Many patients with reversed diastolic flow require transplant nephrectomy. Renal vein thrombosis may be more frequent in patients with this finding. It carries a poor outlook for graft survival, but does not reliably distinguish between acute rejection and acute tubular necrosis.

▶ These 2 thorough analyses (Abstracts 1–24 and 1–25) undertaken at UCLA confirm my prejudice that Doppler sonography cannot be used as an incisive means to diagnose rejection.—T. Strom, M.D.

Renal Transplants: Can Acute Rejection and Acute Tubular Necrosis Be Differentiated With MR Imaging?
Liou JTS, Lee JKT, Heiken JP, Totty WG, Molina PL, Flye WM (Washington Univ, St Louis)
Radiology 179:61–65, 1991   1–26

Background.—Authors disagree on the clinical usefulness of MRI in differentiating acute tubular necrosis (ATN) from acute rejection in renal transplant recipients.

Methods.—Forty renal transplant recipients underwent MR imaging for differentiation of ATN and acute rejection by means of corticomedullary differentiation (CMD). Each patient had an initial MRI after allograft renal transplantation. Twenty-nine patients also had subsequent MRI.

Findings.—Seventeen studies were obtained during episodes of ATN. Twelve studies, or 71%, showed poor CMD. Eleven studies were obtained during episodes of acute rejection. Eight, or 73%, showed poor CMD. Six of 7 studies, or 86%, showing various combinations of renal disease, also demonstrated poor CMD.

Conclusions.—Loss of CMD is reversible after ATN and acute rejection improves. Loss of CMD is a nonspecific though sensitive sign reflecting renal transplant dysfunction; thus MRI is of limited value in differentiating ATN from acute rejection.

▶ Ditto for MRIs! "Corticomedullary differentiation" (CMD) correlates poorly with the clinical diagnosis. Obliteration of CMD occurs in both rejection and ATN (see Table 3 in the original article). Magnetic resonance imaging is costly and adds little, if anything, to resolution of the differential diagnosis of rejection.—T. Strom, M.D.

Miscellaneous Topics in Clinical Kidney Transplantation

▶ ↓ The following potpourri of articles is an interesting and diverse group dealing with clinical topics.—Terry Strom, M.D.

Is Preliminary Binephrectomy Necessary in Patients With Autosomal Dominant Polycystic Kidney Disease Undergoing Renal Transplantation?
Rayner BL, Cassidy MJD, Jacobsen JE, Pascoe MD, Pontin AR, van Zyl Smit R
(Groote Schuur Hospital, Cape Town, South Africa)
Clin Nephrol 34:122–124, 1990   1–27

Background.—Agreement is lacking as to the indications for preliminary binephrectomy before transplantation in patients with end-stage renal failure caused by autosomal dominant polycystic kidney disease (ADPKD). The outcome of ADPKD patients who did and did not have pretransplant binephrectomy was evaluated.

Patients.—Nineteen AKPKD patients underwent renal transplantation during a 20-year period. Ten were male and 9 were female, with a mean age of 43 years at end-stage chronic renal failure. Conventional immunosuppression was used in all patients except 9 who received cyclosporin A and steroids for the first 3 months. Preliminary binephrectomy was done in 6 patients and no pretransplant surgery was performed in 13.

Outcome.—A total of 21 allografts was performed in 18 patients. Ten of the grafts were functioning at a mean of 20 months. Seven patients died of sepsis, and 5 grafts were rejected. One patient returned to dialysis. Binephrectomy was done because of recurrent pyelonephritis in 3 patients and for undetermined indications in the rest. None of the nonbinephrectomy patients had a history of urinary tract infection or recurrent hemorrhage into a cyst. Combination of morbidity and mortality data showed that patients who did not have binephrectomy did significantly worse because of septic complications of polycystic kidney disease.

Conclusions.—Binephrectomy before renal transplantation appears to reduce morbidity and mortality in patients with ADPKD by reducing sepsis related to polycystic kidneys. The indications for bilateral nephrectomy should be reconsidered.

▶ The authors advocate routine removal of polycystic kidneys because 7 of 18 patients with polycystic kidney disease that did not undergo pretransplant or peritransplant nephrectomies died as a consequence of sepsis "related to polycystic kidney disease." This experience was dreadful, but almost certainly not representative. I have not witnessed anything like this ghastly experience, and several previous analyses have reached diametrically opposing conclusions regarding the need for nephrectomy. Keep the scalpels in their sheaths!—T. Strom, M.D.

Outcome of Renal Transplantation After Urinary Diversion and Enterocystoplasty: A Retrospective, Controlled Study

Nguyen DH, Reinberg Y, Gonzalez R, Fryd D, Najarian JS (Univ of Minnesota, Minneapolis)
J Urol 144:1349–1351, 1990   1–28

Objective.—Complications were examined in 17 patients with intestinal urinary diversion or enterocystoplasty who underwent renal transplantation into an intestinal conduit, enterocystoplasty, or defunctionalized native bladder. Control patients were matched with the study group for age, transplant date (± 3 years), donor type, nondiabetic disease, and immunosuppression.

Outcome.—In 10 patients, 2 of whom required retransplantation, the graft ureter was implanted into an ileal or colonic conduit or enterocystoplasty. In 7 other patients, 1 of whom required a second transplant, the diversion was taken down and the graft ureter was placed in the defunctionalized bladder. The respective graft survival rates were 58% and 87%; this was not a significant difference. Complications such as ureteroileal anastomotic leakage and stenosis, stone formation, and urosepsis occurred only when the graft ureter was placed in an intestinal conduit or enterocystoplasty.

Conclusions.—Although it is feasible to perform renal transplantation into an intestinal conduit or augmented bladder, the associated complication rate is relatively high. However, graft survival is not compromised when the complications can be effectively treated. Implantation of the ureter into the native bladder is preferable.

▶ The sample size is small, and the message (also made in other reports) is quite simple: whenever possible, plug the ureter into the bladder (see Figure 1 in the original article). Implantation into the gut is associated with leaks, extravasation, stenosis, stones, severe acidosis, wound infection, and urosepsis. That is a hell of a long list of complications for such a small number of transplants. Intestinal urinary diversion is fraught with trouble—big trouble!—T. Strom, M.D.

Adult Height Achieved in Children After Kidney Transplantation
Aschendorff C, Offner G, Winkler L, Schirg E, Hoyer PF, Brodehl J (Children's Hospital Hannover Medical School, Germany)
Am J Dis Child 144:1138–1141, 1990   1–29

Background.—Children with chronic renal failure, particularly those requiring dialysis, may have growth retardation. Use of cyclosporine, which allows reduction of steroid dose, improves growth rate after kidney transplantation in comparison with conventional azathioprine and high-dose steroid treatment. The effect on ultimate height is unknown. Twenty adolescents who had received kidney transplants were studied to assess their linear growth, bone maturation, and adult height.

Patients.—The patients received kidney transplants as adolescents over a 12-year period. Eleven were boys and 9 were girls; age at operation ranged from 10.5 years to 17 years. Eleven patients treated between 1974 and 1982 received azathioprine and high-dose prednisolone; the remainder, treated between 1982 and 1986, received cyclosporine and low-dose prednisolone. Bone age, estimated by the radius-ulna-short bones method of Tanner and Whitehouse, was 15 years for boys and 13.3 years for girls in the cyclosporine group and 14.6 years and 13.1 years, respectively, in the azathioprine group. At the time of operation, the investigators predicted adult height by the Tanner-Whitehouse Mark II method. The definitions of adult height were 18 years in male and 16 years in females.

Results.—The cyclosporine group received cumulatively less steroid after transplantation. That group had a normal rate of bone maturation— .92 bone-age years per chronologic year—compared with a significantly slower rate of .57 bone-age years per year for the azathioprine group. Yearly growth rate was 3 cm for the cyclosporine group vs. 1.4 cm for the azathioprine group. As adults, the cyclosporine group exceeded their predicted adult heights by a mean of 1.3 cm; the azathioprine group was a mean of 3.9 cm beneath the prediction. Neither group achieved their target heights. The cyclosporine group had significantly lower kidney function, but none of the patients had severe renal insufficiency.

Conclusions.—In children receiving kidney transplants, cyclosporine and low-dose prednisolone treatment results in normal bone maturation and a better prognosis for final height. Patients who receive azathioprine do not reach their predicted height, but their renal function appears better. Cyclosporine does not accelerate bone maturation; azathioprine delays it.

▶ Growth retardation is a serious problem in children afflicted with end-stage renal disease. Whereas several studies have indicated a more favorable growth rate in childhood recipients of renal transplants treated with CsA and low dose steroids than with azathioprine plus steroids, an analysis of final adult height in patients treated with these regimens has not been established. This study confirms the value of the CsA-based protocol.—T. Strom, M.D.

Systemic Lupus Erythematosus After Renal Transplantation: Patient and Graft Survival and Disease Activity

Nossent HC, Swaak TJG, Berden JHM, Dutch Working Party on Systemic Lupus Erythematosus (Dr Danielden Hoed Clinic, Rotterdam, The Netherlands; University Hospital, Nijmegen, The Netherlands)
Ann Intern Med 114:183–188, 1991   1–30

Background.—End-stage renal failure now is a major problem in patients with systemic lupus erythematosus because high-dose steroid therapy frequently controls extrarenal manifestations of the disease. Most patients benefit from dialysis, and successful renal transplantation may allow the return of a full, active life.

Series.—Twenty-eight patients received renal transplants for systemic lupus erythematosus and end-stage renal failure during an 8-year period. Six of the patients had undergone dialysis for less than 1 year before transplantation. All but 3 patients were given cadaveric grafts. The median age at the time of renal transplantation was 34 years, and the median follow-up of patients with viable grafts was 31.5 months.

Outcome.—Actuarial graft survival is 71% at 6 months after transplantation, 68% at 1 year, and 54% at 5 years. The respective actuarial patient survival rates are 91% at 6 months, 87% at 1 year, and 87% at 5 years after transplantation. Disease activity, as reflected by Systemic Lupus Erythematosus Disease Activity Index scores, declined during dialysis and further after renal transplantation.

Conclusions.—A moderate-to-good renal graft survival rate is found in patients who undergo transplantation for renal failure caused by systemic lupus. The precise reasons why disease activity declines after renal transplantation warrant further investigation. Lupus nephritis recurred in only 1 of the study patients.

▶ It is interesting that neither a short duration of dialysis nor a high rate of disease activity during dialysis were noted to affect graft survival. Lupus nephritis recurred in only 1 of 28 patients. Clearly the immunosuppressive regimens used in the posttransplant period have a favorable influence on systemic lupus erythematosus disease activity in those patients whose disease activity does not "burn out" as a consequence of uremia.—T. Strom, M.D.

The Recurrence of Focal Segmental Glomerulosclerosis in Kidney Transplant Patients Treated With Cyclosporine

Banfi G, Colturi C, Montagnino G, Ponticelli C (Ospedale Maggiore, Milan, Italy)
Transplantation 50:594–596, 1990   1–31

Characteristics of Patients With and Without Recurrence of Focal Segmental
Glomerulosclerosis

	Cyclosporine			Azathioprine		
	Recurrence	P	Nonrecurrence	Recurrence	P	Nonrecurrence
Number of patients	10		8	2		4
Age at onset of FSGS	11.5±7.5	NS	14.5±12.5	7.2±1.2	NS	12.5±7.2
Age at transplantation	18.5±7.7	NS	22.7±11.5	10±2	NS	23.5±6
Duration of disease	41.6±31.5	NS	68.0±37.5	24±12	NS	117±93
Duration of dialysis	28.7±30	NS	30.3±18.5	10.5±5.5	NS	26.5±8.0

(Courtesy of Banfi G, Colturi C, Montagnino G, et al: *Transplantation* 50:594–596, 1990.)

Background.—Cyclosporin A (CsA) might protect against recurrence of focal segmental glomerulosclerosis (FSGS) and improve the clinical course of this disease in patients who have renal transplantation. However, other studies have shown similar recurrence rates in patients treated with CsA or azathioprine. In this study, recurrence and clinical course of FSGS in patients who have renal transplantation treated with CsA or azathioprine were examined.

Patients.—The study was comprised of 837 transplants performed during 19 years. Roughly the first half of this series was treated with azathioprine and prednisolone, whereas the second half was treated with CsA with or without prednisolone or with CsA, prednisolone, and azathioprine. The current report concerns 24 patients who had uremia as a result of biopsy-proven FSGS. Six of these received azathioprine and prednisolone and 19 received CsA, 14 in combination with prednisolone and 5 with prednisolone and azathioprine. Mean follow-up was 42 months in the azathioprine group and 30 months in the CsA group.

Findings.—There were 2 cases of recurrent FSGS and nephrotic syndrome in the azathioprine group, a rate of 33%. Focal segmental glomerulosclerosis caused graft loss in both of these patients, 1 at 24 and 1 at 25 months after transplantation. Recurrent FSGS occurred in 55% of the CsA group, including 1 patient who had recurrence in an initial graft treated with azathioprine. There was 1 graft loss because of acute rejection a few weeks after transplant and 3 because of FSGS 4–28 months after nephrotic syndrome occurred. There was 1 death in a patient with nephrotic syndrome because of pneumonia at 14 months after transplantation. At 15–37 months, 3 patients had nephrotic syndrome, with plasma creatinine levels of 1.9–2.4 mg/dL. At 10 and 31 months, the final 2 patients had nephrotic syndrome and normal renal function. Nephrotic syndrome tended to occur in the first postoperative week in both groups. Those who had recurrence tended to be younger at the onset of disease and to have a shorter duration of disease, although these differences were not significant (table).

Conclusion.—The outcome of FSGS recurring in patients who have renal transplantation does not seem to be affected by treatment with either CsA or azathioprine. A 44% incidence of graft loss is reported in patients

Steinhoff/Feddersen/Wood/et al

Patient	IgG	Tf	Alb	α₁AT	β₂MG	RBP	α₁MG	Diagnosis
Pat. Ze.	++	++	++	+	=	–	– –	* interstitial Rejection
Pat. He.	++	++	++	+	=	+	=	* interstitial Rejection
Pat. Ba.	++	+++	++	+	=	=	=	* interstitial Rejection
Pat. Ja.	+++	+++	+++	++	– –	– –	– –	* interstitial Rejection
Pat. Wi.	+++	+++	+++	+++	=	=	– –	* interstitial Rejection
Pat. Jo.	+++	+++	+++	=	–	– –	– –	* interstitial Rejection
Pat. Fr.	++	+++	+++	++	=	– –	– –	* interstitial Rejection
Pat. Öt.	+++	+++	+++	+++	=	=	=	* interstitial Rejection
Pat. Hö.	++	++	++	+	=	– –	–	* interstitial Rejection
Pat. Bl.	+++	+++	+++	++	=	+	+	* interstitial Rejection
Pat. Gr.	++	++	++	++	–	–	–	* interstitial Rejection
Pat. Be.	++	++	+++	++	=	=	+	* interstitial Rejection
Pat. St.	+++	++	++	++	=	=	–	* interstitial Rejection
Pat. Lub.	+++	++	++	++	=	=	=	* interstitial Rejection
Pat. Sei	++	++	++	++	–	–	– –	* interstitial Rejection
Pat. Fed.	+++	+++	++	++	=	=	=	* interstitial Rejection
Pat. Lew.	++	++	++	+	=	=	+	* interstitial Rejection
Pat. Len.	+++	+++	+++	+++	=	–	–	* interstitial Rejection
Pat. Ris.	+++	+++	+++	++	=	–	– –	* interstitial Rejection
Pat. Un.	++	++	++	+	+	+	+	* vascular Rejection
Pat. Jo.	++	++	++	+	+	=	=	* vascular Rejection
Pat. Sch.	++	++	++	+	+	+	–	* vascular Rejection
Pat. Gür.	+++	+++	+++	+++	+	+	+	* vascular Rejection
Pat. Baa.	+++	+++	+++	+++	+	+	+	* vascular Rejection
Pat. Zap.	+++	+++	+++	+++	+	+	+	* vascular Rejection
Pat. Wa.	=	=	=	=	=	=	=	uncomplicated course

Patient	TF	Alb	α₁AT	β₂MG	RBP	α₁MG	Course
Pat. Ku.	=	=	=	=	=	=	uncomplicated course
Pat. Ja.	=	=	=	=	=	=	uncomplicated course
Pat. Fe.	=	=	=	=	=	=	uncomplicated course
Pat. Eh.	=	=	=	=	=	=	uncomplicated course
Pat. Kö.	=	=	=	=	=	=	uncomplicated course
Pat. Bac.	=	=	=	=	=	=	uncomplicated course
Pat. Tim.	=	=	=	=	=	=	uncomplicated course
Pat. Dür.	=	=	=	=	=	=	uncomplicated course
Pat. Kra.	=	=	=	=	=	=	uncomplicated course
Pat. Schl.	=	=	=	=	=	=	uncomplicated course
Pat. Sev.	=	=	=	=	=	=	uncomplicated course
Pat. Bad.	=	=	=	=	=	=	uncomplicated course
Pat. Wal.	=	=	=	=	=	=	uncomplicated course
Pat. Wul.	=	=	=	=	=	=	uncomplicated course
Pat. Schm.	=	=	=	=	=	=	uncomplicated course
Pat. Gla.	=	=	=	=	=	=	uncomplicated course
Pat. Lie.	=	=	=	=	=	=	uncomplicated course
Pat. Kru.	=	=	=	=	=	=	uncomplicated course
Pat. La.	=	=	=	=	=	=	acute Ciclosporin-Tox.
Pat. Ro.	=	+	+	=	=	=	acute Ciclosporin-Tox.
Pat. Bal.	+++	+++	++	=	+	=	Urosepsis after Ntx
Pat. Ehl.	=	=	=	=	=	=	Anal abscess
Pat. He.	=	=	=	=	=	=	bact. gastro enteritis
Pat. Bä.	=	++	++	=	=	=	CMV-infection

Abbreviations: CMV, cytomegalovirus; TF, transferrin; Alb, albumin; α₁AT, α₁-antitrypsin; β₂MG, β₂-microglobulin; RBP, retinol-binding protein; α₁MG, α₁-microglobulin.

Note: + = rise in quotient value up to 2x, compared with previous day; ++ = rise in quotient from 2–5x, compared with previous day; +++ = rise in quotient from greater than 5x, compared with previous day; − = drop in quotient by up to ⅓, compared with previous day; − − = drop in quotient by up to ½, compared with previous day; = = no change when compared with previous day.
*Result confirmed histologically.

(Courtesy of Steinhoff J, Feddersen A, Wood WG, et al: *Clin Nephrol* 35:255–262, 1991.)

with recurrent FSGS. There is currently no valid treatment for recurrent FSGS in patients who have transplantation.

▶ This disappointing report indicating that CsA treatment fails to prevent recurrent FSG mirrors our experience. As noted by others, patients with rapidly progressive ("malignant") FSG in their native kidney appear to be at higher risk of developing recurrent disease (table). It is frustrating not to have a reliable marker to rely on in advising patients about the merits and pitfalls of transplantation, especially given the lack of effective treatment. Rumor has it that extracorporeal treatment with protein A immunoabsorption columns can grossly diminish albuminuria in FSG patients. This information, if confirmed, offers a flicker of hope that we can understand and treat this common and serious disorder.—T. Strom, M.D.

Glomerular Proteinuria as an Early Sign of Renal-Transplant Rejection
Steinhoff J, Feddersen A, Wood WG, Hoyer J, Sack K (Medizinische Universität, Lübeck, Germany)
Clin Nephrol 35:255–262, 1991   1–32

Background.—The advent of cyclosporine immunosuppression in renal transplantation created the problem of distinguishing between acute transplant rejection and toxicity from cyclosporine. Assays for specific proteins in urine may provide a noninvasive solution to this problem.

Methods.—Fifty-five patients given allogenic renal transplants had daily determinations of urinary IgG, transferrin, albumin, β_2-microglobulin, retinol-binding protein, α_1-microglobulin, and α_1-antitrypsin. All the proteins were estimated by immunoluminometric assay, and the results were related to the actual creatinine clearance.

Findings.—Acute rejection was consistently accompanied by peaks of IgG, transferrin, and albumin in 24-hour urine specimens (table). There was no peak in the "tubular" proteins, retinol-binding protein, β_2-microglobulin, and α_1-microglobulin. Protein excretion returned to baseline when rejection was effectively treated. Urinary levels of α_1-antitrypsin increased in bacterial infection of the urogenital tract and declined after effective antibiotic therapy. Neither patient with cyclosporine toxicity excreted abnormal amounts of glomerular or tubular proteins.

Conclusions.—Quantitative immunoluminometric assays for urinary proteins make possible the timely differentiation between cyclosporine toxicity and rejection or urosepsis, thereby allowing proper treatment at an early stage.

Atrial Natriuretic Factor Does Not Improve the Outcome of Cadaveric Renal Transplantation
Sands JM, Neylan JF, Olson RA, O'Brien DP, Whelchel JD, Mitch WE (Emory Univ, Atlanta)
J Am Soc Nephrol 1:1081–1086, 1991   1–33

Background.—In animal studies of acute ischemic renal failure, atrial natriuretic factor (ANF) lessens renal damage. Atrial natriuretic factor might be able to blunt the ischemic acute tubular necrosis that is commonly seen in cadaveric kidney transplants. A randomized, double-blind, placebo-controlled study was done to determine whether administration of ANF immediately after cadaveric renal allografts in humans could benefit renal function.

Methods.—Twenty patients received 10 pairs of cadaveric kidneys. Recipients were paired to receive either α-human ANF (hANF) or vehicle alone. When the graft was revascularized, the hANF or placebo was given intravenously in a 50 μg bolus, followed by a 4-hour infusion at a rate of .1 μg/kg/minute. Four to 7 days and 14–21 days posttrans-plant, glomerular filtration rate was measured by (^{125}I)iothalamate clearance. Each hospital day and twice weekly in the outpatient clinic, serum creatinine measurement was done. The 2 groups had no significant differences in donor or recipient age, cold ischemia time, or HLA matching.

Results.—There were no adverse effects of hANF infusion. No significant differences in serum creatinine or glomerular filtration rate were seen between the hANF and placebo groups; glomerular filtration rate at 4–7 days posttransplant was 33.9 in hANF patients and 27.9 in placebo patients. All patients but 1 had allograft function at 1 month; the remaining allograft, in a patient in the hANF group, never functioned.

Conclusions.—With the protocol studied, hANF appears to have no benefit in the outcome of cadaveric renal transplantation in humans. No adverse effects were seen. A longer infusion or higher dose could still prove beneficial.

▶ In a group of patients receiving vigorous excellular volume expansion with saline solution, albumin and mannitol plus furosemide, the addition of ANF infusions were without effect despite evidence that ANF can prevent ATN in animal models. Why did ANF fail to aid these subjects? The aggressive volume-expanding protocol used in the control arm of the study is almost certain to stimulate maximal release of endogenous ANF.—T. Strom, M.D.

Redevelopment of Hepatitis B Surface Antigen After Renal Transplantation

Marcellin P, Giostra E, Martinot-Peignoux M, Loriot M-A, Jaegle M-L, Wolf P, Degott C, Degos F, Benhamou J-P (Hôpital Beaujon, Clichy; INSERM U24; Hôpital de Hautepierre, Strasbourg, France)
Gastroenterology 100:1432–1434, 1991   1–34

Introduction.—Immunosuppressive therapy in patients with hepatitis B surface antigens (HBsAg) can reactivate hepatitis B virus (HBV) infection and cause the reappearance of serum hepatitis B e antigen (HBeAg) and/or HBV DNA. In 1 patient who was free of detectable HBsAg but had HBsAg antibodies (anti-HBs) and hepatitis B core antibodies (anti-HBc), chronic hepatitis B developed after renal transplantation.

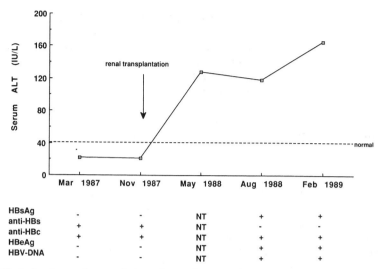

Fig 1–5.—Course of serum alanine aminotransferase (ALT), HBsAg, anti-HBs, anti-HBc, HBeAg, and HBV DNA (*dot-blot*) before and after renal transplantation. *NT* indicates not tested. (Courtesy of Marcellin P, Giostra E, Martinot-Peignoux M, et al: *Gastroenterology* 100:1432–1434, 1991.)

Case Report.—Man, 42, had HBsAg-positive chronic active hepatitis and cirrhosis with renal failure treated by hemodialysis. In March 1987, before receiving a transplant, he was HBsAg-negative and anti-HBs positive with normal transaminase levels (Fig 1–5). In November 1987, he received a renal allograft, followed by immunosuppressive therapy. By May 1988, the patient had an extremely elevated transaminase level and was positive for HBsAg and HBeAg and negative for anti-HBs, anti-HBe, and immunoglobulin M (IgM) anti-HBc. In August 1988 and later, he was tested for HBV DNA by dot-blot analysis. Sera from the pretransplantation time did not demonstrate the presence of HBV DNA by dot-blot analysis, but the HBV DNA was found using polymerase chain reaction (PCR) followed by Southern blot hybridization. The serum levels of the HBV DNA were 10^{-4} to 10^{-3} pg/mL. During the posttransplantation period, the HBV DNA was documented with dot-blot analysis and PCR, resulting in an estimated HBV DNA serum level of 10–50 pg/mL.

Discussion.—The findings in this patient suggest chronic hepatitis B did not develop after kidney transplantation, but that reactivation of the virus resulted from the immunosuppressive therapy accompanying transplantation. However, because PCR results can be contaminated with nonspecific signals, cautious interpretation of these results is recommended.

▶ This study dramatically emphasizes the powerful debilitating effects of antirejection therapy on anti-HBV immunity. Immunosuppressive therapy caused enhanced viral replication and reactivation of viral hepatitis. Apparently, transplantation cannot be done in HBV carriers with any certainty that the infection will remain latent.—T. Strom, M.D.

Effects of Theophylline on Erythropoietin Production in Normal Subjects and in Patients with Erythrocytosis After Renal Transplantation

Bakris GL, Sauter ER, Hussey JL, Fisher JW, Gaber AO, Winsett R (Ochsner Med Insts, New Orleans; Tulane Univ School of Medicine; Univ of Tennessee School of Medicine, Memphis)

N Engl J Med 323:86–90, 1990   1–35

Background.—Erythrocytosis, the rise in red blood cells with normal plasma volume, occurs after kidney transplantation, although the mechanism of its initiation remains unknown. Adenosine stimulates A_1 and A_2 receptor activity and has been implicated in erythropoietin production and adenylate cyclase action.

Objective.—Whether adenosine alters the production of erythropoietin in patients with erythrocytosis receiving renal transplants was tested prospectively with the use of theophylline in 8 patients with erythrocytosis and 5 controls.

Study Plan.—After review of the records of 100 kidney transplant recipients, 8 male patients between 48 and 55 years of age were found with erythrocytosis requiring a weekly phlebotomy. Urinary and plasma concentrations of cyclic adenosine monophosphate were measured for 4 consecutive weeks before theophylline treatment. Each kidney transplant recipient participated in the study for 28 weeks, receiving a starting dose of 8 mg of theophylline per kilogram of body weight per day.

Findings.—The findings from the treatment phase demonstrated that normal subjects had significant decreases in their hematocrit and erythropoietin levels from baseline after theophylline (Fig 1–6). The mean plasma theophylline level in the 5 normal subjects was 49 μmol/L, much below the usual therapeutic concentration. All 8 renal transplant recipients had decreases in their hematocrit 8 weeks after the beginning of

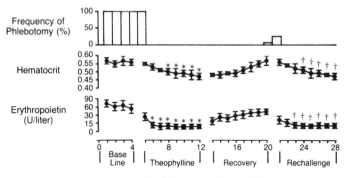

Study Period and Week of Treatment

Fig 1–6.—Effect of theophylline treatment on the frequency of phlebotomy, the serum erythropoietin level, and the hematocrit in 8 renal transplant recipients. *Asterisks* indicate measurements with a significance level less than .05 in the comparison with baseline measurements, and *daggers* measurements with a significance level less than .05 in the comparison with the measurements during the recovery period. *Vertical bars* represent means ± 1 SEM. (Courtesy of Bakris GL, Sauter ER, Hussey JL, et al: *N Engl J Med* 323:86–90, 1990.)

therapy. Their requirement for a weekly phlebotomy was totally eliminated after 1 week of theophylline treatment. The drug therapy, however, produced significant reduction of erythropoietin even at the end of the first week of treatment. Serum ferritin was also significantly lowered. Iron supplementation had no effect on hematocrit at the end of 8 weeks. Urinary and plasma concentrations or cyclic adenosine monophosphate demonstrated no significant increases during theophylline intake, which often caused headache, nervousness, and insomnia.

Conclusion.—Theophylline aids erythropoietin production in normal individuals and in kidney transplant recipients. Theophylline thus provides a useful alternative treatment to phlebotomies for some recipients of renal transplant.

▶ Other workers previously demonstrated that theophylline, a nonselective adenosine antagonist, can inhibit renal erythropoietin production, whereas an A_2 receptor agonist increases EPO production and often "overshoots" in the posttransplant period. Therefore it was of interest to study the effect of theophylline on posttransplant patients. A subset of posttransplant patients develops erythrocytosis for months to years. The authors provide evidence that theophylline administration does indeed temper erythropoietin production. No evidence is provided that this theoretically interesting approach offers an advantage over phlebotomy for patients with hematocrits above .55.—T. Strom, M.D.

Preemptive Transplantation: An Analysis of Benefits and Hazards in 85 Cases
Katz SM, Kerman RH, Golden D, Grevel J, Camel S, Lewis RM, Van Buren CT, Kahan BD (Univ of Texas Med School at Houston)
Transplantation 51:351–355, 1991   1–36

Background.—Preemptive renal transplantation—the use of transplantation as primary renal replacement treatment in the absence of preoperative dialysis—is done to optimize the potential benefits of transplantation compared with dialysis. Whether a preemptive procedure was associated with risks to the patient or graft survival was investigated in 85 patients who received transplants without prior dialysis and 84 transplant recipients who had at least 6 months of dialysis.

Methods.—The groups were matched for donor type, gender, age, disease, immunologic risk factors of HLA mismatch, and percent panel-reactive antibody. All patients were given cyclosporine and prednisone. Minimum follow-up was 1 year.

Findings.—Survival rates in the preemptive group were 94% at 1 year, 93% at 2 years, and 91% at 5 years. Corresponding rates for the control group were 96%, 96%, and 93%, respectively, which was not significantly different. The actuarial graft survival rates in the preemptive group were 83% at 1 year, 81% at 2 years, 76% at 3 years, 73% at 4 years, and 73% at 5 years. Those rates were not significantly different from control group rates, which were 90%, 81%, 80%, 77%, and 76%. Cyclosporine nephrotoxicity and rejection episodes were comparable among the groups. Seven episodes of irreversible rejection in the preemptive group were the result of noncompliance, compared with none in the control group. Patients in the preemptive group were more likely to be employed full time before and after transplantation than patients in the control group. Patients requiring chronic dialysis who had been employed before transplantation had a higher incidence of delayed rehabilitation beyond 6 months after surgery than the patients undergoing preemptive transplantation.

Conclusions.—The faster rehabilitation and avoidance of dialysis in patients undergoing preemptive renal transplantation are not associated with an increased risk of death or graft failure. However, patients receiving transplants preemptively appear to be at increased risk of noncompliance.

A Cadaveric Kidney Transplant Functioning for a Quarter of a Century—A Case Report
Stevens LE (LDS Hosp, Salt Lake City)
Transplantation 50:874–884, 1990   1–37

Introduction.—An unusual case of a cadaveric kidney transplant that has functioned for 25 years, despite being done without the benefit of ABO and HLA matching, was examined. This appears to be the longest continuously functioning cadaveric renal graft.

Case Report.—Man, 37, with progressive renal failure from chronic pyelonephritis, was admitted in 1965 with perforated duodenal ulcer that surprisingly healed. The patient was held on intermittent peritoneal dialysis until a cadaveric kidney became available, about 1 month later. This was the physician's first experience with human kidney transplant, having previously done a number of operations in dogs. The donor was ABO-type A and the recipient type was O, and no HLA tissue typing was available at the time. The new kidney promptly began to function, reaching high urine volumes probably because of a treatment program that replaced volume losses with intravenously administered crystalloids. The patient had seizures, a subcutaneous wound infection, and severe bilateral pneumonitis, but all responded to treatment, and he was discharged 34 days postoperatively. The patient was given azathioprine and methylprednisone and then prednisone, but he was only marginally compliant and at 15 years had stopped taking his medications for 3½ years. In this time, his creatinine level increased from 1.2 to 2.4 mg/dL; and in another 2-month period, of stopping medications, it reached to 3.2 mg/dL. Since his transplant, he had squamous cell cancers of his forearms and left ear that did not recur after excision. About 21 years postoperatively, after his horse fell, he had broken ribs, hemothorax, and bilateral pneumonia, that healed gradually. He was also treated for reflux esophagitis about 24 years postoperatively. At most recent follow-up, his serum creatinine level was 3.2 mg/dL.

Discussion.—An unusually fortunate case of cadaveric kidney transplant surviving for 25 years is studied. The donor and recipient must have had a fortuitously close histocompatibility match.

▶ The report celebrates the 25th anniversary of a successful cadaver donor transplant. The patient received his graft in 1965 at age 37. The patient had severe renal failure and underwent transplantation without access to hemodialysis. The graft was grafted across an ABO barrier. The patient survived an extensive postoperative wound infection and bilateral pneumonia requiring tracheotomy. During one 3½-year period (commencing at about posttransplant year 15), he stopped taking his immunosuppressive drugs, but his serum creatinine level rose only from 1.2 to 2.4 mg/dl. He has had multiple squamous cell cancers and several other intercurrent problems. Nonetheless, the graft continues to function reasonably well (creatinine level is 3.2 mg/dl). As Dr. Stevens concludes "This patient, with a cadaveric graft continuing to function now more than a quarter of a century, surviving under distinctly adverse conditions, offers hope to all present-day patients who may be facing kidney failure and the daunting prospects of a kidney transplant." Amen. Some recipients are born lucky!—T. Strom, M.D.

Acute Colitis in Renal Transplant Recipients
Indudhara R, Kochhar R, Mehta SK, Chugh KS, Yadav RVS (Postgraduate Institute of Medical Education and Research, Chandigarh, India)
Am J Gastroenterol 85:964–968, 1990   1–38

Background.—In kidney transplant recipients, gastrointestinal complications may cause serious morbidity or death. Early and vigorous treatment is essential. Severe acute colitis in the posttransplant period was evaluated.

Patients.—Two hundred seventy-six renal allotransplants were performed during a 15-year period. Ten patients had colitis, an incidence of 3.6%. Maintenance immunosuppression consisted of prednisone and azathioprine, with acute rejection treated by orally administered prednisolone. Symptoms occurred from 2 months to 5 years after transplantation. Two patients had graft dysfunction before the onset of colitis. Each patient received an extensive diagnostic work-up to identify a specific cause, but 7 had nonspecific colitis. However, 6 of these patients responded to broad-spectrum antibiotics and might have had an unrecognized infective colitis. There was 1 patient with tubercular colitis resulting from atypical mycobacteria. No patient had a positive toxin assay or stool culture for *Clostridium difficile* or any pseudomembranes. All patients had *Candida albicans* in stool and were given orally administered nystatin. However, serologic studies for *C. albicans* were negative and no pseudohyphae were found. Two cases of ischemic colitis were found at autopsy. Six patients died in the acute stage of colitis. The last 3 patients responded quickly to broad-spectrum antibiotics and blood transfusions.

Conclusions.—Acute colitis in kidney transplant patients was studied.

The importance of a vigorous search for the cause of the disease, aggressive medical treatment, and if there is no response, prompt surgical intervention is stressed. Tubercular causes of this condition should be sought vigorously in developing countries, because this is a salvageable entity.

▶ This article is a poignant reminder that I do not want to run a transplant unit in India. I'm not up to the challenge! I have some notion about the causes of enteropathy in my own patient population. Microbes, (e.g., viruses, *Clostridium dificile,* and ischemia) come to mind. Clearly, infection with agents that I can barely remember hearing about and cannot spell are common in India. These mystery agents can cause much grief in immunosuppressed hosts. Most of these patients with acute colitis died! The Indian patients received a vigorous and thoughtful work-up and a specific cause could not be found in most individuals. The course and apparent response of some patients to broad antimicrobial coverage indicates an infectious agent was causal. The authors recommend vigorous, rapid work-up and consideration of total colectomy or mutliple colostomies in seriously ill patients. I admire the skill and courage of the Indian physicians; they face daunting problems that I have not needed to consider.—T. Strom, M.D.

2 Liver Transplantation

Technical Advances in Liver Transplantation

▶ ↓ These papers represent important technical advances in the field of liver transplantation. The use of pared down, split and liver donor livers are all techniques used to expand the donor pool. The introduction of the TIPS procedure is a method to delay or avoid liver transplantation.—Nancy L. Ascher, M.D., Ph.D.

Evolution and Future Perspectives for Reduced-Size Hepatic Transplantation
Broelsch CE, Whitington PF, Emond JC (Univ of Chicago; Wyler Childrens Hosp, Chicago)
Surg Gynecol Obstet 171:353–360, 1990   2–1

Introduction.—Pediatric liver transplantation often reduces the size of a donor's liver to accomodate the smaller size of the recipient. Studies have shown that the reduced-sized hepatic allograft works, promoting long-term liver replacement equal to that seen with whole liver transplants. The development of the reduced-sized liver method from research status to clinical use was reviewed.

Methods.—Animal research in reduced-sized liver transplantation began about 20 years ago with auxiliary transplantation methods that did not remove part or all of the recipient's liver during the transplant procedure. Portal blood flow through the graft was apparent. Since this time, it has been determined that portal venous blood contains hepatotrophic factors necessary for normal hepatocyte turnover and replacement. How much to reduce the whole liver for the small-sized transplant remains an inexact procedure, with acceptable donors weighing sometimes more than 8 times the recipient. The transplant procedures include simultaneous hepatectomy of the recipient while the donor liver is undergoing surgical reduction by a second surgical team. In general, parenchymal dissection is along the anatomical line through the gallbladder fossa and the falciform ligament toward the left median hepatic vein. Use of the right or total left lobe of the liver allows the surgeon to leave the inferior vena cava intact along with the graft so that the common hepatic duct can serve for biliary drainage.

Results.—The chief use of reduced-sized liver grafts is in children because of the low availability of size-matched livers. Reduced-sized liver transplant procedures were used in nonemergency conditions in 49 pediatric liver transplant patients; 13 received reduced-sized grafts, and 39 received full-size grafts. Of the 49 patients, 40 (82%) were alive 6–30 months after surgery. The use of the reduced-size livers did not increase

45

postsurgical mortality compared with that of patients receiving whole-liver grafts.

Conclusion.—Reduced-sized liver grafts can serve as a permanent hepatic transplant, as the reduced-sized organ grows to fill the hepatic fossa. If the graft is too large, the graft remains the same size until the patient grows to accomodate the organ. Ethical issues include the questions about using full-sized organs for children while older children and adults are bypassed for liver transplantations. However, the knowledge gained through the use of reduced-sized hepatic transplants may lead to liver transplantation using living donors who contribute only part of the organ, which could alleviate the donor shortage problem.

► The group from the University of Chicago has made a major contribution to the field of liver transplantation with the use of liver-related donors and the extensive study of reduced-size hepatic grafts. Patients receiving reduced size grafts enjoy the same results as those receiving whole organs. The use of living-related grafts is currently limited; their usefulness in adult transplantation is as yet unknown but holds promise. The field of liver transplantation is increasingly donor limited as indication for transplantation expands.—N.L. Ascher, M.D., Ph.D.

Intrahepatic Portocaval Shunt for Variceal Hemorrhage Prior to Liver Transplantation
Roberts JP, Ring E, Lake JR, Sterneck M, Ascher NL (Univ of California-San Francisco)
Transplantation 52:160–162, 1991   2–2

Background.—There have been reports of creation of an intrahepatic portocaval shunt by use of angiographic techniques. This technique should decompress the portal system and prevent variceal hemorrhage in patients who do not respond to endoscopic sclerotherapy and require emergency liver transplantation. Creation of an intrahepatic portocaval shunt was used as a temporary measure in a patient with variceal hemorrhage before transplantation.

Case Report.—Woman, 46, had cirrhosis resulting from presumed non-A, non-B hepatitis. She had side-to-side portocaval shunt for massive variceal hemorrhage at another hospital. She needed a peritoneovenous shunt for ascites, recurrent hemorrhage, and a thrombosed H graft. The patient was transferred with recurrent variceal hemorrhage.

Endoscopy and sclerotherapy were done twice after stabilization. When bleeding from multiple gastric erosions was noted at the second attempt, intrahepatic portocaval shunt was attempted. Intravenous sedation and local anesthetic were given, then a 3-F catheter was placed percutaneously and transhepatically into the portal vein. A 9-F sheath was then placed into the middle hepatic vein, a long, curved needle was inserted and used to puncture into the intrahepatic portal vein, and a guidewire was introduced (Fig 2–1). After a 10-mm balloon dilatation of

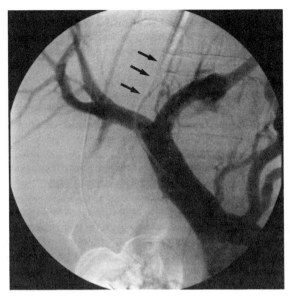

Fig 2–1.—Portal vein angiogram. The transhepatic catheter can be seen in portal vein. *Arrows* point to transjugular catheter passing from hepatic vein to portal vein. (Courtesy of Roberts JP, Ring E, Lake JR, et al: *Transplantation* 52:160–162, 1991.)

the track, a 10 × 42-mm expanding stent was placed. Portal venous pressure fell immediately from 35 to 23 cm of H_2O, and the gastrointestinal hemorrhage stopped. The patient was well until variceal hemorrhage recurred 3 months later. At that time, the shunt was found to be occluded and was replaced. The patient did well after orthotopic liver transplantation.

Conclusions.—An intrahepatic shunt may be used to control portal hypertension temporarily. Liver transplantation may be made easier and portal hypertension may be diminished by reopening of the stent. Transplantation should be done within 3 months of shunting.

▶ The refinement of the technique of percutaneous hepatic portal caval shunt (TIPS) to treat portal hypertension had modified the indications and urgency of liver transplantation. Successful TIPS allows for thorough assessment and treatment in the alcoholic recipient. Long-term patency and encephalopathy may be the limiting factors in the use of the TIPS procedure. To date, experience in more than 100 TIPS patients at UCSF indicates an encephalopathy rate of 24%; all incidences of encephalopathy could be adequately managed with lactulose.—N.L. Ascher, M.D., Ph.D.

Predictors of Function in Liver Transplantation

▶ ↓ These articles attempt to predict when patients require transplantation and which livers are likely to work. These questions have not been studied systemically.—Nancy L. Ascher, M.D., Ph.D.

Symptom Development and Prognosis in Primary Biliary Cirrhosis: A Study in Two Centers

Mitchison HC, Lucey MR, Kelly PJ, Neuberger JM, Williams R, James OFW (University of Newcastle Upon Tyne, England; King's College Hospital, London; Univ of Michigan, Ann Arbor)

Gastroenterology 99:778–784, 1990

2–3

Background.—Some patients may have biochemical, immunologic, and histologic evidence of primary biliary cirrhosis (PBC) without having symptoms of liver disease. However, it is uncertain what proportion of such patients may develop symptoms later and whether some may have a different, more benign disease from which symptoms and complications may never arise.

Methods.—Investigators studied 70 patients with asymptomatic PBC from a regional referral center and 25 similar patients from an international tertiary referral center. Patients had a similar mean age at diagnosis and duration of follow-up, which was a median of 12 months. Patients' records were reviewed retrospectively and, when any of the following symptoms appeared on the records, patients were considered symptomatic: pruritus; at least 2 of the triad of anorexia, fatigue, and otherwise unexplained abdominal pain; jaundice; portal systemic encephalopathy; ascites; or bleeding esophageal varices.

Results.—Thirty-four of 95 asymptomatic patients developed hepatic symptoms during follow-up. A higher proportion of these patients were from the tertiary referral hospital than from the regional referral center. The time to appearance of symptoms was significantly longer at the latter institution. Twenty-five patients died. Of these, 15 had developed symptoms and died of liver-related disease. Ten who died remained asymptomatic and died of non–liver-related causes. Hepatic mortality was greater than among the population at large. In a comparison of study patients with already symptomatic patients at both institutions, there was no difference in survival once hepatic symptoms were detected.

Conclusions.—Asymptomatic PBC is not necessarily presymptomatic: 11 patients were followed for 8 or more years without developing symptoms. However, if symptoms do appear, it is likely that patients will die of liver disease rather than of unrelated causes. Once patients develop symptoms, the rate of survival is similar to that of patients who had symptoms initially. The mortality rate in these patients is approximately 50% in 85 months.

▶ In a significant number of patients with asymptomatic primary biliary cirrhosis, the disease does not progress. Once patients develop symptoms of pruritus, anorexia, fatigue, jaundice, or signs of portal systemic, survival is limited. Data from the Mayo Clinic in a larger patient population suggest that once bilirubin reaches a certain level, a patient's life span is limited. Taken together, symptomatic patients or patients with serum bilirubin greater than 8 mg/L should be referred for liver transplant evaluation.—N.L. Ascher, M.D., Ph.D.

The Predictive Value of Donor Liver Biopsies for the Development of Primary Nonfunction After Orthotopic Liver Transplantation

D'Alessandro AM, Kalayoglu M, Sollinger HW, Hoffmann RM, Reed A, Knechtle SJ, Pirsch JD, Hafez GR, Lorentzen D, Belzer FO (Univ of Wisconsin School of Medicine, Madison)
Transplantation 51:157–163, 1991   2–4

Introduction.—Primary nonfunction (PNF) after orthotopic liver transplantation causes significant morbidity and mortality. Improved preservation methods, the use of UW solution in particular, have allowed histologic analysis of liver tissue before transplantation. To assess the value of donor liver biopsy specimens to predict PNF, data on 124 donor liver biopsy specimens were reviewed.

Methods.—In 1987–1990, 170 liver transplants were performed in 147 patients; 124 donor liver biopsy specimens were obtained and divided into 3 groups. The 77 biopsy specimens in group 1 were obtained 2–4 hours after revascularization. The 19 specimens in group 2 were obtained before dissection but not re-examined until after transplantation. The 28 specimens in group 3 were obtained before dissection but were re-examined before transplantation. All livers were preserved in UW solution with a mean preservation time of 12.5 hours (13.1 hours for livers with an available biopsy specimen).

Results.—Histologic findings were normal in 89 livers; PNF developed in 3 (3.4%) of these livers and demonstrated macrovesicular steatosis (table). Of the 26 biopsy specimens with a minimal or moderate amount of fatty infiltration, PNF developed in 1 (3.8%). In addition, PNF developed in 3 livers with severe fatty infiltration, 3 with hydropic degeneration, and in 1 with centrilobular necrosis. Of the 89 patients with hydropic degeneration and poor function, retransplantation was necessary in 1 after 8 weeks. Donor age and weight were significantly higher in those livers with fatty infiltration compared with normal livers.

Conclusion.—Prospective liver biopsies are important in assessing abnormal hepatic pathology in livers available for transplantation. Severe fatty infiltration and hydropic degeneration indicate a high degree of pri-

Development of PNF According to Histology

	Group 1		Group 2		Group 3		Total	
	n	PNF	n	PNF	n	PNF	n	PNF
Normal	57	2	14	1	18	0	89	3 (3.4%) *
Minimal fatty infiltration	11	1	0	0	4	0	15	1 (6.7%)
Moderate fatty infiltration	6	0	1	0	4	0	11	0
Severe fatty infiltration	0	0	3	3	1	Discarded	3	3
Hydropic degeneration	2	2	1	1	1	Discarded	3	3
Centrilobular necrosis	1	1	0	0	0	0	1	1

*P < .01 compared with all other histologic patterns. (Courtesy of D'Alessandro MA, Kalayoglu M, Sollinger HW, et al: *Transplantation* 51:157–163, 1991.)

mary nonfunction. Although the cost of discarding the organ is high, it is ultimately much less than retransplantation.

▶ Primary nonfunction is an important clinical problem in liver transplantation. The incidence of primary nonfunction ranges between 2% and 20% in spite of the uniform use of University of Wisconsin (UW) solution. The Wisconsin group confirms previous observation that macrovesicular fat correlated with primary nonfunction. An unsolved issue is whether the cause of the steatosis is significant in terms of reversibility and association with poor initiation function. This distinction may be important to minimize wastage of potentially usable livers.— N.L. Ascher, M.D., Ph.D.

Characteristics of Biliary Lipid Metabolism After Liver Transplantation
Ericzon BG, Eusufzai S, Kubota K, Einarsson K, Angelin B (Karolinska Institutet at Huddinge University Hospital, Stockholm)
Hepatology 12:1221–1228, 1990.   2–5

Introduction.—Although bile production is monitored as the earliest sign of function in the transplanted liver, little has been published characterizing the biochemical composition of this early bile. The developing pattern of biliary lipid secretion in the transplanted liver is described and perturbations of this pattern that might indicate impending rejection or malfunction are described.

Methods.—Nine patients received rapidly in situ-cooled livers for 10 orthotopic transplants from cadaveric donors. Drainage and continuous collection of bile samples for 3 weeks was through a T tube in 7 choledochocholdochostomy patients, and through a choledochus catheter in 3 choledochojejunostomy patients. Patients were immunosuppressed with cyclosporine and prednisolone. Biliary lipid analysis was done on morning samples after the overnight fast.

Results.—The concentrations of cholesterol, bile acids, and phospholipids initially were low, but had increased to previously reported values for T tube bile in nontransplanted cholecystectomized patients by 3 weeks. Phospholipids were secreted at .22 μmol and cholesterol at .08 μmol/μmol of bile acids, and release was entirely dependent on bile salts. There was a substantial amount of bile acid–independent bile flow, amounting to 63 mL/day, with a linear, rather than the normal human curvilinear, relationship between bile acid output and bile flow. As expected, only the primary bile acids, cholic acid, and chenodeoxycholic acid were present in the bile; however, the relative proportion of the latter was greater during the first few days after surgery. In a patient with hepatic artery thrombosis, the problem was reflected in a sharp decline in biliary lipids, but 2 days later, severe liver dysfunction was indicated by standard serum liver tests. In contrast, impending rejection or failure of antirejection treatments in 2 patients was heralded first by a decline in biliary lipids and later by increased bilirubin.

Discussion.—The present series is small, but it appears that, although biliary lipids react briskly to disturbances of function in the transplanted liver, their analysis adds little to the information gained from measurements of bile flow or serum tests. One exception may be in the diagnosis of rejection, when changes in biliary lipids provided the first sign of trouble in this study.

▶ A number of noninvasive parameters have been used as early predictors of liver transplant dysfunction caused by rejection, vascular compromise, or primary malfunction. Perturbation in bile lipid secretion preceded abnormal liver function tests in 2 patients with rejection and in 1 patient with hepatic artery thrombosis. The bile lipid profile does not distinguish the specific liver pathology and does not add to the current tests, which are the mainstay of evaluation. These are liver biopsy, doppler ultrasound and cholangiography.—N.L. Ascher, M.D., Ph.D.

Liver Transplant Outcome in Select Recipient Populations

▶ ↓ Indications for liver transplantation have expanded over the past 5 years, but outcome remains troubling in certain subgroups. Patients with hepatitis B infection and cancer have had a high incidence of recurrence and death from recurrent disease. Can we achieve better results by selection or specific therapy?—Nancy L. Ascher, M.D.

Passive Immunoprophylaxis After Liver Transplantation in HBsAg-Positive Patients
Samuel D, Bismuth A, Mathieu D, Arulnaden J-L, Reynes M, Benhamou J-P, Brechot C, Bismuth H (Paris South University; Hôpital Paul Brousse, Villejuif; Hôpital Beaujon, Clichy, France; Institut Pasteur, Paris)
Lancet 337:813–815, 1991   2–6

Introduction.—Survival rates in patients undergoing orthotopic liver transplantation because of cirrhosis or fulminant hepatitis caused by hepatitis B virus (HBV) have been disappointing. High rates of HBV infection of the transplanted liver have been implicated as a cause for the poor survival. The efficacy of long-term passive immunoprophylaxis against HBV in the prevention of graft reinfection and its effect on survival in orthotopic liver recipients was prospectively studied.

Patients.—During a 3-year study period, 85 men and 25 women, aged 15–56 years, with end-stage liver disease who tested positive for hepatitis B surface antigen (HBsAg) received an orthotopic liver transplant. All patients were given 10,000 IU of anti-HBs immunoglobulin intravenously during the anhepatic phase and on every postoperative day until HBsAG disappeared from the serum.

Results.—During a mean follow-up of 19.6 months, all patients became HBsAg negative and anti-HBs positive by the end of the first

TABLE 1.—HBsAg Reappearance After Transplant Related
to Initial Liver Disease

Initial liver disease	HBsAg positive after transplant	Actuarial rate of HBV recurrence	
		1 year	2 years
Posthepatitis B cirrhosis	19/40 (47·5%)	46%	59%
Fulminant hepatitis B	0/17 (0%)	0%	0%
Posthepatitis B-δ cirrhosis	5/49 (10·2%)	0%	13%
Fulminant hepatitis B-δ	1/4 (25%)	..	..
Total	25/110 (22·7%)	17%	29%

(Courtesy of Samuel D, Bismuth A, Mathieu D, et al: *Lancet* 337:813–815, 1991.)

postoperative week. Circulating HBsAg reappeared in the serum of 25 (22.7%) patients after a mean delay of 9.1 months (Table 1). The overall actuarial rate of HBV recurrence was 17% at 1 year and 29% at 2 years. Patients with HBV cirrhosis who initially were HBV-DNA positive were at much greater risk of HBsAg recurrence than were those who were initially HBV-DNA negative (Table 2). The overall actuarial survival after transplantation was 83.6% at 1 year and 74% at 2 years.

Conclusion.—Long-term passive anti-HBV immunoprophylaxis in patients undergoing orthotopic liver transplantation significantly reduces the HBV reinfection rate and improves survival.

▶ Recurrent hepatitis B is a major problem after orthotopic liver transplantation for this disease. The group was shown a remarkably low incidence of disease recurrence after the use of hyperimmune HBs immunoglobulin after transplantation to maintain high antibody titers. This therapy was not effective in patients who had evidence of active viral replication, that is, who were HbeAg positive. Many centers consider positive antigen status to be a contraindication to transplantation. The presence of delta coinfection, on the other hand, is not considered to be a contraindication.—N.L. Ascher, M.D., Ph.D.

TABLE 2.—HBsAg Reappearance in Posthepatitis B
Cirrhosis Related to Pretransplant HBV Status

Initial HBV status	HBsAg positive after transplant	Actuarial rate of HBV recurrence	
		1 year	2 years
HBV-DNA positive	13/16 (81·2%)	71%	96%
HBeAg positive	5/7 (71·4%)	82%	82%
HBeAg negative	8/9 (88·8%)	42%	100%
HBV-DNA negative	6/24 (25%)	29%	29%
HBeAg positive	2/6 (33·3%)	40%	40%
HBeAg negative	4/18 (22·2%)	25%	25%
Total	19/40 (47·5%)	46%	59%

(Courtesy of Samuel D, Bismuth A, Mathieu D, et al: *Lancet* 337:813–815, 1991.)

Orthotopic Liver Transplantation for Patients With Hepatitis B Virus-Related Liver Disease
Todo S, Demetris AJ, Van Thiel D, Teperman L, Fung JJ, Starzl TE (Univ of Pittsburgh)
Hepatology 13:619–626, 1991   2–7

Introduction.—Liver transplantation in patients with hepatitis B virus (HBV) can be risky, with possibly recurring hepatitis and impaired recovery. Patients who had chronic or fulminant HBV when undergoing liver transplantation were followed for at least 19 months.

Methods.—Fifty-nine patients with positive hepatitis B surface antigen (HBsAg) were studied after liver transplantation and 38 patients with anti-HBs but not HBsAg in their serum were used as the control group. Orthotopic liver transplantation was done with the use of a venovenous bypass, and immunosuppressive therapy was administered postoperatively. Adjuvant immunotherapy was administered during operation and 1 month later in an effort to eliminate the HBV and to avoid recurrent disease.

Results.—There was no significant difference in mortality between the HBV-infected group and HBV-immune control group during the first 60 days after transplantation. After 60 days, mortality, rate of graft loss, retransplantation, and increased incidence of abnormal liver function were significantly higher in the HBV-infected group. Six of 22 patients living longer than 60 days and treated with active plus passive immunization were cleared of HBsAg, as was 1 of 16 patients treated with α-interferon, and 1 of 4 patients receiving no treatment. Of 3 patients treated with only passive immunization, none were cleared of HBsAg. Patients undergoing a second retransplantation were more vulnerable to HBV.

Conclusion.—The efficacy of treatment used in this study is not conclusive. Combined active plus passive immunization and better designed α-interferon should be further investigated because they might allow long-term serologic conversions.

▶ The appropriate pretransplant treatment for the recipient with hepatitis B disease is unknown. Given the huge patient pool of HBV+ and the poor results after transplant, measures to decrease viral recurrence are important. A number of European groups have used passive immunization, with good results in delaying viral recurrence. This study is less optimistic but points to the need for large multicenter trials.—N.L. Ascher, M.D., Ph.D.

Primary Hepatic Malignancy: The Role of Liver Transplantation
Ismail T, Angrisani L, Gunson BK, Hübscher SG, Buckels JAC, Neuberger JM, Elias E, McMaster P (Queen Elizabeth Hospital, Birmingham, England)
Br J Surg 77:983–987, 1990   2–8

Orthotopic Liver Transplantation (OLT) for Primary Hepatic Malignancy

OLT number	Age	Sex	Tumour type	CT +ve	IO +ve	HIST +ve	Size (cm)	CE	Survival (months)	Cause of death
Cirrhotic										
1	54	F	NF HCC	n.a.	Y	N	11	Y	0	Sepsis
6	55	M	NF HCC	n.a.	N	N	m.f.	Y	0	Infarction
9	13	M	NF HCC	N	Y	Y	m.f.	N	2	Recurrence
48	59	M	NF HCC	N	Y	N	10	Y	12	Recurrence
60/62	56	M	NF HCC	N	Y	N	1	Y	0	Bleed
78	22	F	NF HCC	N	N	N	1·5	Y	0	Rejection, necrosis
79	45	M	NF HCC	N	N	N	m.f.	Y	0	Bleed
117	46	M	NF HCC	N	N	N	m.f.	Y	3	Hepatitis B recurrence
119	55	M	NF HCC	N	N	N	m.f.	Y	0	MOF
126	65	M	NF HCC	N	Y	N	m.f.	Y	0	Bleed
Non-cirrhotic										
2	39	M	NF HCC	n.a.	Y	N	22	Y	87	
5	44	M	NF HCC	N	Y	Y	m.f.	N	6	Recurrence
7	60	F	NF HCC	N	N	N	16	Y	71	
146	49	M	NF HCC	Y	N	N	15	Y	13	
226	38	F	NF HCC	N	N	N	m.f.	N	5	Recurrence

25	21	M	FL HCC	Y	Y	Y	Y	15	N	18	Recurrence
28	27	F	FL HCC	N	Y	Y	Y	15	N	0	Bleed
32	19	F	FL HCC	N	Y	Y	Y	18	Y	20	Recurrence
70	23	F	FL HCC	N	N	N	Y	16	Y	34	
131	21	F	FL HCC	Y	Y	Y	Y	16	N	19	
214	18	M	FL HCC	N	Y	Y	Y	18	N	8	
16	47	F	EHE	N	N	N	Y	m.f.	Y	55	Recurrence
39	53	F	CholCa	Y	Y	Y	Y	m.f.	N	12	Recurrence
43	46	F	CholCa	Y	Y	Y	Y	m.f.	N	11	Recurrence
65	33	F	AS	Y	Y	N	N	m.f.	N	5	? recurrence
139	40	M	CholCa	Y	N	N	N	m.f.	N	7	Recurrence
237	37	M	AS	N	N	N	Y	m.f.	Y	4	
241	3	F	IHE	N	N	N	Y	20	Y	4	

Note: Three patients were node negative but had incomplete excision of tumor (OLT 32 and 226 had tumor in the portal vein, OLT 139 had tumor in the extrahepatic bile duct; OLT 60/62 had a second liver graft 1 month after the first transplant. CT/IOHIST relate to presence (Y) or absence (N) of enlarged nodes on CT and intraoperatively (IO) and to tumor-positive nodes at postoperative histology (HIST)

Abbreviations: n.a., not available; *m.f.,* multifocal; *CE,* complete excision; *MOF* multiorgan failure; *NF HCC,* nonfibrolamellar hepatocellular carcinoma; *FL HCC,* fibrolamellar hepatocellular carcinoma; *CholCa,* cholangiocellular carcinoma; *AS,* angiosarcoma; *EHE,* epithelioid hemangioendothelioma; *IHE,* infantile hemangioendothelioma.

(Courtesy of Ismail T, Angrisani L, Gunson BK, et al: *Br J Surg* 77:983–987, 1990.)

Introduction.—Complete surgical excision is the best chance of cure for patients with primary liver malignancy. Total hepatectomy and liver replacement have been used as a method to clear all malignancy, but a high incidence of tumor recurrence has deterred use of this method.

Methods.—The preoperative and intraoperative assessment of disease were determined and the stage of disease was correlated with patient outcome after liver transplantation.

Results.—Of 134 patients with suspected liver neoplasm, 105 (78%) had a histologically confirmed diagnosis of primary liver tumor (table). Primary hepatocellular carcinoma was found in 47 (45%) patients; 29 orthotopic liver transplants were performed in 28 (27%) of these patients. Of the patients, 20 (71%) survived 30 days or longer; the median survival was 11.5 months (range, 2–87 months). In diagnosing tumor-positive nodes, CT was superior to intraoperative assessment (86% vs. 58%). Patients with tumor-negative lymphadenopathy and noncirrhotic patients with hepatocellular carcinoma had the best prognosis. The worst outcome was for patients with cholangiocellular carcinoma and cirrhotic patients with hepatocellular carcinoma.

Conclusion.—If there is an advanced stage of disease at time of presentation, the value of liver transplantation is limited. However, in patients with advanced disease confined to the liver (stage I/II) in whom conventional hepatic resection is not possible, liver transplantation may provide significant benefit.

▶ This study confirms findings from Starzl and Pichylmayr that in a limited subgroup of patients with hepatic malignancy, liver transplantation may be beneficial palliation. In noncirrhotic patients, extended survival may be achieved; death in general is from recurrence. There has not been an adequate study to prospectively compare liver transplantation with resection for early disease.—N.L. Ascher, M.D., Ph.D.

Orthotopic Liver Transplantation in Patients 60 Years of Age and Older

Pirsch JD, Kalayoglu M, D'Alessandro AM, Voss BJ, Armbrust MJ, Reed A, Knechtle SJ, Sollinger HW, Belzer FO (Univ of Wisconsin)
Transplantation 51:431–433, 1991   2–9

Background.—With the use of cyclosporine, renal transplantation can be performed successfully in patients ≥60 years old, but the success of liver transplantation in this age group is unknown. The results of orthotopic liver transplantation in 23 patients ≥60 years old, who received transplants under a quadruple immunosuppression protocol are reported.

Patients.—Patient records were analyzed retrospectively and compared with those of 84 patients aged 18 to 59 years who also received liver transplants. In the older group, indications for transplantation included 6 for alcoholism, 6 for postnecrotic cirrhosis, 4 for cancer, 3 for primary biliary cirrhosis, 2 for sclerosing cholangitis, and 1 for polycystic liver disease.

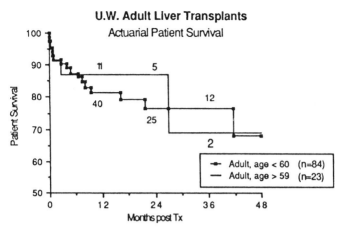

Fig 2–2.—Patient survival in recipients of primary liver transplants 60 years of age and older compared to recipients 18 to 59 years of age. (Courtesy of Pirsch JD, Kalayoglu M, D'Alessandro AM, et al: *Transplantation* 51:431–433, 1991.)

Results.—The 2 groups were similar in initial transplant hospitalization and in the incidence of infection and rejection. In the older group, no patient required retransplantation. At 2 years, actuarial patient survival was 83% in recipients ≥ aged 60 years, 76% in adult recipients < age of 60 years (Fig 2–2).

Conclusions.—Patients older than age 60 years have excellent survival and liver-graft survival and postoperative morbidity similar to that of younger adult patients. These findings suggest that advanced age is not a contraindication to orthotopic liver transplantation.

▶ Recipient age should not be considered a contraindication to liver transplantation. The older patients had no higher incidence of postoperative complications. It is not clear whether the cardiac evaluation of the older patient needs to be more extensive to avoid cardiovascular complications. Bone disease in the elderly patient may be a major problem and requires the aggressive use of calcium and etidronate.—N.L. Ascher, M.D., Ph.D.

Liver Transplantation—Histopathology

▶ ↓ These articles expand our understanding of liver transplant rejection and causes of death after transplant.—Nancy L. Ascher, M.D., Ph.D.

The Effects of Tissue-Associated and MHC Class II Antigen Presentation on In Vitro Lymphoproliferative Responses Against Canine Liver and Kidney Cell Subpopulations

Ranjan D, Roth D, Esquenazi V, Carreno M, Fuller L, Leif RC, Burke G, Miller J (Univ of Miami, Fla)

Transplantation 51:475–480, 1991   2–10

Effect of Class II MHC Antigen Induction on the Stimulating Capacity of Liver Cells[a]

Responding cells	Incubation with no inducer[b]			Incubation with MLC supernatant[c]			Incubation with INF-γ[d]		
	LH	LKu	LD	LH	LKu	LD	LH	LKu	LD
Autologous lymphocytes (n=3)	895±229	403±89	494±188	413±126	33±98	340±92	417±148	276±59	354±67
Allogeneic lymphocytes (n=3)	735±146	1940±295	2829±737	604±123	3567±649	5268±1106	897±233	3056±847	8261±1716
Percent positive class II cells[e]	10.1±1.1 (n=8)	22.9±3.4 (n=8)	30.5±4.2 (n=10)	11.4±0.7 (n=10)	31.4±2.1 (n=10)	40.4±3.8 (n=12)	12.0±0.8 (n=8)	29.9±2.8 (n=8)	41.7±4.2 (n=10)

B. Freshly isolated stimulating cells[f]

	LH	LKu	LD
Autologous lymphocyte	637±137	495±147	591±199
Allogeneic lymphocyte	988±433	2621±884	12,597±2636
Percent positive class II cells[e]	10.7±2.9	40.5±9.2	39.7±7.5

[a] ^{3}H-thymidine uptake of 9-day cultures; mean cpm of triplicate cultures ± SE.
[b] Liver cells cultured for 48 hours in tissue culture medium only.
[c] Liver cells cultured for 48 hours in diffusion chambers against 2-way MLC cultures. In control cultures, ^{3}H-thymidine uptake of 9-day cultures (responding vs. x-irradiated stimulating lymphocytes) using 1×10^5 responding cells was 8,424 ± 1,010 (n = 3) for the allogeneic mongrel lymphocytes and 20,426 ± 4,415 (n = 3) for the beagles' lympocytes. The background of cpm of the autologous cultures were 2,169 ± 300 and 674 ± 112, respectively.
[d] Liver cells cultured for 48 hours in .16% interferon gamma.
[e] Quantation of class II-positive cells was determined by fluorescence-activated cell sorter using B1F6 anticanine class II mab (mean ± SE).
[f] Obtained from the same animal as in A, but 48 hours later.
(Courtesy of Ranjan D, Roth D, Esquenazi V, et al: *Transplantation* 51:475–480, 1991.)

Background.—After allografting, there is increased expression of class II genes by the grafted organ. As transplanted organs differ in the frequency of rejection, it has been thought that differences in expression of class II antigens may be responsible. The apparent difference in the immunogenicity of canine liver and kidney cells in vitro was examined as it related to expression of class I and II MHC antigens.

Methods.—Purified hepatocytes (LH), Kupffer cells (LKu), interhepatic biliary duct cells (LD), and kidney tubular cells were isolated. These cells were incubated for 48 hours in a 2-compartment diffusion chamber opposite 2-way mixed lymphocyte cultures or canine interferon-gamma. Class II expression was detected by monoclonal antibody-derived cell sorting.

Results.—Incubation of LH, LKu, and LD with lymphocyte cultures or interferon resulted in significantly increased class II expression. Interferon-gamma preinduction of canine class II expression by LKu and LD cells amplified allogenic mixed lymphocyte liver cultures twofold (table). However, there was no autologous response. There was both an allogeneic and an autogenous response to kidney tubular cells, which was stimulated further by interferon-gamma. Antibody to class II antigens blocked uptake of labeled thymidine, indicating dependence of amplification in all cases on class II antigen gene expression. An antibody against tubular cells had no effect.

Conclusion.—Normal canine liver cells are significantly different in immunogenicity from normal canine kidney tubular cells. Cells of the normal canine liver do not stimulate a primary lymphoproliferative autoimmune reaction in vitro despite class II amplification. Therefore, autoreactivity is less important in immune recognition of purified cellular components of liver tissue than of kidney tissue.

▶ These authors have addressed the issue of whether some organs are more immunogenic than others by using an in vitro system of mixed lymphocyte parenchymal cell culture in the canine model. They note low proliferative response to lymphocytes and, in increasing order, higher proliferative responses to Kupffer cells and liver duct cells. These responses are elucidated with gamma-interferon exposure of the stimulating cells to increase class II expression. They also note a strong proliferative response to renal tubular cells. These data support the histologic pattern of rejection seen in liver allografts.—N.L. Ascher, M.D., Ph.D.

Neutrophil Activation—An Important Cause of Tissue Damage During Liver Allograft Rejection?

Adams DH, Wang LF, Burnett D, Stockley RA, Neuberger JM (Queen Elizabeth Hospital; General Hospital Birmingham, England)
Transplantation 50:86–91, 1990   2–11

Introduction.—Approximately 70% of patients who have undergone liver transplantation have allograft rejection. Liver biopsy specimens taken during rejection suggest that neutrophil activation may play a part in the mechanism of graft damage. Peripheral neutrophil activation was assessed in 16 patients to determine the role of this process in rejection after liver transplantation.

Methods.—Venous blood samples were taken from 4 men and 12 women on several occasions after the operation. There was no evidence of clinical rejection in 3 patients. In the remaining 13 patients in whom rejection developed, samples were studied on the day rejection was diagnosed histologically, and in 11 patients, once graft function was stable. Studies measured the ability of neutrophils to respond to the chemotactic peptide FMLP, to release superoxide radicals, and to cause extracellular proteolysis.

Results.—All 3 aspects of neutrophil function showed a significant increase during rejection compared with prerejection and stable samples. These functions increased 1–2 days before the episodes of acute rejection and returned to normal only after treatment with high-dose corticosteroids. No increase in neutrophil function was noted in the 3 patients in whom rejection did not develop. Stable patients and healthy controls showed similar values of neutrophil chemotactic activity compared with patients with rejection (Fig 2–3).

Conclusion.—Neutrophil-mediated mechanisms may contribute to the tissue damage of acute rejection. Neutrophil activation may occur in re-

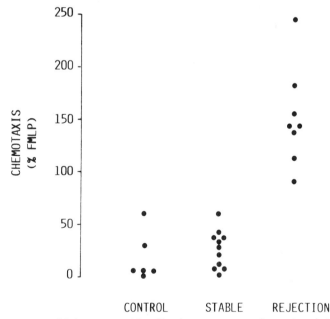

Fig 2–3.—Neutrophil chemotactic activity of lymphocyte supernatants from patients during episodes of acute rejection, during stable graft function, and from healthy controls. Chemotactic activity is expressed as a percentage of the activity with the chemotactic peptide FMLP. (Courtesy of Adams DH, Wang LF, Burnett D, et al: *Transplantation* 50:86–91, 1990.)

sponse to lymphokine secretion, suggesting a previously unrecognized mechanism of graft damage during liver allograft rejection.

▶ Neutrophils are frequently noted in biopsy specimens of patients with liver allograft rejection. This group noted neutrophil activation in the peripheral blood of patients with liver allograft rejection. The authors hypothesize that polymorphonuclear neutrophils become activated in response to cytokines released by activated lymphocytes. The majority of cells accumulating at the graft site manifest nonspecific inflammatory response. To further support their hypothesis, it would be important to determine whether neutrophils that accumulate at the allograft site also demonstrate evidence of activation.—N.L. Ascher, M.D., Ph.D.

Differentiation of Liver Graft Dysfunction by Transplant Aspiration Cytology
Schlitt HJ, Nashan B, Ringe B, Bunzendahl H, Wittekind C, Wonigeit K, Pichlmayr R (Medizinische Hochschule Hannover, Germany)
Transplantation 51:786–792, 1991   2–12

Introduction.—Liver graft dysfunction after transplantation is a common complication. Episodes of dysfunction can be from different causes, each requiring specific therapy. Liver biopsy provides a differential diagnosis, but the procedure is not without risk and may require several

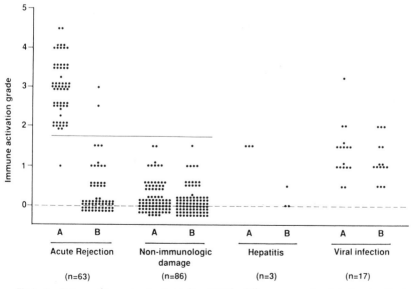

Fig 2–4.—Patterns of immune activation in liver TAC for different causes of graft dysfunction. Semiquantitative scoring (0–5) of immune activation in liver graft aspirate *(A)* and blood *(B)* was analyzed, showing clearly different patterns for acute rejection and nonimmunologic graft damage, and also typical patterns in hepatitis and systemic viral infection. (Courtesy of Schlitt HJ, Nashan B, Ringe B, et al: *Transplantation* 51:786–792, 1991.)

hours for results. Clinical usefulness and safety of transplant aspiration cytology (TAC) for diagnosing liver graft dysfunction were assessed.

Methods.—In a 2-year period, 123 patients experienced 292 episodes of liver dysfunction or fever after transplantation. All patients underwent routine TAC 2 to 3 times a week during the first 3 weeks and once a week thereafter. Biopsies were performed percutaneously, without local anesthesia, and were usually obtained from the right lobe of the liver using a 25-g spinal needle. Immune activation and parenchymal damage in the aspirates were determined cytologically.

Results.—Marked immune activation was present in aspirate but not in blood in 63 episodes of acute rejection; varying degrees of hepatocyte damage and cholestasis were noted. In 86 cases of toxic, ischemic, or septic liver damage, little or no immune activation was observed; there was, however, considerable parenchymal damage and cholestasis. Slight-to-moderate immune activation with large granular lymphocytes was found in the aspirate in 3 cases of hepatitis. In 17 cases of viral infection there was slight-to-moderate immune activation in aspirate and blood (Fig 2–4).

Conclusion.—Although TAC gives only a morphological description of parenchymal damage and immune activation, the method is very useful in the differential diagnosis of several of the more important causes of liver graft dysfunction. In addition, TAC is easily performed, has good patient acceptance, and the risk of complications is low.

▶ Aspiration cytology has the potential to be a safer method to determine intragraft events in liver transplantation. Disease states are assumed based on activation state of the aspirated cell. Recent findings of activated donor lymphocytes within stable liver allografts may provide misleading information about graft status.—N.L. Ascher, M.D., Ph.D.

Neuropathological Findings in Autopsies After Liver Transplantation
Boon AP, Adams DH, Buckels JAC, McMaster P (University of Birmingham, Birmingham, England)
Transplant Proc 23:1471–1472, 1991   2–13

Introduction.—Reports in the literature indicate the incidence and pattern of neurologic alterations in patients who had liver transplantation significantly differ from those who undergo other organ transplants. The results of a prospective autopsy survey of the neuropathology from 52 patients who died after undergoing orthotopic liver transplantation were reviewed.

Methods.—Of the 117 (41.9%) of 279 patients who received orthotopic liver transplants who died in 1983–1989, autopsies were performed on 71 (60.7%). In 47 patients, whole brains were studied prospectively and 5 were available in paraffin blocks.

Results.—There was severe cerebral edema along with increased intracranial pressure in 15 (29%) patients (table). In 7 patients, the edema

Summary of Neuropathologic Findings	
Severe hypoxic damage	
Global	19
Watershed infarcts	2
Cystic infarction	1
Venous infarction	1
A2 astrocytosis	18
Severe cerebral oedema	15
Cerebral mycosis	
Aspergillosis	10
Candidosis	2
Central pontine myelinolysis	5
Sterile haemorrhages	4
Focal white matter damage	4

(Courtesy of Boon AP, Adams DH, Buckels JAC, et al: *Transplant Proc* 23:1471–1472, 1991.)

was associated with cerebral mycosis, infarction, and hemorrhage. In the remaining 8 patients, edema resulted from hepatic encephalopathy. In 4 patients, there was intracerebral hemorrhage without any signs of an infection, 4 had established infarcts, and 10 had cerebral aspergillosis. In the 10 patients with invasive microbiology, infection significantly occurred 1–4 weeks after transplantation and appeared significantly related to high doses of steroids and to surgery during the winter and spring months. Focal lesions, particularly in the white matter, occurred in 4 patients.

Conclusion.—There is a high incidence of significant cerebral pathology occurring after liver transplantation, with the pattern of the disease process differing from that reported after other organ transplants. Patient management procedures have been changed accordingly, and the patient's cyclosporine A levels are carefully monitored, large perisurgical sodium shifts are avoided, and antifungal drugs are used aggressively. These changes in protocol have reduced neurologic morbidity in liver transplant patients.

▶ The autopsies, including neuropathology studies, of 52 patients who died after liver transplantation yield a few surprises. Unsuspected fungal infection (10 cerebral aspergillosis and 2 candidosis) was present in 20% of patients, and 10% of patients had central pontine myelinolysis in the absence of severe electrolyte perturbation. This incidence of cerebral pathology in liver transplant recipients is much higher than in recipients of other solid organ transplants. It is unclear whether this represents preexisting pathology; for example, central pontine myelinolysis is seen in the alcoholic without transplantation. It may be that these patients represent such a complex set of complications that these important premorbid conditions are overlooked.—N.L. Ascher, M.D., Ph.D.

3 Heart Transplantation

Heart Transplantation—General

▶ ↓ These articles deal with pretransplant management of patients, posttransplantation complications, and results in patients with cancer.—Nancy L. Ascher, M.D., Ph.D.

Univentricular Versus Biventricular Assist Device Support
Pennington DG, Reedy JE, Swartz MT, McBride LR, Seacord LM, Naunheim KS, Miller LW (St. Louis Univ Med Ctr)
J Heart Lung Transplant 10:258–263, 1991   3–1

Background.—The success of circulatory support for postoperative cardiogenic shock is often limited by impaired right ventricular function. This realization led to the use of biventricular support for biventricular failure. A controversy continues over whether to use selective univentricular assist devices (UVADs) or biventricular assist devices (BVADs) in heart surgery. A retroactive review compared the morbidity and mortality of patients who had received UVADs or BVADs after heart surgery, an acute myocardial infarction, or as an interim device for heart transplant.

Methods.—Only patients supported with a ventricular assist device for longer than 48 hours were considered. The Thoratec ventricular assist device (VAD) was used to provide temporary circulatory support for patients with cardiogenic shock that did not respond to inotropic therapy and an intra-aortic balloon pump (IABP). Attempts were made to determine the presence of right ventricular, left ventricular, or biventricular failure before insertion of the VAD. If the ventricular failure was judged balanced, the BVADs were inserted. If failure was left-sided, a left VAD was inserted and drugs administered to support the right ventricle. If failure was considered right-sided, a right VAD was used in conjunction with an IABP and inotropic support.

Results.—Thirty-nine patients required support with the VADs for more than 48 hours, with 23 patients receiving UVADs, and 16 receiving BVADs. Twenty-four patients had VAD insertion after coronary artery bypass grafting, valve replacement, repair of congenital anomaly, or heart transplantation; 3 received VADs after myocardial infarction, and 12 received the device as a bridge to heart transplantation. All patients had adequate VAD support and blood flow. Complications affected both patient groups in a similar manner. Bleeding was the most frequent complication (in 7 UVAD patients and 9 BVAD patients). Although anticoagulation therapy was used, thrombus developed in the VAD in 7 UVAD and 3 BVAD patients. Cannulation problems developed in 2 BVAD patients.

Conclusions.—Similar mortality and morbidity were found in patients with UVADs or BVADs. The type of ventricular failure should be determined before selecting the method of treatment. The BVAD is not intended for all patients. Its use should be based on a consideration of the patient's hemodynamic requirements.

▶ Both ventricular and biventricular assist device support are associated with a high incidence of complications and mortality. Few guidelines are available about which device is appropriate, and the authors suggest the choice be individualized. The high mortality (21/49) suggests that additional solutions are needed for this very high risk group of patients, and whether early and aggressive transplantation improves results remains to be seen.—N.L. Ascher, M.D., Ph.D.

High-Risk Heart Surgery in the Heart Transplant Candidate
Blakeman BM, Pifarré R, Sullivan H, Costanzo-Nordin MR, Zucker MJ (Loyola Univ Med Ctr, Maywood, Ill)
J Heart Transplant 9:468–472, 1990   3–2

Introduction.—Because of the limited supply of hearts for transplantation, some patients referred for heart transplantation may undergo a more conservative procedure to delay heart transplantation or stabilize the patient's condition while waiting for a heart. Data on 174 patients were retrospectively reviewed to define the predictors of outcome and prognosis to identify patients who would benefit from conventional procedures.

Methods.—Of the 174 patients who were accepted as heart transplant recipients, 104 had a heart transplant and 23 died while waiting for a heart. Of 20 patients who were considered for traditional heart operations, 18 had elective operations and 2 had emergency operations. Surgery was repeated in 10 patients, 5 had revascularization only, and 1 had aneurysmectomy with revascularization.

Results.—Of the 20 patients, 17 survived their hospitalization, and 11 avoided transplantation or placement on the transplant waiting list; these patients constituted a high-risk subset. Patients for whom conventional heart surgery was beneficial included those with poor ventricular function and ventricular arrhythmias, we well as those with poor ventricular function who had first-time vascularization; all 10 of these patients survived their operation. A poor result was obtained in 6 patients with poor ventricular function who needed repeated bypass operation, 3 of whom died.

Conclusion.—In carefully selected high-risk patients, conventional heart surgery can be performed even in those with severe left ventricular dysfunction. A 50% mortality rate may be acceptable in this group. Patients with poor ventricular function and life-threatening ventricular arrhythmias may have 35% to 50% mortality as a result of sudden cardiac death.

▶ Temporizing operations may be necessary in some patients awaiting heart transplantation. This group has defined a subset of patients who can be safely revascularized and for whom heart transplantation may be avoided. With the increasing shortage of donor hearts, identification of this subset of patients is important. It is likely that this approach requires greater technical and management skills than required for the heart transplantation.—N.L. Ascher, M.D., Ph.D.

Influence of Preoperative Transpulmonary Gradient on Late Mortality After Orthotopic Heart Transplantation

Erickson KW, Costanzo-Nordin MR, O'Sullivan EJ, Johnson MR, Zucker MJ, Pifarré R, Lawless CE, Robinson JA, Scanlon PJ (Loyola Univ Med Ctr, Maywood, Ill; Hines VA Med Ctr, Hines, Ill)
J Heart Transplant 9:526–537, 1990   3–3

Background.—Pulmonary hypertension is associated with a poor perioperative outcome in patients undergoing heart transplantation. This serious pulmonary condition appears to be a result of the dilation and failure of the donor right ventricle when it is placed abruptly into a high-resistance vascular bed. Comparisons were made of different preoperative measures of pulmonary hypertension to determine which most accurately predicted a poor outcome after orthotopic heart transplantation (OHT).

Method.—The medical records of 109 heart recipients (aged 44.6 ± 13.5 years) between March 1984 and March 1988 were reviewed for pulmonary arterial systolic pressure, pulmonary vascular resistance (Wood units), transpulmonary gradient, and pulmonary vascular resistance index (Wood units × body surface area). These patients were followed for up to 57 months after their transplant procedure.

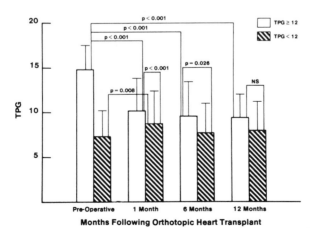

Fig 3–1.—Sequential changes in transpulmonary gradient after OHT. (Courtesy of Erickson KW, Costanzo-Nordin MR, O'Sullivan EJ, et al: *J Heart Transplant* 9:526–537, 1990.)

Findings.—Of the 109 patients, 19 died within 1 year after OHT. Causes of death included acute rejection (8), chronic rejection (1), infection (2), nonspecific OHT failure (4), bowel ischemia (1), pancreatitis (1), lymphoma (1), and liver failure (1). Preoperative pulmonary vascular resistance and its index, and pulmonary arterial systolic pressure were not predictive of 1-month, 6-month, or 1-year mortality. The 6-month mortality rate of OHT patients with transpulmonary gradient $\geq$12 mm Hg was 5 times higher than that of patients with <12 mm Hg (24% vs. 5%; p = .003). The 12-month mortality among these patients with transpulmonary gradient $\geq$12 mm Hg was 7 times greater than that of patients with transpulmonary gradient <12 mm Hg (36% vs. 5%; p = .0005) (Fig 3–1).

Conclusion.—These findings suggest that the present measures of pulmonary hypertension do not aid in predicting mortality during the first month after OHT. Patients with increased preoperative transpulmonary gradient had significantly higher mortality 6 and 12 months after surgery. Multicenter, randomized trials are needed to determine which hemodynamic measures would best identify patients at risk of dying early and late after OHT.

▶ Graft failure secondary to pulmonary hypertension after cardiac transplantation is a disastrous complication. This study failed to correlate preoperative pulmonary vascular resistance, the restive index, and pulmonary arterial systolic pressure with short- and long-term outcomes. This underscores the need for development of more predictive hemodynamic measurements. The small number of patients who died of pulmonary hypertension in this series underscores the need to combine results at multiple centers.—N.L. Ascher, M.D., Ph.D.

Cyclosporine-Induced Sympathetic Activation and Hypertension After Heart Transplantation
Scherrer U, Vissing SF, Morgan BJ, Rollins JA, Tindall RSA, Ring S, Hanson P, Mohanty PK, Victor RG (Univ of Texas, Dallas; Univ of Wisconsin, Madison; Med College of Virginia; McGuire VA Med Ctr, Richmond)
N Engl J Med 323:693–699, 1990   3–4

Background.—Although cyclosporine has greatly enhanced long-term survival after organ transplantation, it has produced a high incidence of hypertension in heart transplant recipients. The mechanism by which cyclosporine causes hypertension is unknown. In anesthetized animals, however, the immunosuppressive agent increases sympathetic-nerve discharge, which may lead to hypertension. A study was undertaken to determine whether cyclosporine-induced hypertension is accompanied by sustained sympathetic neural activation in humans.

Methods.—Microelectrode recordings of postganglionic sympathetic action potentials were performed in 19 heart transplant recipients, 16 patients with myasthenia gravis, 5 patients with essential hypertension, and 9 normal controls. Fourteen transplant recipients and 8 patients with myasthenia gravis were receiving cyclosporine.

Heart-Transplant Recipient Taking Cyclosporine

Heart-Transplant Recipient Not Taking Cyclosporine

Patient with Essential Hypertension

Normotensive Control

|——— 15 sec ———|

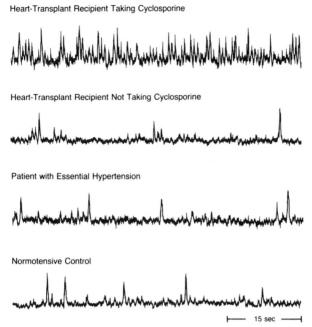

Fig 3–2.—Recordings of muscle sympathetic nerve activity in heart transplant recipient taking cyclosporine, heart transplant recipient not taking cyclosporine, patient with essential hypertension, and normotensive control subject. Each peak represents a spontaneous burst of sympathetic discharge. Frequency of sympathetic neural firing was much higher than normal in heart transplant recipient treated with cyclosporine. Sympathetic activity was normal in heart transplant recipient not taking cyclosporine and in patient with essential hypertension. (Courtesy of Sherrer U, Vissing SF, Morgan BJ, et al: *N Engl J Med* 323:693–699, 1990.)

Findings.—Heart transplant recipients treated with cyclosporine had a rate of muscle sympathetic discharge that was 2.9 times that of normal controls and 2.7 times that of the recipients not treated with cyclosporine (Fig 3–2). Both the heart transplant recipients who did not receive cyclosporine and the patients with essential hypertension showed sympathetic activity that was normal. In patients with myasthenia gravis, sympathetic discharge was 1.8 times higher in patients who received cyclosporine than in those given placebo. Similar doses of cyclosporine resulted in significantly higher mean arterial pressure (112 vs. 100 mm Hg) and sympathetic activity (80 vs. 46 bursts per minute) in heart transplant recipients than in patients with myasthenia gravis.

Discussion.—Cyclosporine treatment results in sustained sympathetic activation in both heart transplant recipients and patients with myasthenia gravis. This sympathetic activation appears to be facilitated by the cardiac denervation that accompanies heart transplantation.

▶ Hypertension is a particular problem in cardiac allograft recipients who are treated with cyclosporine. Cardiac denervation results in removal of the ventricular-baroreceptor restraint on sympathetic outflow and compounds with hypertension seen with cyclosporine after cardiac transplantation. Cyclosporine treatment was associated with sustained increased sympathetic activation in patients who had not received heart transplantation. Increased sympathetic activation appears to be one of the mechanisms by which cyclosporine causes hypertension.—N.L. Ascher, M.D., Ph.D.

Heart Transplantation in Patients With Malignant Disease
Armitage JM, Kormos RL, Griffith BP, Fricker FJ, Hardesty RL (Univ of Pittsburgh)
J Heart Transplant 9:627–630, 1990   3–5

Background.—Heart transplantation is usually reserved for patients with end-stage heart disease, but some studies indicate the aged, the diabetic, and the mortally ill may benefit from this procedure. Preliminary results were reviewed in 11 cancer patients undergoing heart transplantation.

Methods.—Eleven patients who had a history of malignant disease or a localized unresectable primary heart tumor were selected for heart transplantation. Of these 11 patients, 7 were adults and 4 were children. A leading acceptance criterion was a 1-year interval free of malignant disease. However, if the patient had less than a 1-year interval free of cancer and had an unresectable primary heart tumor or good prognostic tumor, he or she could be accepted. Minimal dosing, multidrug immunoprophylaxis was used in these transplant patients, as well as close endomyocardial biopsy surveillance during follow-up.

Findings.—The 11 patients had 12 transplants; 1 patient had acute graft dysfunction that required regrafting 3 days later. All patients survived and have been followed for 4–41 months (mean, 18 months). Two technical challenges related to tumors occurred: an angiosarcoma of the right atrium required removal of the entire right atrium and two thirds of the atrial septum, and dissection was difficult in a patient who had undergone a mastectomy, skin grafting, irradiation therapy, sternotomy, and partial pericardiectomy.

Comment.—The initial requirement for a 1-year cancer-free period before transplantation may be modified on an individual basis, depending on the nature of the tumor, anatomical constraints, and the urgency of surgery. Experience with patients with Ewing's sarcoma and heart angiosarcoma who were in active chemotherapy programs has shown that both chemotherapy and immunotherapy can be given together; however, doxorubicin and immunoprophylaxis should be avoided in these patients.

▶ This is a very interesting review from a number of aspects. Certainly the group from Pittsburgh is expanding the indications for heart transplantation to patients with previous or current malignancy. Although these authors deliberately administered less immunosuppression, it remains to be determined whether the proper level of immunosuppression in terms of rejection vs. tumor recurrence can be achieved. The issue of whether immunosuppression used in transplantation enhances growth of quiescent preexisting tumor is argued. This is important in potential renal transplant recipients and in potential liver transplant recipients with hepatoma.—N.L. Ascher, M.D., Ph.D.

The Use of Myocytes as a Model for Developing Successful Heart Preservation Solutions
Schmid T, Landry G, Fields BL, Belzer FO, Haworth RA, Southard JH (Univ of Wisconsin, Madison)
Transplantation 52:20–26, 1991   3–6

Background.—Preservation of hearts for transplantation is affected by many factors, and it is nearly impossible to study them all systematically. Isolated myocyte preparation is a useful model for studying the way in which different factors affect the preservation of heart cells. The effect of cold storage for up to 24 hours on viability of rabbit heart myocytes was measured.

Methods.—Isolated myocytes were stored at 5° C for 5 minutes, 12 hours, or 24 hours in 1 of 6 solutions: EuroCollins (EC), the Stanford (ST) and Bretschneider's (HTK) cardioplegic solutions, and University of Wisconsin (UW) solution alone and with added polyethylene glycol mol wt 8,000 or 20,000. Viability was assessed by the percentage of rod-shaped cells, adenosine triphosphate concentration, and lactic dehydrogenase release after preservation and rewarming.

Results.—After 12 and 24 hours, the cells stored in cardioplegic solutions were the least well preserved. Decreased in percentage of rod-shaped cells at these times was greater with EC than with UW solutions. Myocyte morphologic structure was best preserved and adenosine triphosphate content was highest for myocytes stored in UW solution with polyethylene glycol.

Conclusion.—The myocyte model of heart preservation suggests that loss of cell integrity is related to the preservation solution. The results are similar to those of other models, so the myocyte model appears to be of use in testing how preservation solutions and other variables affect heart cell metabolism.

▶ Development of optimal organ preservation solutions is complicated by the differential effects of different cell types and the complex transplant models required for testing. Use of myocyte cultures to screen cardiac preservation solutions may prove time and cost savings. The interplay between cell types that are manifested after reperfusion may limit the ability of these cell cultures to reflect adequately the beneficial or harmful effects of a given preservation solution.—N.L. Ascher, M.D., Ph.D.

Heart Transplantation—Rejection

▶ ↓ These articles summarize novel approaches to the avoidance and treatment of heart transplant rejection. Graft atherosclerosis is a common problem after heart transplantation, which likely represents chronic rejection. Immunosuppressive strategies will be aimed toward reducing the incidence of this important complication.—Nancy L. Ascher, M.D., Ph.D.

The Role of Anti-HLA Antibodies in Heart Transplantation
Suciu-Foca N, Reed E, Marboe C, Harris P, Xi YP, Yu-Kai S, Ho E, Rose E, Reemtsma K, King DW (Columbia Univ, New York)
Transplantation 51:716–724, 1991   3–7

Background.—Heart transplantation is now a therapeutic option for individuals with end-stage heart disease. Long-term survival among these patients is threatened by the rejection of the heart graft. To determine the role of the anti-HLA antibodies in the heart allograft rejection process, the survival of 107 heart transplant patients was compared between those in whom these antibodies did or did not develop.

Methods.—All 107 patients had received cyclosporine-based immunosuppression treatment and, at study entry, showed no antidonor HLA antibodies in serum. Endomyocardial biopsies were taken once a week for the first 3 weeks, then every 10 days during the next month, and once every 3 weeks for the next 6 weeks, then monthly throughout the first year. The patients' serum was monitored for various HLA antibodies.

Results.—The presence of mononuclear cell infiltrates in the biopsy material provided evidence of acute cellular rejection. Of the 107 patients, 47 had no signs of rejection in any of the serial biopsies. In the remaining 60 patients, evidence of cellular rejection was demonstrated in 129 of the 1,477 first-year biopsies. The actuarial survival at 4 years remained at the 90% level in patients who did not produce anti-HLA antibodies, while patients who did manufacture anti-HLA antibodies showed a survival rate of 80.9%, 73.3%, 67.5%, and 38.1% after 1, 2, 3, and 4 years, respectively. The difference in the survival rates was significant between these 2 groups, indicating that anti-HLA antibody production is associated with graft rejection. In a study of 65 patients determining the amount of anti-HLA antibodies in sera depleted of HLA antigens, 28 patients died after 1 year or more and 37 continued to live 2 years or more after the graft. In these poor outcome patients, the anti-HLA antibodies increased from 28% before depletion to 56% after the procedure. The significance of the differences was much higher between these patients and those with good outcomes when the sera were depleted of soluble HLA antigens than when the sera was tested before the depletion. The frequency of sera with anti-HLA antibodies was significantly lower in patients who tolerated the heart transplant than in those who died. The donor HLA antigens and antigen-antibody complexes had significantly higher frequency in sera from those who rejected, rather than accepted, transplants.

Conclusions.—These findings indicate that a relatively high proportion of sera from heart graft patients contain complexes of HLA antigens and anti-HLA antibodies. It may be that the amount of anti-HLA antibodies can be used as a prognostic factor in graft rejection, with the lower frequency of the anti-HLA antibody determining whether the patient will develop anti-idiotypic antibodies.

▶ This group has undertaken the difficult study of the development of anti-idiotypic antibodies in clinical heart transplantation. This study supports the notion that anti-idiotypic antibody, manifest by low levels of anti-HLA antibody may be adaptive in heart allograft acceptance.—N.L. Ascher, M.D., Ph.D.

Production of Antiidiotypic Antibodies in the Rat: In Vitro Characterization of Specificity and Correlation With In Vivo Specific Suppression of Cardiac Allograft Immune Reaction Across Major Histocompatibility Complex
Wasfie T, Reed E, Suciu-Foca N, Hardy MA (Columbia Univ, New York)
Surgery 108:431–441, 1990   3–8

Background.—Although it has been demonstrated that preadministration of donor-specific blood transfusions has a beneficial effect on allograft survival, the mechanism is not known. It has been suggested that the development of anti-idiotypic antibodies may play a role in increased allograft survival. This hypothesis was examined in Lewis rats receiving ACI cardiac allografts.

Methods.—Lewis anti-ACI hyperimmune sera were obtained from rats that had rejected successive ACI skin grafts. Purified IgG fractions (idiotypic antibodies) were used to immunize 5 naive Lewis rats, 15, 7, and 3 days before and at the time of ACI cardiac allografting. Serum was obtained from these rats before allografting.

Results.—In pretreated rats, the median allograft survival was approximately 11 days, whereas in untreated rats, it was approximately 6 days. Use of purified IgM fractions did not affect survival. Purified sera from the rats immunized with idiotypic antisera were obtained before transplantation and used in a complement-mediated cytotoxicity assay to test for anti-idiotypic activity. Strain-specific blocking activity was demonstrated in the rats that had received idiotypic immunization.

Conclusion.—Lewis rats treated with anti-ACI sera exhibited impaired anti-ACI reactivity and prolonged ACI allograft survival. This suggests that pretreatment of graft recipients with idiotypic antibodies leads to the development of anti-idiotypic antibodies that modulate alloreactivity and suppress allograft rejection.

▶ One mechanism by which host adapt to allografts in the development of anti-idiotypic antibodies. The deliberate induction of these antibodies may prove useful in prolonging allografts. It will be essential to develop a technique of reliably inducing anti-idiotypic antibodies and avoid induction of a sensitized state. The specific signals for these 2 pathways are not yet known.—N.L. Ascher, M.D., Ph.D.

Total Lymphoid Irradiation for Treatment of Intractable Cardiac Allograft Rejection

Hunt SA, Strober S, Hoppe RT, Stinson EB (Stanford Univ Med Ctr, Calif)

J Heart Lung Transplant 10:211–216, 1991   3–9

Background.—Current immunosuppressive treatments maintain graft function and reverse graft rejection in most patients, but with considerable toxicity. Some patients continue to reject their grafts despite a host of different immunosuppressants. Another immunosuppressive modality, total lymphoid irradiation (TLI), was used to reverse recurrent cardiac allograft rejection that was refractive to conventional therapy.

Methods.—Heart transplant recipients had between 1 and 6 rejection episodes before TLI was used. The TLI regimen followed was that described by Levin et al. (1989), and used treatment with an upper and lower field. The upper field covered all major supraradiaphragmatic lymphoid regions and is known as the "mantle." The heart is not specifically shielded during the procedure. The lower, or subdiaphragmatic, field is an inverted "Y." Peripheral blood samples were assayed for T cells using flow cytometry.

Results.—Ten heart transplant patients received a complete TLI course. The patients included 2 women and 8 men ranging in age from 1 to 51 years. All had received maintenance immunosuppression with cyclosporine, azathioprine, prednisone, and an initial 10-day regimen of intravenous OKT3 monoclonal antibody. The TLI therapy was interrupted in 5 patients because of complications; 4 patients experienced neutropenia and 1 suffered pneumocystis and cytomegalovirus pneumonitis. Six patients received the full TLI course and 4 received a partial TLI course. The mean duration of TLI was 47 days. Graft rejection occurred in 6 patients after an initial resolution of the rejection episode, with recurrence appearing 40 to 769 days after the initiation of TLI. Three patients had no recurrence of rejection after TLI therapy. Two of the 10 patients died, one from cardiogenic shock during TLI and one from rejection recurrence after unadvised cessation of immunosuppressive therapy. The clinical courses of the 3 living patients who did not complete the full TLI course appeared similar to that of the other patients.

Conclusions.—These preliminary findings suggest that TLI may aid in salvage therapy of heart transplants in cases when conventional immunosuppressive agents do not appear to work. Total lymphoid irradiation should also be investigated as an adjunct to immunosuppression therapy in patients susceptible to the side effects of immunosuppressive drugs.

▶ The cardiac transplant recipient with recurrent acute rejection is fortunately a rare but vexing problem. The need for more potent prophylaxis is clearly underscored by these patients and those who develop graft atherosclerosis. New immunosuppressive agents such as FK 506, RS 61443 and Rapamycin may obviate the need for such treatment as total lymphoid irradiation.—N.L. Ascher, M.D., Ph.D.

Regeneration of Adult Human Myocardium After Acute Heart Transplant Rejection
McMahon JT, Ratliff NB (Cleveland Clinic Found, Cleveland)
J Heart Transplant 9:554–567, 1990   3–10

Background.—Previous observations have shown that the myocyte injury seen in human heart transplant rejection can be reversed, rarely leaving myocyte necrosis. Normal myocardial ultrastructure recovers rapidly after the acute rejection phase. Data were reviewed on the ultrastructure of cell repair and regeneration in adult myocytes after acute heart transplant rejection.

Methods.—From August 1984 to March 1989, 1,535 endomyocardial biopsy specimens from 79 heart transplant patients were assessed for evidence of rejection. One third of the specimens were preserved in Hollande's fixative and studied by light microscopy. Another one third of the biopsies were snap frozen and studied by immunolabled antibodies, and the final one third of the specimens were prepared for analysis by high-resolution light microscopy and electron microscopy. All samples were studied for rejection.

Findings.—Of the 1,535 specimens, 388 showed signs of accelerating, moderate, severe, or resolving acute rejection. Twenty-two specimens demonstrated regeneration of adult human myocardium after the acute rejection phase. Regeneration was identified in myocytes having ultrastructural and light microscopic evidence of nuclear division and cytoplasmic dedifferentiation. Cytoplasm had characteristics of embryonic growth such as rough endoplasmic reticulum, numerous ribosomes, and abundant mitochondria. Cytoplasmic and subsarcolemmal clumps of Z band material were evidence of sarcomerogenesis. Myofibrillogenesis appeared throughout the cytoplasmic and subsarcolemmal areas. Intercalated disks had a primitive appearance, but nexus junctions were not found.

Conclusion.—Myocytic regeneration observed during the resolution of heart transplant rejection supports the concept that this injury is usually reversible and without necrosis in cases of moderate and severe acute rejection in cyclosporine-treated heart transplant patients. These findings indicate that adult myocardium has the capacity to regenerate, a new concept in cardiac physiology.

▶ These authors have summarized the ultrastructural features of regenerating myocytes recovering from acute cardiac allograft rejection. These features are shared by embryologic myocytes. The ability of adult myocytes to regenerate has enormous implications for the field of cardiac transplantation, but is perhaps more important in terms of recovering from other insults. An understanding of the triggers for regeneration is an essential next step to make this work clinically applicable.—N.L. Ascher, M.D., Ph.D.

Multidrug Resistance in Heart Transplant Patients: A Preliminary Communication on a Possible Mechanism of Therapy-Resistant Rejection
Kemnitz J, Uysal A, Haverich A, Heublein B, Cohnert TR, Stangel W, Georgii A (Hannover Medical School, Germany)
J Heart Lung Transplant 10:201–210, 1991   3–11

Background.—Multidrug resistance in heart transplant patients is a complex cellular phenomenon comprising many intracellular changes. The overexpression of P-glycoprotein has been linked to multidrug resistance and is related to the changes in P-glycoprotein structures that result in an altered multidrug resistant (mdr) phenotype in cells transfected with mutant P-glycoprotein. There are considerable differences between heart transplantation patients for the number of rejection episodes. The results of immunocytochemical staining of peripheral blood mononuclear cells (PMNs) for P-glycoprotein were evaluated.

Methods.—Peripheral blood from 49 patients with heart transplantation were obtained 0 to 872 days after the operation. The observers were blinded to the patients' clinical course. The control group consisted of 1,026 healthy blood donors with no history of drug therapy that could induce multidrug resistance. Rejection was diagnosed according to the "Hannover Classification." Immunosuppressive therapy included azathioprine, methylprednisolone, and cyclosporine.

Results.—Three percent to 21% of peripheral blood mononuclear cells were mdr cells in 39 patients (3.8%) of the control group. In the heart transplantation group of 49 patients, mdr cells were found in 3 of 13 patients sampled on the day of transplantation. Overall, 32 of 49 patients had mdr cells, with 16 showing nearly constant amounts of mdr cells and 16 others with significantly increasing values of mdr cells. Seventeen of 49 heart transplant patients demonstrated no detectable mdr cells. The increase in the frequency of acute rejection episodes was significantly correlated with the increasing values of mdr cells compared to the transplant patients with no mdr cells.

Conclusions.—The mechanisms for induction and development of mdr relate to rejection in heart transplantation. These findings suggest that patients with a positive mdr phenotype before transplantation and those showing a gradual increase in mdr cells during immunosuppressive therapy may be expected to have a higher frequency of rejection episodes.

▶ This study addresses the issue of recurrent heart rejection from a different angle. The presence of a specific white blood cell phenotype is associated with both drug resistance and increased evidence of heart allograft rejections. This may be an important predictive host factor in the pathogenesis of rejections. The validity of this observation will require the study of large numbers of recipients.—N.L. Ascher, M.D., Ph.D.

4 Lung Transplantation

▶ ↓ The growing field of lung transplantation is represented by these articles.— Nancy L. Ascher, M.D., Ph.D.

Cardiopulmonary Exercise Testing After Single and Double Lung Transplantation
Miyoshi S, Trulock EP, Schaefers H-J, Hsieh C-M, Patterson GA, Cooper JD
(Toronto General Hospital, University of Toronto, Ont; Washington Univ)
Chest 97:1130–1136, 1990   4–1

Background.—Results of formal cardiopulmonary exercise testing after either single lung transplantation (SLT) or double lung transplantation (DLT) have not been reported. Exercise performance was evaluated in SLT and DLT recipients and physiologic factors that influenced transplant patients' exercise capacities were studied.

Methods.—Six SLT and 6 DLT recipients, who had been participating in a structured rehabilitation program that included cycle and treadmill exercise, underwent an incremental exercise test on a cycle ergometer 1 week after undergoing a routine pulmonary function test. Oxygen saturation and pulse rate were monitored continuously, inspired and expired gases were analyzed, and venous blood was sampled for lactate determination.

Results.—Maximum $\dot{V}O_2$ averaged 44.2% of predicted maximum $\dot{V}O_2$ in the SLT group and 48.5% in the DLT group. There was no evidence of ventilatory exercise limitation in either group; however, circulatory factors, such as submaximal heart rate and anemia, might have limited exercise capacity. In the SLT group, there was a strong correlation between $\dot{V}O_2/kg$ at a venous blood lactate level of 2.2 mEq/L and vital capacity/body surface area, but this correlation was not found in the DLT group.

Conclusions.—In these lung transplant recipients, maximum $\dot{V}O_2$ was comparable to that reported previously in heart-lung transplant recipients. Maximum oxygen uptake remained below normal in long-term survivors of both SLT and DLT, but there was no evidence of ventilatory limitation. In most patients, chronic anemia contributed to circulatory limitation. Cardiac denervation in the DLT group and limited pulmonary vascular capacitance in the SLT group also might contribute to reduced oxygen uptake, but these factors require further study.

▶ An important parameter in assessing the value of a given transplant procedure is quality of life after transplantation. Exercise capacity after single- or double-lung transplant remains far below predicted levels, but is comparable to that of heart-lung transplant recipients. Conditioning to increase heart rate and correction of other factors such as anemia may enhance exercise capacity. For lung transplant recipients to resume leisure or work activity, exercise capacity should be maximized.—N.L. Ascher, M.D., Ph.D.

Life in the Allogeneic Environment After Lung Transplantation
Paradis I, Rabinowich H, Zeevi A, Yousem S, Noyes B, Hoffman R, Griffith B, Dauber J (Univ of Pittsburgh, Pa)
Lung 168:11725–11815, 1990   4–2

Background.—The presence of numerous macrophages in the transplanted lung helps explain why it is more susceptible to rejection than is the transplanted heart. In addition, alveolar macrophages (AMs) are critical to pulmonary defense against infection.

Methods.—The ability of AMs and lymphocytes to generate an immune response against transplantation antigens from the donor was examined using the primed lymphocyte test (PLT). Responsiveness to antigens from unrelated allogeneic persons was tested using the mixed lymphocyte reaction (MLR). The study included 12 lung transplant recipients and 14 normal subjects having bronchoalveolar lavage.

Findings.—Peak chemotactic responses were increased soon after lung transplantation. Both the phagocytic and killing properties of AMs from lung recipients were impaired in vitro. Monocyte- and AM-related support of mitogen-induced lymphocyte proliferation were impaired in lung recipients. Patient AMs were as efficient as autologous monocytes in stimulating an MLR. A PLT with AMs and lung lymphocytes occurred chiefly when acute or chronic rejection was present.

Conclusions.—Some antimicrobial functions of AMs seem to be impaired in the transplanted lung. At the same time, functions related to transplant immunity are upregulated. In lung transplantation, AMs are faced with protecting against infection while not destroying their home. Neither of these mutually exclusive tasks is performed efficiently.

▶ This important study separates the antimicrobial function from the immunogenic function of alveolar macrophages in lung transplant recipients. Whereas some antimicrobial functions are impaired in the transplant situation, the ability of these cells to elicit an immune response is intact. Inhibition of this immunogenic function may further inhibit the ability of these cells to defend against infection and compound infectious complications in these patients.—N.L. Ascher, M.D., Ph.D.

Growth Potential of the Immature Transplanted Lung: An Experimental Study
Hislop AA, Odom NJ, McGregor CGA, Haworth SG (Institute of Child Health, London; Mayo Clinic, Rochester, Minn)
J Thorac Cardiovasc Surg 100:360–370, 1990   4–3

Introduction.—Combined heart-lung transplantation is the sole treatment for children with a congenital heart condition in whom inoperable pulmonary vascular disease develops. Although children as young as 3 years have undergone this procedure, the effects of the surgery remain to be seen. Because children younger than 4 years continue to experience rapid alveolar multiplication, the growth of both the transplanted and contralateral lungs after single lung transplantation were investigated.

Methods.—Male Lewis and Brown Norway (BN) rats were used in 4 groups in the following experimental design: groups 1 and 2 underwent a single left lung transplant each, but group 1 had syngeneic transplants between Lewis rats, whereas group 2 had allogeneic transplants between BN and Lewis animals; group 3 used Lewis rats in which the hilar section of the extrapulmonary bronchus, artery, and vein of the left lung were denervated and devascularized for transplantation; and group 4 consisted of both Lewis and BN animals serving as controls. Under general anesthesia, the left lung was removed from donor rats, usually with hilum of the left lung. The left lung was removed from the recipient animal and the donor organ was then implanted by anastomosing the vein and artery. The lung was reperfused.

Results.—Animals receiving organ transplants at first had slower weight gain than normal. At 2 weeks after surgery, no difference was observed between experimental animals and controls. No right ventricular hypertrophy or pulmonary hypertension was found in the experimental animals. Rats that received allogeneic transplants showed an early inflammatory response in the form of mononuclear cells and some eosinophils in groups surrounding the airway 2 weeks after surgery. A sustained immune response could still be seen 6 months after transplantation. Control and syngeneic and allogeneic transplant animals showed lung growth, but the syngeneic transplant animals demonstrated a significantly greater increase in lung volume than even normal rats. In denervated animals, the left lung increased in size normally no matter when the transplant occurred (at ages 4 or 6 weeks). The right lung did not grow normally in these animals. The right lung was larger than normal in all transplant animals 2 weeks after surgery; 6 months after surgery, the right lung was twice normal size in the syngeneic transplant rats. Alveolar multiplication occurred at a normal rate and the diameter of the left main extrapulmonary bronchus at the hilum and at the terminal bronchiolar level increased 2 weeks after transplantation.

Conclusion.—The immature rat lung will grow after transplantation through the formation of normal new structures and an increase in size of the remaining structures.

▶ Denervation does not adversely affect the growth of immature transplanted lungs in the rat allograft model. These data are important in the consideration of the use of fetal tissue for transplantation. The model demonstrates development of new alveoli and increase in airway diameter. The limiting factors in human lung transplantation using fetal tissue would be expected to be anastomotic sites.—N.L. Ascher, M.D., Ph.D.

5 Progress in Pancreas and Islet Transplantation

▶ ↓ In recent years, there has been a gratifying increase in the success rate of pancreatic transplantation. Tefveson et al. noted that the success rate of combined renal and pancreatic transplantation rivals that of renal transplantation alone. The success rate of pancreatic retransplantation is now quite acceptable. Although the long-term rate of pancreatic transplant engraftment is now acceptable, it is still an unpleasant reality to note that the morbidity of pancreatic transplantation adds greatly to the overall morbidity of the combined renal and pancreatic transplantation procedure.

As these improvements in whole organ pancreatic transplantation have progressed, inroads have been made in human islet cell transplantation. Improved methods for islet cell procurement and preservation have been accomplished. Several groups have now succeeded in transplanting freshly isolated and cryopreserved pancreatic islets in humans afflicted with diabetes mellitus. New methods of encapsulation and incorporation into biohybred devices hold great promise.—Terry Strom, M.D.

Renal Transplantation in Diabetic Patients With or Without Simultaneous Pancreatic Transplantation 1986: Data from the EDTA Registry
Tufveson G, Brynger H, Dimeny E, Brunner FP, Ehrich JHH, Fassbinder W, Geerlings W, Rizzoni G, Selwood NH, Wing AJ (EDTA Registry, St Thomas' Hospital, London)
Nephrol Dial Transplant 6:1–4, 1991   5–1

Introduction.—The combined grafting of the pancreas and kidney in patients with diabetic nephropathy has led to controversy over the double organ procedure, focusing on the survival of the patient and of the transplanted kidney. The results of 90 combined kidney and pancreas grafts performed in 1986 were surveyed using data from the European EDTA Registry.

Survey.—The EDTA Registry showed that 122 combined organ transplants were performed in Europe in 1986. In 1988, 96 questionnaires were sent to all of the centers performing this operation, requesting information about each patient and outcome of the transplantation. Ninety of the 96 (93.8%) questionnaires were returned. Controls included 389 patients receiving kidney grafts in 1986 in Belgium, Denmark, Germany, Finland, France, Switzerland, and England.

Findings.—This uncontrolled survey indicated that combined trans-

81

plants occurred relatively predominantly in Sweden and Norway and relatively few transplants in France, England, and Italy. Thus, the control group of kidney recipients did not match the study group, necessitating the omission of all data on patients from Sweden and Norway. Recipients of combined grafts were younger, with a median age at transplantation of 36 years, than recipients of kidney grafts alone, who had a median age of 39 years. Survival was nearly equal for the 2 patient groups (89% for combined transplants vs. 90% for kidney-only transplants).

Conclusions.—Pancreas plus kidney transplantation can have the same success rate as kidney-only transplantation if performed by experienced surgeons in properly selected patients. However, this report is an uncontrolled study that did not establish whether patients' characteristics such as cardiovascular disease and age at transplant were equivalent.

▶ This analysis suggests—perhaps too boldly—that combined kidney-pancreas transplantation can be performed as safely as kidney transplantation. Survival of kidney graft recipients was comparable in both groups. This brief analysis of an uncontrolled study does not provide any assurance that the patients undergoing kidney and patients undergoing combined transplantation were equivalent in terms of age, cardiovascular disease, etc. This report is encouraging, but hardly convincing that "two grafts are as safe as one." By the way, I'm not against combined transplantation. It's hard to rationalize isolated kidney transplantation as a means to rehabilitate a patient with type I diabetes who has end-stage renal disease.—T. Strom, M.D.

Pancreas Retransplants Compared With Primary Transplants
Morel P, Schlumpf R, Dunn DL, Moudry-Munns K, Najarian JS, Sutherland DER (Univ of Minnesota Hosp, Minn)
Transplantation 51:825–833, 1991   5–2

Introduction.—Results of pancreas transplantation are generally improving, and evidence suggests that this procedure positively affects the course of secondary diabetic complications. Thus, there is an impetus to perform a subsequent transplant in patients whose initial grafts have failed. Whether such a retransplant policy would be justified was examined.

Methods.—The results of 327 pancreas transplants performed in 261 patients between 1978 and 1989 were analyzed. Of these, 79% were primary procedures and 21% were retransplants. The latter included 48 second, 18 third, and 2 fourth transplants.

Findings.—The overall patient survival rates at 1 month and 1 year were 98% and 91%, respectively, after primary transplantation. After retransplantation, these rates were similar—94% and 89%, respectively. The overall rates of graft function also were similar. At 1 month they were 76% for all primary transplants and 79% for all retransplants; at 1 year the rates were 46% and 43%, respectively. Causes of graft loss at 1 month were similar in patients with primary and second, third, or fourth transplants. When analyzed according to surgical technique, there were generally no significant differences between the results of primary transplantation and retransplantation. However, when pancreas and kidney transplantation was done simultaneously, the results of the primary transplants were significantly better than those of retransplants, with 1-year pancreas graft function rates of 68% and 32%, respectively.

Conclusions.—Except for patients who need a kidney in addition to a pancreas transplant, pancreas retransplantation can yield results as good as those of primary transplantation. Such retransplantation should be offered to selected diabetic patients after a previous graft has failed.

▶ The authors present some rather sobering data in an upbeat manner. They correctly point out that primary and retransplantation with isolated pancreatic grafts result in a similar rate of patient survival and engraftment. That's the good news. The bad news is that the rate of successful engraftment in recipients of isolated grafts is quite low. Data from the large multicenter registers reveal that simultaneous kidney-pancreas transplantation results in a far superior rate of pancreatic engraftment compared with rates in recipients of isolated grafts. My own modest clinical experience has taught me just how difficult it is to detect early reversible pancreatic rejection. Apparently, the administration of antirejection therapy to patients sustaining obvious kidney graft rejection serves to eradicate otherwise undetected bouts of early pancreatic graft rejection.—T. Strom, M.D.

Morbidity of Pancreas Transplantation During Cadaveric Renal Transplantation

Rosen CB, Frohnert PP, Velosa JA, Engen DE, Sterioff S (Mayo Clinic, Rochester, Minn)
Transplantation 51:123–127, 1991   5–3

Background.—Diabetics who require renal transplantation may undergo simultaneous pancreas transplantation to limit diabetic complications; however, the additional risk that this procedure poses is unclear. Pancreas transplantation may halt the progression of peripheral vascular disease, coronary artery disease, neuropathy, and retinopathy.

Objective.—A group of 18 consecutive recipients of combined pancreas and kidney transplants was followed for at least a year after operation. The group was then compared with 18 consecutive patients who were given kidney transplants only. All of the patients received cadaver kidney allografts, and all had type I diabetes with chronic renal failure.

Outcome.—Both groups of patients had 94% survival up to 18 months after transplantation. In both groups, more than 80% of the renal allografts functioned satisfactorily. Pancreatic graft function was satisfactory in 81% of the recipients at 18 months. Wound complications, particularly infection, were substantially more frequent in the pancreas-kidney recipients, and the same was true for infectious complications in general. Acute rejection was nearly twice as frequent in the pancreas-kidney group. These patients required more time in hospital during the first posttransplant year than those given kidneys only.

Conclusion.—Morbidity is substantially greater after pancreas-kidney transplantation than after renal allografting. This will have to be considered when advising diabetics with renal failure.

▶ What are the transplant-related therapeutic options for patients with type I diabetes mellitus and end-stage renal disease? The options are combined pancreas-kidney transplantation or kidney transplantation alone with or without delayed pancreatic transplantation. Isolated pancreatic transplantation has an immunologic failure rate that is twice that of combined pancreas-kidney transplantation because of the difficulties in prompt diagnosis of pancreatic graft rejection. Thus, we rarely recommend isolated pancreatic transplantation. What are the risks of adding pancreas to kidney transplantation? Patient survival and graft survival were not compromised in this uncontrolled analysis, although it is likely that the "best" patients were selected for combined transplantation. There is no doubt, however, that combined transplantation adds considerable morbidity. Forty-four additional days of hospitalization in the first posttransplant year is one price that is exacted for pancreatic transplantation. Is this steep toll in morbidity worth the price? The jury is still out. Yet there is little doubt that a functioning pancreatic graft does aid in ameliorating diabetes-related tissue damage. It is not easy to advise patients on the merits of combined transplantation because detailed information on the pros and cons is not yet available.—T. Strom, M.D.

Reversal of Diabetic Somatic Neuropathy by Whole-Pancreas Transplantation
Orloff MJ, Greenleaf G, Girard B (Univ of California, San Diego)
Surgery 108:179–190, 1990   5–4

Background.—It has been demonstrated previously that whole-pancreas transplantation, performed early in the course of alloxan-induced diabetes mellitus (DM) in rats, can confer precise, lifelong metabolic control and prevent development and progression of diabetic lesions of the somatic nerve. Further rat pancreas transplant experiments were performed to determine whether this procedure can reverse diabetic somatic neuropathy.

Methods.—Three groups of highly inbred Lewis-strain rats were studied: 47 nondiabetic controls, 90 untreated alloxan-induced diabetic controls, and 230 rats that, 6–21 months after induction of DM, had syngeneic pancreaticoduodenal transplants. Animals were monitored monthly for 2 years by metabolic studies and electron microscopic morphometry of the sciatic and testicular nerves. According to a "blind" protocol, the lesions evaluated were loss of myelinated axons, intra-axonal glycogen deposits, axons with glycogen deposits, demyelinated axons, degenerating axons, and loss of intact axoglial junctions in paranodal terminal myelin loops. Nerve samples were taken before transplantation and at death

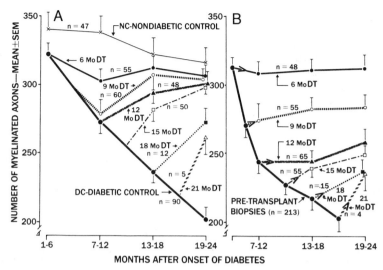

Fig 5–1.—**A,** mean number of myelinated axons in the sciatic nerve of the 3 groups of rats and (**B**) in the testicular nerve of the group of diabetic rats given syngeneic pancreaticoduodenal transplants before and after pancreaticoduodenal transplantation. The *n* at each time interval after onset of diabetes mellitus for the nondiabetic controls and the untreated alloxan-induced diabetic controls, respectively, was: 12 and 25 at 1–6 months, 12 and 25 at 7–12 months, 11 and 24 at 13–18 months, and 12 and 16 at 19–24 months. (Courtesy of Orloff MJ, Greenleaf G, Girard B: *Surgery* 108:179–190, 1990.)

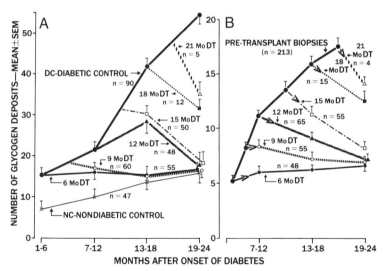

Fig 5–2.—**A,** mean number of glycogen deposits in the sciatic nerve of the 3 groups of rats and (**B**) in testicular nerve of diabetic rats given syngeneic pancreaticoduodenal transplants before and after pancreaticoduodenal transplantation. The *n* at each time interval after onset of diabetes mellitus for the nondiabetic controls and the untreated alloxan-induced diabetic controls, respectively, was: 12 and 25 at 1–6 months, 12 and 25 at 7–12 months, 11 and 24 at 13–18 months, and 12 and 16 at 19–24 months. (Courtesy of Orloff MJ, Greenleaf G, Girard B: *Surgery* 108:179–190, 1990.)

in the transplantation group so that the animals could serve as their own controls.

Results.—In the animals with untreated diabetes, all 6 types of nerve lesions progressed relentlessly throughout the study period. Rats that received pancreas transplantation attained lifelong, complete control of DM and reversal of all 6 types of lesions in both the testicular and sciatic nerves (Figs 5–1 and 5–2). Nerve lesions reversed even when transplantation was done as late as 15 months after the induction of DM.

Conclusions.—Whole pancreas transplantation, the first form of DM therapy to achieve reversal of diabetic somatic neuropathy, was studied. Such reversal does not necessarily mean that lesions in other organs and tissues could be reversed by this treatment. There appears to be a rational basis for whole pancreas transplantation in patients with advanced insulin-dependent DM.

▶ OK. This is a study of rats, not people. OK. Neuropathy did not result from a spontaneous autoimmune form of diabetes—it was created by chemical ablation of islet function. Nonetheless, this study does offer controlled data showing a beneficial effect of pancreatic transplantation on diabetic neuropathy (Figs 5–1 and 5–2). Clinical data are also slowly accruing, indicating a rehabilitative role for successful pancreatic transplantation. If we only could learn how to successfully transplant before end organ diabetic damage becomes severe.—T. Strom, M.D.

Long-Term Metabolic and Quality of Life Results With Pancreatic/Renal Transplantation in Insulin-Dependent Diabetes Mellitus
Nathan DM, Fogel H, Norman D, Russell PS, Tolkoff-Rubin N, Delmonico FL, Auchincloss H Jr, Camuso J, Cosimi AB (Massachusetts Gen Hosp; Harvard Med School, Boston)
Transplantation 52:85–91, 1991   5–5

Background.—Assessing whole-organ pancreas transplantation in the treatment of insulin-dependent diabetes mellitus (IDDM) has been difficult because of generally poor graft survival and significant complications. A simultaneous pancreas and kidney transplantation program has been technically successful in 33 patients with IDDM.

Patients and Outcomes.—From 1986 to 1989, 33 patients with IDDM and renal failure received simultaneous cadaver renal and pancreas transplants. Patient and graft survival at a mean follow-up of 21 months was 85%. In all but 1 recipient, glucose metabolism was normalized without need for exogenous insulin immediately after transplantation, and it remained normal in 85%. Outcomes in these 33 recipients were compared with those in 18 patients with insulin-dependent diabetes who received kidney transplants only in the same period. General quality of life improved significantly in both groups of recipients, but the diabetes-specific quality of life improved only in those receiving both pancreas and kidney. Pancreas and kidney recipients required twice the length of stay in the hospital for the transplantation and 2 times as many re-admissions for various complications. Of the 5 deaths in the pancreas-kidney group, 2 were attributed to pancreas transplantation.

Conclusions.—Pancreas transplantation in patients with IDDM can now be done with a high degree of success. Glucose metabolism can be normalized, and overall mortality can be comparable to that associated with kidney transplantation alone. Successful pancreas transplantation improves diabetes-specific quality of life, although patients undergoing both pancreas and kidney transplantation must stay in the hospital longer and have complications related to the transplanted pancreas. The effect of this procedure on the long-term complications of insulin-dependent diabetes is not yet known.

▶ Pancreatic transplantation is a double-edged sword. Most studies note that complications arising from pancreatic transplantation result in a significant increase in short morbidity for type I diabetic patients undergoing combined pancreatic-kidney transplantation as compared to kidney transplantation. On the other hand, indices of well being suggest that successful pancreatic transplantation does provide important benefits for diabetic subjects.—T. Strom, M.D.

Percutaneous Biopsy of Bladder-Drained Pancreas Transplants
Allen RDM, Wilson TG, Grierson JM, Greenberg ML, Earl MJ, Nankivell BJ, Pearl TA, Chapman JR (Westmead Hospital, Sydney, Australia)
Transplantation 51:1213–1216, 1991   5–6

Introduction.—Biopsy is a frequent practice in most areas of organ transplantation, but percutaneous biopsy of pancreatic transplants has

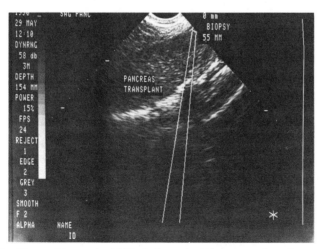

Fig 5–3.—Ultrasound image using 3-MHz duplex mechanical sector transducer. Pancreas transplant is demonstrated, together with biopsy guide lines between which biopsy needle tracks. (Courtesy of Allen RDM, Wilson TG, Grierson JM, et al: *Transplantation* 51:1213–1216, 1991.)

not been previously described, presumably because of the fear of complications. The safety of fine-needle aspiration biopsy and needle core biopsy was evaluated in 18 patients with end-stage renal disease and insulin-dependent diabetes mellitus who received combined cadaveric kidney-pancreas transplants. An additional patient received a pancreas transplant only.

Methods.—Percutaneous needle core biopsies were taken 1 and 3 weeks and 3 months after transplantation by using an 18-gauge needle. Biopsy was done under local anesthesia and ultrasonic guidance, and a 3-MHz duplex mechanical sector transducer with biopsy guide attached was used (Fig 5–3). If practicable, fine-needle aspiration biopsy was done at the same time by using a 22-gauge needle. The distal half of the organ was sampled.

Results.—Actuarial survival rates at up to 40 months were 84% for pancreas grafts and 95% for kidney grafts. Three functioning pancreas grafts were lost because of venous thrombosis. Seventy percent of attempts at fine needle aspiration biopsy were successful. All but 7% of core biopsies were suitable for histopathologic evaluation. The serum level of amylase often rose transiently after biopsy. One patient had gross hematuria on 2 occasions. In 11 episodes of pancreas graft rejection the urinary level of amylase was a most unreliable marker. The pancreas graft exhibited signs of rejection in 69% of cases of renal graft rejection, but not in the absence of kidney rejection.

Conclusions.—Percutaneous biopsy of the pancreatic transplant is a safe and useful procedure. It is less complicated and less costly than either open biopsy or cystoscopic transduodenal biopsy.

▶ These fearless investigators have performed percutaneous pancreatic allograft biopsies. The safety and diagnostic reliability of percutaneous 20-gauge pancreatic needle biopsies were assessed. To obtain the biopsy, the biopsy needle was attached to an ultrasound instrument transducer (see Fig 5–3). This technique provided the visual support required to undertake biopsies of this enzyme-producing (flesh-digesting), fistula prone organ. Thirty-seven of 40 attempts were successful. By way of comparison, 33 of 47 fine needle aspiration biopsies yielded diagnostic information. Monitoring of urinary amylase levels was extremely unreliable in indicating rejection. Many rejections were evident in the absence of reduced amylase excretion. The technique appears to be relatively safe, although 29% of biopsied individuals experienced a transient hyperamylasemia. It is most interesting to note that pathologic evidence of pancreatic rejection was not noted in the absence of renal graft rejection. The message: (1) monitoring of urinary amylase is a near useless means of detecting pancreatic rejection, (2) it is not outrageous to biopsy the pancreas transplant, but (3) pancreatic biopsy may not be necessary if a renal biopsy is obtained.—T. Strom, M.D.

Pancreatic Transplants: CT-Guided Biopsy
Bernardino M, Fernandez M, Neylan J, Hertzler G, Whelchel J, Olson R (Emory Univ, Atlanta)
Radiology 177:709–711, 1990   5–7

Background.—Percutaneous pancreatic biopsies are less accurate than other types of percutaneous biopsies. An initial experience with an automated biopsy device for obtaining tissue from pancreatic transplants was assessed.

Methods.—Ten biopsies of pancreatic allografts were performed under CT guidance in 4 patients to determine the cause of pancreatic dysfunction. An 18-gauge biopsy needle and a biopsy gun were used in all of the biopsies. Simultaneous biopsies of the pancreatic head and tail were done on 4 occasions.

Results.—The specimens obtained in 9 of the 10 biopsies were adequate for diagnosis. Important histological differences were seen between specimens from the head and the tail of the allograft in 2 of the 4 simultaneous procedures. There were no complications immediately after the procedure or during the 48-hour follow-up period. The procedure was well tolerated by all of the patients.

Conclusions.—Computed tomography-guided biopsies of pancreatic transplants performed with a biopsy gun appear to be safe and accurate. The procedure is easy to perform. Simultaneous sampling of the pancreatic head and tail may provide important data that may not be available with cytoscopically guided biopsy of the head only.

▶ Biopsy gun biopsies have been used to investigate the nature of suspect pancreatic masses. Armed with that piece of information, this intrepid group initiated paired head and tail pancreatic allograft biopsies with the biopsy gun and CT guidance (see Figure 1 in the original article). Noninvasive measures to promptly and reliably diagnose pancreatic graft rejection don't exist. Many have feared undertaking pancreatic graft biopsies. They did not get into trouble, and useful information was obtained. I would have had to premedicate myself to get the courage to launch this interesting approach.—T. Strom, M.D.

Histologic Diagnosis of Rejection by Using Cytoscopically Directed Needle Biopsy Specimens From Dysfunctional Pancreatoduodenal Allografts With Exocrine Drainage into the Bladder
Carpenter HA, Engen DE, Munn SR, Barr D, Marsh CL, Ludwig J, Perkins JD (Mayo Clinic and Mayo Found, Rochester, Minn)
Am J Surg Pathol 14:837–846, 1990   5–8

Background.—The diagnosis of pancreatoduodenal allograft rejection is based primarily on indirect evidence. Needle biopsy specimens obtained under cystoscopic direction were studied to determine the histologic features of rejection and to identify nonrejection causes of human pancreatic allograft dysfunction.

Methods.—The study included 17 pancreatic and 14 duodenal biopsy specimens obtained from 15 dysfunctional pancreatoduodenal allografts with exocrine drainage into the bladder. Rejection was diagnosed in the presence of diffuse mixed inflammatory infiltrates of pancreatic acinar tissue, diffuse mixed inflammatory infiltrates of the duodenal mucosa with necrosis of individual epithelial cells in the crypts, or diffuse mixed inflammatory infiltrates of the duodenal muscularis propria.

Findings.—Only 8 of the 15 dysfunctional allografts demonstrated the most common histological features of rejection including diffuse mixed inflammatory infiltrates of pancreatic acinar tissue and the duodenum wall. The earliest histological change in rejection was the diffuse infiltration of pancreatic acinar tissue by the neutrophils. A group of 7 dysfunctional allografts with nonrejection demonstrated a normal pancreas or various changes including acinar dilation with inspissation of secretions, fibrosis, cytomegalovirus inclusions, and enzymatic necrosis. In both rejection and nonrejection, the histological changes in the duodenum paralleled those in the pancreas.

Conclusions.—The histological features of rejection in pancreatoduodenal allografts appear to be distinctive. The biopsy specimen changes reflect the state of the graft accurately, and they can be used to diagnose rejection and other causes of graft dysfunction. Biopsy samples from both the duodenum and pancreas are helpful diagnostically, and the biopsy findings can be used to guide clinical management of rejection and to develop other noninvasive rejection tests.

▶ Reflecting the need to develop an accurate and prompt means to diagnose pancreatic graft rejection, these authors undertook a different approach to graft biopsy. This technique limits the target area available for biopsy because access to the graft is achieved through the exocrine drainage into the bladder. Useful data were usually achieved (see Table 1 of the original article). The principle attributes of pancreatic graft rejection resemble those of graft rejection in other organs, except for a curious propensity to attack acinar ducts or islets. It is interesting that similar changes were usually noted in both the duodenal and pancreatic samples. The correlation was not tight enough, however, to exclude the diagnosis of pancreatic rejection if the duodenum appeared normal.—T. Strom, M.D.

Comparison of Automated and Manual Methods for Islet Isolation
Warnock GL, Kneteman NM, Evans MG, Dabbs KD, Rajotte RV (University of Alberta, Edmonton)
Can J Surg 33:368–371, 1990   5–9

Background.—Although progress has been made in the isolation of islets of Langerhans from the pancreas of human donors, islet yields must be improved to reverse the insulin-dependent state. Improvements can be made in collagenase digestion of the fibrous connective tissue stroma of the pancreas, gentle mechanical dissociation of islets from exocrine constituents, and purification. The principal features of a collagenase perfusion method and an automated dissociation technique were used to determine whether islets could be isolated from the large mammal pancreas and to compare the effects of the 2 methods on isolated islets.

Methods.—Sixteen dogs were used. Their pancreata were cannulated and perfused with collagenase at 4° C, then warmed to 37° C. The pancreata of the 8 dogs in group 1 were perfused at 37° C until digested, then dissociated manually by teasing and trituration. The pancreata of the 8 dogs in group 2 were transferred to a closed chamber for continued collagenase digestion and dissociation at 37° C. Identical Ficoll gradients were used to purify the islets. Aliquots were stained with dithizone and assessed, and total islet volume was determined.

Results.—Pancreata in group 2 were thoroughly digested, leaving only a few residual ducts. However, undigested fragments persisted in group 1 pancreata. Both groups had similar islet sizes. Group 2 had a greater islet volume before and after Ficoll purification, but the difference was nonsignificant. In both groups, purity was greater than 90%. Perfusion with 28mM glucose produced a biphasic insulin release from islets in both groups of dogs.

Conclusions.—The combined protocol enables mass isolation of purified islets from the pancreas in dogs. The automated protocol for pancreas dissociation tends to improve the yield of islets compared with the manual method, without compromising islet size and viability. It also offers the advantages of a close system with increased control over the extent of collagenase digestion.

▶ Two techniques have been developed to harvest islet cells. A duct method for collagenase perfusion through the pancreas aims to digest the fibrous stroma and liberate islets. This technique was used in concern with gentle mechanical dissociation. Recordi previously reported on a method that uses a simultaneous collagenase digestion and mechanical islet cell dissociation. This report confirms that combined collagenase treatment and gentle mechanical dissociation are beneficial for purifying viable islets.—T. Strom, M.D.

A Simple Method for the Release of Islets by Controlled Collagenase Digestion of the Human Pancreas
London NJM, Lake SP, Wilson J, Bassett D, Toomey P, Bell PRF, James RFL
(University of Leicester, England)
Transplantation 49:1109–1113, 1990   5–10

Background.—The most efficient way to obtain islets from the human pancreas is collagenase digestion of the gland. An automated method of digestion has been described previously, but it is very complex. A simpler technique for liberating islets from the human pancreas that is similar to the automated method was evaluated.

Technique.—The pancreas is distended with collagenase and a biopsy is obtained. The specimen is divided into 5 pieces that are placed in Universals containing minimal essential medium and dithizone at 39° C. The pancreas is incubated at 39° C in MEM. At 5 minutes and at intervals thereafter, a Universal is removed from the water bath and shaken for 30 seconds. The contents are then examined by microscopy. When free cleaved islets are seen, the pancreas is placed into 1 compartment of a kidney bowl divided in half by a 1-mm mesh. The pancreas is then gently teased apart. The fluid digest in the empty half of the bowl is aspirated and passed through a 500 μm mesh into ice cold MEM containing 20% newborn calf serum. The process is repeated until digestion has ceased.

Results.—This method was used on 20 consecutive pancreata with a median weight of 53.9 g. A total of 131,672 islets were counted in the digest. This is equivalent to a median of 2,394 islets/g pancreas. The median volume of islet tissue in the digest was 299 mm³, equivalent to 5.81 mm³/g pancreas.

Conclusions.—A potential advantage of using an automated method of islet isolation is a decreased risk of bacterial contamination. All of the islet cultures produced using the less complex method were sterile. With strict attention to aseptic technique, the risk of infection is low. This method is a simple, effective way to produce large numbers of cleaved islets from the collagenase-digested human pancreas.

▶ Because pure islets evoke a weak immune response in rodents and because the exocrine pancreas is the source of much grief in pancreas transplant recipients, it would be nice to begin larger scale islet cell transplantation in man. A catch-22–like problem haunts this effort. It has proven more difficult to harvest islets from humans than from rodents. What else is new? It's always harder in the clinic. In mice we know which strains give us a high or low yield of islets. This paper describes a rational and apparently effective means of increasing the yield of islets (see Figure 1 in the original article). This work won't win a Nobel Prize, but thank goodness that several groups are devoted to making headway in solving this vexing problem.—T. Strom, M.D.

Successful Banking of Pancreatic Endocrine Cells for Transplantation
Tze WJ, Tai J (University of British Columbia, Vancouver)
Metabolism 39:719–723, 1990   5–11

Background.—Difficulties in collecting enough donor pancreatic islets for transplantation pose a major obstacle in the clinical application of islet transplantation. Cryopreservation is a potentially useful way to bank islet tissues until adequate quantities are obtained, but there is some reduction in islet cell function after the freezing and thawing process. Five different cryopreservation protocols were compared to determine optimal freezing and thawing conditions for rat pancreatic endocrine cells (PEC) and insulinoma cells.

Methods.—Pancreatic endocrine cells and insulinoma cells were cooled at rates of −.3° C/min to −70° C/min in the presence of 10%, 15%, or 20% dimethylsulfoxide (DMSO) with a programmable temperature controller. The cells were then transferred to liquid nitrogen for storage. Frozen cells were thawed by the rapid thawing procedure in a 37° C water bath or the slow thawing procedure in air. An hour after thawing, trypan blue dye exclusion was done to test cellular viability.

Results.—The viability results for PEC and insulinoma cells were similar. A slow cooling rate at −.3° C/min combined with a rapid thawing gave the best results, with up to 80% cellular viability. Cryoprotectant DMSO at 10% concentration was the most effective concentration. Using the best protocol, intraportal transplantation of cryopreserved Wistar strain PEC into allogeneic ACI diabetic recipients normalized their blood glucose for 8.3 days, which was comparable to the outcome using noncryopreserved preparations. Cytotoxic antibody titers in the ACI recipients of cryopreserved and noncryopreserved Wistar PEC grafts were also comparable. Intrathecal transplantation of frozen-thawed Wistar PEC into allogeneic ACI diabetic recipients ameliorated the diabetic state in the long term in all animals.

Conclusions.—Cryopreservation is an effective procedure for banking PEC before transplantation. The best protocol is −5° C/min to 4° C, held for 3 minutes; −.3° C/min to −7° C, held for 3 minutes; −.3° C/min to −40° C; and −5° C/min from −40° C to −70° C in 10% DMSO with a programmable temperature controller, then transfer to liquid nitrogen for storage.

▶ The inability to harvest enough islet cells from an individual pancreas donor to render a transplant recipient englycemic has prevented development of clinical islet cell transplantation. It is now well recognized that islets must be procured from at least 2 donors to harvest a sufficient islet cell mass for successful transplantation. Cryopreservation of harvested islets has emerged as the best bet to cope with this awful problem. Several methods have been analyzed in this study, and the data clearly demonstrate the value of cryopreservation in DMSO for this purpose.—T. Strom, M.D.

Normoglycaemia After Transplantation of Freshly Isolated and Cryopreserved Pancreatic Islets in Type 1 (Insulin-Dependent) Diabetes Mellitus
Warnock GL, Kneteman NM, Ryan E, Seelis REA, Rabinovitch A, Rajotte RV (University of Alberta, Edmonton)
Diabetologia 34:55–58, 1991   5–12

Background.—Initial islet transplants in patients with insulin-dependent diabetes led to sustained insulin production, but it was not possible to withdraw exogenous insulin therapy. Apparently, an increased β-cell mass is necessary in the setting of long-term diabetes. One approach is to collect and store islets in a bank until enough are available to treat an individual recipient effectively.

Case Report.—Woman, 36, with complications of type I diabetes, received both a renal transplant and pancreatic islets. The islet graft contained nearly 250,000 fresh islets with a mean diameter of 150 μm, which were syngeneic with the kidney graft. In addition, she received 368,000 cryopreserved islets from 4 other donors. The patient received approximately 10,000 islets per kilogram of body weight, infused into her liver through umbilical venous catheter. She received antilymphocyte globulin, prednisone, cyclosporine, and azathioprine for immunosuppression. Insulin secretion returned postoperatively. Plasma C-peptide levels rose from less than .12 to 4–5 ng/mL, and further to 7.1 ng/mL when Sustacal was given. Mean daily glucose levels ranged from 5.5 to 8.1 mmol/L in the first 2 months after transplantation. When exogenous insulin was withdrawn, a mean 24-hour glucose of 6.6 mmol/L was maintained with Sustacal. Renal transplant function remained stable.

Discussion.—In this patient, long-standing type I diabetes was effectively treated by the infusion of both fresh and cryopreserved islets, the latter from multiple donors. Cases such as this are a necessary step in evaluating islet transplantation for the treatment of serious diabetic complications.

▶ This case report catalogues a successful outcome using cryopreserved islets harvested from multiple donors. This patient is one of several patients who have undergone successful short-term islet cell transplantation in other centers. Can these results be obtained consistently?—T. Strom, M.D.

Results of Our First Nine Intraportal Islet Allografts in Type 1, Insulin-Dependent Diabetic Patients

Scharp DW, Lacy PE, Santiago JV, McCullough CS, Weide LG, Boyle PJ, Falqui L, Marchetti P, Ricordi C, Gingerich RL, Jaffe AS, Cryer PE, Hanto DW, Anderson CB, Flye MW (Washington Univ, St Louis)
Transplantation 51:76–85, 1991   5–13

Introduction.—A new era of clinical islet transplantation will begin when the first patient becomes insulin independent after intraportal islet transplantation. Data were reviewed on 9 consecutive portal vein islet transplants in 7 diabetic recipients.

Methods.—The first 3 procedures were performed in nonrenal failure diabetics, with 6,319 islets/kg processed from a single pancreas and cultured for 7 days at 24° C. Before transplantation, prednisone, azathioprine, and cyclosporine were administered. Although C-peptide function was seen in all patients after operation, all rejected their grafts at 2 weeks. Although OKT3 was given for 5 days, it failed to recover more than 10% of grafts. Thereafter, established kidney transplant (EKI) recipients were studied. Their basal immunosuppression was maintained, and 7 days of Minnesota antilymphoblast globulin was given using islets from single donor pancreas that had been cultured for 7 days at 24° C. An average of 6,161 islets were transplanted intraportally in 3 recipients.

Results.—In all patients, a C-peptide response was seen, but none achieved independence from insulin. The graft was rejected at 2 weeks by 1 patient; the other 2 had islet function up to 10 months. C-peptide responsiveness with a delayed pattern was seen on Sustacal challenge testing, suggesting that insufficient islet mass was transplanted. The next 3 patients received an average of 13,916 islets/kg from more than 1 donor pancreas. One achieved insulin independence from days 10—25. The other 2 achieved partial islet function from a single pancreas donor, and were retransplanted with islets from multiple donors; 1 was demonstrating long-term partial function at 184 days but was not insulin independent, and the other was demonstrating insulin independence for 154 days, with a glycated hemoglobin value of 5.6%. Total stimulated C-peptide response to Sustacal challenge was 155 pmol/mL at 4 months compared with 148 pmol/mL for normal controls and 425 pmol/mL for EKI recipients who received triple immunosuppression.

Conclusion.—Insulin independence in type I patients is feasible with islet transplantation. Studies should be continued to document how many recipients can achieve insulin independence and for how long.

▶ The group at Barnes Hospital has led efforts to apply clinical islet transplantation. Although the intraportal injection of human islets was feasible in humans, insulin independence requires multiple donors. This decreases the practicality of human islet transplantation, although the use of multiple donors may be advantageous from the point of view of inducing tolerance. Many groups have shifted attention to the application of xenogeneic islet transplantation.—N.L. Ascher, M.D., Ph.D.

Successful Treatment of Diabetes With the Biohybrid Artificial Pancreas in Dogs
Maki T, Ubhi CS, Sanchez-Farpon H, Sullivan SJ, Borland K, Muller TE, Solomon BA, Chick WL, Monaco AP (New England Deaconess Hosp; Harvard Med School, Boston; BioHybrid Technologies, Inc, Shrewsbury; WR Grace & Co-Conn, Lexington, Mass)
Transplantation 51:43–51, 1991   5–14

Introduction.—Attempts to control blood glucose levels by diet, insulin, and exercise in patients with insulin-dependent diabetes mellitus do not stop the development of serious neurologic and vascular problems. Pancreatic islet transplantation in contrast to whole pancreas transplantation is an attractive possible treatment for these patients, with the use of a biohybrid pancreas as an alternative. A new hybrid artificial pancreas device to transplant islet allografts without concomitant immunosuppression was used in diabetic dogs.

Methods.—The biohybrid pancreas instrument resembles a hollow fiber cell culture device. The prototype is a single coiled, hollow fiber membrane within a disk-shaped, acrylic housing. The special ultrafiltration membrane has a molecular weight maximum of 80,000 daltons. For each experiment in this series, an in vitro device was seeded at the same time under the same conditions and then placed in a perfusion culture. Seeded devices were implanted in 6 female mongrel dogs in the first series and in 13 animals in the second series. Later, unseeded devices were planted in other dogs. Device implantation occurred 2–3 weeks after pancreatectomy, when the animals received daily insulin injections.

Results.—Dogs in the first seeded device series did not have long-term functioning, whereas 10 of the 13 dogs in the second series did have a reversal of hyperglycemia. Of the first series of 12 animals with unseeded devices, 2 still remain patent at 388 and 421 days after implantation, respectively. In the second series of 8 animals receiving unseeded devices in which arterial and venous anastomoses were performed end-to-side in 6 dogs, all 8 continued to maintain the unseeded devices. No animal had significant weight loss. Removal of the device caused a required insulin increase from 16 to 32 units per day.

Conclusion.—The seeded biohybrid artifical pancreas device can maintain reasonable diabetic control in dogs without the use of immunosuppressive agents. The use of 2 devices per animal to improve insulin secretion is under investigation.

▶ The hybrid artificial pancreas device marks a major breakthrough in the treatment of diabetes mellitus. The physical separation of islets from the vascular system inhibits cellular and antibody mediated rejection but allows for diffusion of insulin from the chamber into the host circulation. Technical improvements will maximize longevity of the islets and the function of this apparatus.—N.L. Ascher, M.D., Ph.D.

Biohybrid Artificial Pancreas: Long-Term Implantation Studies in Diabetic, Pancreatectomized Dogs
Sullivan SJ, Maki T, Borland KM, Mahoney MD, Solomon BA, Muller TE, Monaco AP, Chick WL (BioHybrid Technologies, Inc, Shrewsbury, Mass; Harvard Med School, Brookline, WR Grace & Co-Conn, Lexington, Mass)
Science 252:718–721, 1991   5–15

Introduction.—Although pancreatic transplantation can produce normoglycemia, many problems attend the use of whole or segmental pancreatic transplants, including limited availability of donor organs. The biohybrid artificial implantable pancreas uses a selectively permeable membrane coiled inside a housing for islet cells and connected to a polytetrafluoroethylene graft that joins the implant to the vascular system as an arteriovenous shunt.

Methods.—Islets from either adult mongrel dogs or bovine calves were seeded into devices for implantation in vivo in dogs and for in vitro perfusion culture. Long-term insulin secretion was examined in vitro for up to 9 months. In vivo function was assessed in pancreatectomized dogs.

Results.—Insulin secretion in vitro peaked within 2 months of culture and then decreased slowly. Insulin secretion responded to shifts in glucose concentration. Implanted dogs exhibited significantly altered needs for exogenous insulin. Implantation of 2 devices totally eliminated the

Exogenous Insulin Requirements and Fasting Blood Glucose (FBG) Concentrations Before and After Device Implantation

Animal	Before implant Injected insulin (units/d)	FBG (mg/dl)	After implant Injected insulin (units/d)	FBG (mg/dl)	Duration of implant (days)	Status
PS22	18	246	0	107	157	Ongoing
PS23	30	279	0	158	141	Ongoing
PS26	30	323	0	165	100	Ongoing
PS28	24	295	0	168	54	Terminated
PS30	18	248	0	130	27	Terminated
PS35	30	222	15	248	38	Terminated
PS36	30	218	0	142	22	Ongoing

(Courtesy of Sullivan SJ, Maki T, Borland KM, et al: *Science* 252:718–721, 1991.)

need for exogenous insulin in most instances (table). Nevertheless, the response to intravenous glucose administration remained abnormal.

Conclusion.—The biohybrid artificial pancreas holds promise as a treatment for diabetes. Improvements in design may allow the device to provide glycemic regulation resembling that normally provided by pancreatic islets.

▶ Further studies in the pancreatectomized dogs reveal that xenoislets and alloislets functioned long-term and that the use of 2 biohybrid devices eliminated the use for exogenous insulin. The abnormal glucose tolerance test indicated persistent lack of appropriate feedback control. The authors suggest that improvement in design will improve the feedback control, which is necessary for clinical application of this important technology.—N.L. Ascher, M.D., Ph.D.

Restoration of Liver Function in Gunn Rats Without Immunosuppression Using Transplanted Microencapsulated Hepatocytes
Dixit V, Darvasi R, Arthur M, Brezina M, Lewin K, Gitnick G (Univ of California Los Angeles School of Medicine)
Hepatology 12:1342–1349, 1990   5–16

Background.—Cell cultures can be transplanted without immunosuppression by the new technique of microencapsulation within synthetic semipermeable membranes. In animals with galactosamine-induced fulminant hepatic failure, transplantation of isolated encapsulated hepatocytes can support metabolic function long enough to improve survival. The feasibility of using this method to restore the ability to conjugate bilirubin was explored in Gunn rats, which lack this ability congenitally.

Methods.—Forty-five Gunn rats underwent intraperitoneal transplantation with free hepatocytes, isolated encapsulated hepatocytes, control microcapsules, or no treatment. The hepatocytes were isolated from male Wistar rats and microencapsulated with collagen within a sodium alginate-poly-L-lysine-sodium alginate membrane. Serum bilirubin levels

In Vivo Studies: Percentage Decrease in Bilirubin Levels After Transplantation of IEH, FHC, and Control (Empty) Microcapsules

Group	Days after transplantation						
	0	1	3	5	7	10	21	28
IEH	0	28.6 ± 4.5*	43.4 ± 4.0*	35.1 ± 3.3*	37.0 ± 4.4*	33.9 ± 5.8*	44.4 ± 6.8*	35.4 ± 4.6*
FHC	0	11.3 ± 4.0	17.4 ± 3.0†	19.3 ± 4.0†	12.7 ± 4.0†	16.0 ± 5.0†	20.4 ± 8.0	16.5 ± 9.0
Control	0	3.5 ± 1.4	11.9 ± 5.0	19.7 ± 7.0	9.5 ± 4.3	18.3 ± 9.0	1.4 ± 1.1	6.7 ± 6.7

Note: Values are means ± 1 SEM.
Abbreviations: IEH, isolated encapsulated hepatocytes; *FHC,* free hepatocytes.
*P < .01 compared with FHC and control groups.
†Not significant compared with control group.
(Courtesy of Dixit V, Darvasi R, Arthur M, et al: *Hepatology* 12:1342–1349, 1990.

were monitored every day for 10 days, then every week for up to 1 month. At that time, the microcapsules were studied by light and electron microscopy.

Results.—In the first week, the isolated encapsulated hepatocyte group had a mean maximum reduction in serum bilirubin level of 45.7%, compared with 18.6% for the free hepatocyte and 14.3% for the control microcapsule group. Mean reductions in the 3 groups were 34.8%, 13.5%, and 3.3%, respectively, for up to 1 month thereafter (table). On microscopic examination, the hepatocytes showed a number of preserved hepatocytes with numerous mitochondria, smooth and rough endoplasmic reticulum, Golgi bodies, and glycogen.

Conclusions.—Isolated encapsulated hepatocyte transplantation can significantly lower serum bilirubin levels in a model of lifelong hyperbilirubinemia. In patients with congenital enzymatic liver deficiency, this technique could restore at least 1 liver function as a therapeutic option.

▶ Microencapsulation techniques offer the promise of decreasing immunogenicity of cellular transplants. Encapsulated materials used previously were associated with progressive fibrosis and loss of function of cellular grafts. Fibrosis can inhibit ingress of nutrients and to the cells and egress of parenchymal cell products to the host. The efficacy of this material composed of collagen within a sodium alginate-poly-L-lysine-sodium alginate membrane must be assessed over the long run in terms of hepatocyte viability, immunogenicity, and function.—N.L. Ascher, M.D., Ph.D.

Progressive Deterioration of Endocrine Function After Intraportal but Not Kidney Subcapsular Rat Islet Transplantation
Hiller WFA, Klempnauer J, Lück R, Steiniger B (Clinic for Abdominal and Transplantation Surgery and Ctr of Anatomy, Medical School, Hannover, Germany)
Diabetes 40:134–140, 1991   5–17

Introduction.—Late endocrine failure of islet isografts from nonimmunologic causes threatens the whole concept of islet transplantation. It is not known whether this is a general phenomenon in islet transplantation or if it relies on implantation site.

Methods.—The long-term endocrine function of isolated islets of Langerhans transplanted into the portal vein was compared with that of those transplanted beneath the kidney subcapsular space in inbred streptozocin-induced diabetic rats. The function of different endocrine pancreatic isografts was monitored for 1 year.

Results.—The function of isolated islets transplanted into the portal vein deteriorated progressively over time. In contrast, islets under the kidney capsule had a constant long-term function, controlling all the clinical signs of diabetes. Kidney subcapsular islet recipients had a normal growth rate, peripheral serum glucose and insulin concentrations, and metabolic parameters. However, functional reserve in these animals was greatly diminished, as shown by reduced glucose tolerance and insulin-

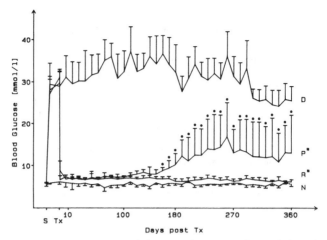

Fig 5–4.—Nonfasting serum glucose in diabetic rats after intraportal *(P)* or kidney subcapsular *(R)* islet transplantation compared with nondiabetic *(N)* and untreated diabetic *(D)* rats expressed as means ± SD. *S* indicates administration of streptozocin; *Tx*, transplantation; *circles*, P < .05 vs. kidney islet graft recipients; *squares*, p < .05 vs. diabetic controls. (Courtesy of Hiller WFA, Klempnauer J, Lück R, et al: *Diabetes* 40:134–140, 1991.)

secreting ability after an intravenous glucose challenge. Vascularized whole-organ pancreatic grafts with portal venous drainage resulted in a complete return to normal parameters (Fig 5–4).

Conclusion.—Adequate long-term graft function must be the goal of clinical islet transplantation. The long-term function of islets transplanted under the kidney capsule is better than islets transplanted into the portal vein.

▶ As the use of pancreatic islet transplant is applied clinically, an important consideration is the optimal site of injection to use to maximize long-term function. It has been suggested that intraportal injection of antigen is beneficial in induction of tolerance. If an intraportal site is not conducive to long-term function but does enhance tolerance, a combination of intraportal and kidney subcapsular sites may be necessary.—N.L. Ascher, M.D., Ph.D.

6 Cell and Small Bowel Transplantation

In Utero Transplantation of Hemopoietic Stem Cells in Humans
Touraine JL, Raudrant D, Royo C, Rebaud A, Barbier F, Roncarolo MG, Touraine F, Laplace S, Gebuhrer L, Bétuel H, Frappaz D, Freycon F, Vullo C (Hôpital Edouard Herriot, Lyon, France; Arcispedale S. Anna, Ferrara, Italy)
Transplant Proc 23:1706–1708, 1991   6–1

Background.—Recently, when no suitable bone marrow donors were available, researchers have treated patients with congenital immunodeficiencies or inborn metabolic errors by transplantation of fetal liver cells. Some 67% of these individuals were cured of their disorder. Three patients who had bare lymphocyte syndrome (BLS) were treated by fetal liver transplant (FLT).

Case 1.—A woman whose first child died of BLS sought prenatal diagnosis at 19 weeks of gestation. The fetus was found to have type III BLS. Both parents chose the earliest possible FLT, which took place at 28 weeks of gestation. Liver and thymic cells were obtained from 2 fetuses that had died at 7 and 7.5 weeks of gestation. At birth, the diagnosis of BLS was confirmed, but some cells with class I HLA antigens were detected. One month after birth, 10% of lymphocytes were normally expressed class I HLA antigens. These cells were shown to be of the donor's type and not inherited from either parent. The infant was placed in a sterile bubble and received 7 additional stem cell transplants from 9 other fetal donors. At 1 year of age, 26% of the infant's peripheral blood lymphocytes were derived from the in utero transplants. The patient was able to leave the isolator after 16 months because of T-cell reconstitution and good health.

Case 2.—The fetus had a complete form of severe combined immunodeficiency disease (SCID). He underwent FLT at 26 weeks of gestation after a prenatal diagnosis of severe immunodeficiency disease. The FLT technique was comprised of intravenous infusion of viable fetal liver cells into the umbilical vein of the fetus by ultrasound monitoring. At birth, the infant continued to have SCID and remained in isolation until the transplanted stem cells could proliferate and differentiate into T lymphocytes.

Case 3.—A pregnant woman with a family history of thalassemia had very early prenatal diagnosis. The fetus underwent FLT at 12 weeks of gestation by intraperitoneal injection of viable cells from a 9-week post-fecundation fetus. Studies performed after the birth indicated that the child had thalassemia, and only a few donor cells were present. No additional transplants were performed in the infant, who was in good health.

Comment.—These results supported the feasibility of performing FLT in utero. The major reasons for in utero FLT include the increased probability of an accepted graft, improved isolation at time of transplant, and a better environment for the development of fetal cells when they are transplanted into the fetus rather than into the infant.

▶ This group has pioneered the use of fetal liver transplantation administered in utero. The fetus has a potential window period during which transplantation easily induces tolerance. The use of fetal hemopoietic cells may also be less immunogenic. The investigators demonstrate the clinical feasibility of the treatment in patients with congenital immunodeficiencies, providing an important milestone for these patients and for other patients who have defects that can be diagnosed prepartum and are amenable to correction with cellular transplantation.—N.L. Ascher, M.D., Ph.D.

A Novel System for Transplantation of Isolated Hepatocytes Utilizing HBsAg-Producing Transgenic Donor Cells

Gupta S, Chowdhury NR, Jagtiani F, Gustin K, Aragona E, Shafritz DA, Chowdhury JR, Burk RD (Albert Einstein College of Medicine, Bronx, NY)
Transplantation 50:472–475, 1990
6–2

Introduction.—Recent transplantation of isolated hepatocytes demonstrated the feasibility of this technique as therapy for acute liver failure and inherited liver diseases. The results of the use of donor cells from a

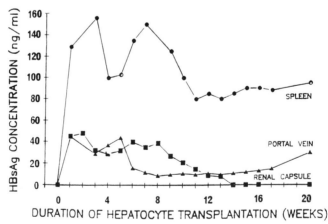

Fig 6–1.—Representative examples showing serum HBsAg levels at various time points after transplantation of 2 × 10⁶ G7 HBV transgenic hepatocytes into splenic pulp, beneath the renal capsule, or into the portal vein of congeneic C57BL/CJ mouse recipients. Stored sera were simultaneously assayed for HBsAg with a radioimmunoassay (Austria II, Abbott Laboratories, North Chicago, IL. Test sera (10 μl) were diluted with HBsAg and anti-HBs negative serum. Samples were considered to be positive when the positive to negative control ratio was greater than 2.1. For quantitative determination of HBsAg expression, a standard curve in a linear range was generated by inclusion of samples containing known concentrations of purified HBsAg standard. (Courtesy of Gupta S, Chowdhury NR, Jagtiani F, et al: *Transplantation* 50:472–475, 1990.)

recently developed transgenic mouse strain were reviewed. These cells contained a uniquely expressed marker gene (a transgene) that secreted its product into the circulation to monitor the fate of transplanted hepatocytes in vivo.

Methods.—Using HBV transgenic mice, the HBV genome was microinjected into on-cell embryos from B6A/F_1 female mice mated to CD1 males. The offspring, G7, had a partially deleted HBV genome integrated into a particular locus in the mouse genome, which was transmitted by way of Mendelian genetics. Hepatocytes from the donor G7 HBV mice secreted the nonpathogenic HBsAg and did not secrete hepatitis B virion particles. Congeneic C57BL/6J mice received 20×10^6 hepatocytes per animal. Splenectomy was performed in recipients at 7 weeks to determine whether transplanted liver cells were retained in the spleen.

Results.—Hepatocytes were found in the spleen by histologic examination 1, 8, and 20 weeks after cell transplantation into the congeneic mice. Serum HBsAg was secreted on day 7 after hepatocyte transplantation into the spleen (Fig 6–1). With splenectomy, no decrease of serum HBsAG secretion was observed, suggesting that the injected hepatocytes migrated out of the spleen to other parts of the body. Serum HBsAg was not detected in allogenic mice who also underwent hepatocyte transplantation, although hepatocytes were found within the splenic pulp. A decrease or total disappearance of serum HBsAg was observed in some animals.

Conclusion.—This technique has the advantage of demonstrating hepatocyte survival easily by simple monitoring serum HBsAg. Therefore, animals do not have to be killed during the early posttransplantation phases, which would allow for study of factors enhancing hepatocellular engraftment and possible modulation of allograft rejection.

▶ The transgenic mouse that secrets HBsAg rather than B virus particles provides the basis for a useful model when used as donor animal for hepatocyte transplantation. This method does not track specific cells but does monitor the functional integrity of cells over the long-term.—N.L. Ascher, M.D., Ph.D.

Refined Technique for Intestinal Transplantation in the Rat
Zhong R, Grant D, Sutherland F, Wang P, Chen H, Lo S, Stiller C, Duff J (University of Western Ontario, London, Ont, Canada)
Microsurgery 12:268–274, 1991   6–3

Background.—Experiments with small intestinal transplantation (IT) have been largely unsuccessful for unknown reasons. A large series of IT procedures in rats was reviewed to describe some technical modifications and demonstrate the results of 1-stage orthotopic intestinal transplantation (OIT).

Methods.—A total of 400 IT procedures were done over a 4-year period. There were 298 heterotopic accessory transplants (HIT), most of them including exteriorization of both ends of the graft as stomas. There

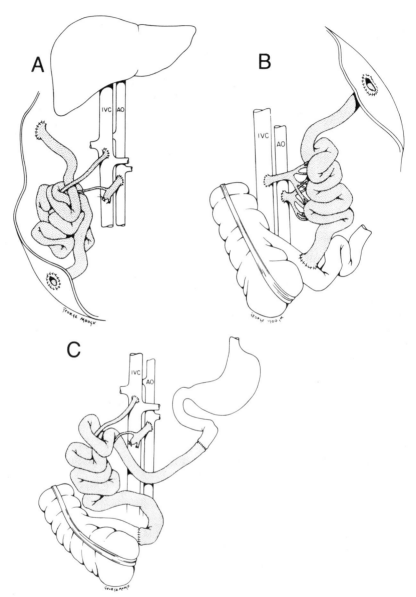

Fig 6–2.—Heterotopic (**A, B**) and orthotopic (**C**) intestinal transplant models. *Abbreviations: IVC,* inferior vena cava; *AO,* aorta. (Courtesy of Zhong R, Grant D, Sutherland F, et al: *Microsurgery* 12:268–274, 1991.)

were 102 OIT procedures in which both ends of the graft were immediately anastomosed to the native small intestine after the jejunum and ileum were excised (Fig 6–2). Care was taken to minimize mechanical and ischemic injury to the graft during the donor operation, and the portal vein and aortic conduit were marked with sutures to ensure correct graft orientation. The intestinal anastomosis was stented with a piece of dry macaroni, and large volumes of crystalloid were given to maintain normal blood pressure during both operations.

Results.—Success rates were 90% in the HIT operations and 86% in the OIT operations. Average time for surgery was 89 minutes. Vascular complication rate was only 2.5%. The most common cause of postoperative death was hypovolemic shock, which occurred in 9.7% of cases. When the rats survived more than 2 days, they generally survived indefinitely. In the OIT group, some animals survived for more than 500 days with normal weight, intestinal function, and histologic features.

Conclusions.—High success rates with HIT and OIT in rats have been achieved. The methods described eliminate most surgical complications, yield high success rates, and allow excellent long-term function. The HIT model, although technically easier, may not be as clinically relevant as the OIT model.

▶ The field of small bowel transplantation has been hampered by difficulties with development of a reliable small bowel transplant model. These investigators outline a number of practical details in the small bowel transplant. The concentrated effort has yielded outstanding results in this model. The outstanding results with the orthotopic technique, which has greater clinical relevance, are encouraging for clinical application. Particularly encouraging is the long-term survival with consistent weight gain.—N.L. Ascher, M.D., Ph.D.

7 Social and Ethical Issues in Transplantation

▶ ↓ The increasing shortage of all types of solid organs for transplantation has led to a number of important analyses. Are we doing all that we might to obtain an ample number of viable, useful organs for clinical transplantation? Once we obtain all these organs, are they distributed in a utilitarian and/or egalitarian manner? The concept of using every organ in a manner to maximize outcome calls for outcome assessment in a variety of different patient populations.— Terry Strom, M.D., Nancy L. Ascher, M.D., Ph.D.

Renal Transplantation From Elderly Living Donors

Sumrani N, Delaney V, Ding Z, Davis R, Daskalakis P, Tejani A, Butt K, Hong J (State Univ of New York, Brooklyn)
Transplantation 51:305–309, 1991
                                                                  7–1

Introduction.—Because the rate of cadaveric donor procurement remains low, transplant centers rely on renal transplantation from living related donors. Both the elderly donor and the recipient may have complications related to adverse events in the posttransplant period and age-associated decline in renal function. To assess the effect of donor age on graft survival, incidence of rejection, and subsequent renal function, clinical results from recipients of living renal transplants were analyzed.

Methods.—A total of 44 of 276 recipients of living related renal transplants received kidneys from donors older than 55 years. Transplants spanned both the cyclosporine and azathioprine eras. Recipients were similar in age, race, haplotype mismatch, number of retransplants, and number of pretransplant transfusions, but there was an increased number of diabetics among the cyclosporine-treated recipients of elderly kidneys.

Results.—The cumulative patient and graft survival rates at 1 and 5 years were independent of donor age when either cyclosporine or azathioprine was used. The incidence of rejection or infection between the older donor group and the younger cohort was not significantly different. Short-term and intermediate-term renal function as assessed by serum creatinine level was significantly worse in the older compared with the younger donor group. However, serum creatinine levels were maintained at a significantly higher, but stable, level 3–9 years posttransplant.

Conclusion.—An identical graft survival rate was achieved in living related renal transplantation whether the kidney was obtained from a younger or older donor. However, when the donor was older than 55

108 / Transplantation

years, serum creatinine levels posttransplant were significantly higher but stable. Renal transplantation from elderly living donors is an acceptable practice, with negligible morbidity to the donors and good graft survival rates.

▶ Whereas the short-term rate of kidney engraftment for primary cadaver and living related donor is smaller, the long-term rate of functional graft attention is heavily influenced by HLA matching. Hence, perfect HLA matched grafts have extraordinary longevity and HLA haploidentical grafts function longer than the prototypic poorly matched cadaver graft. Given the grieveous shortage in kidney donor procurement, I'm a big fan of HLA identical or haploidentical living related donor transplants.

Oftentimes parents—individuals who have a powerful urge to donate—are not approached for organ donation because they are "too old." How old is "too old"? When the potential older donor enjoys good overall health and fine kidney function, I approve of "going ahead" with living related transplantation. —T. Strom, M.D.

Availability of Transplantable Organs From Brain Stem Dead Donors in Intensive Care Units

Gore SM, Taylor RMR, Wallwork J (MRC Biostatistics Unit, Cambridge; Organ Grafting Unit, Royal Victoria Infirmary, Newcastle Upon Tyne; Papworth Hospital, Cambridge, England)
BMJ 302:149–153, 1991   7–2

Background.—The Department of Health in England has estimated that 1,700 possible brain stem deaths and 1,200 confirmed brain stem deaths occur annually in that country. A 30% rate of donation refusal by relatives was reported. Another audit was done to quantify the possible increases in transplantable organs from brain stem dead potential donors for heart, kidneys, liver, lungs, and corneas.

Methods.—Fifteen regional and special health authorities in England participated. All deaths in intensive care units were audited prospectively from January to June of 1989. A subsequent case study of the impact of publicity on offers and donations in October and November of that year was also done.

Results.—Of 5,803 patients dying in the intensive care units during the study period, 497 were confirmed brain stem dead and had no general medical contraindications to organ donation. Of those brain stem dead patients, organ specific suitability was estimated in 63% for the heart, 95% for the kidneys, 70% for the liver, 29% for the lungs, and 91% for the corneas. Relatives refused organ donation in 30% of the cases. For kidneys, this loss was equivalent to 44% of brain stem dead actual kidney donors. The second most important reason for missed kidney donors was that organ donation was not discussed. The second most notable cause of lost liver and lung donors was nonprocurement or difficulties with allocating organs. Nonprocurement of suitable, offered organs was rare for kidneys and modest for heart and corneas. Restricted offers, non-procurement, and no discussion of donation accounted for equal numbers of lost heart donations. Rates of refusal and nondiscussion dropped in October and November when there was intense, positive publicity about transplantation. Offers of suitable donors rose significantly, most notably for heart and kidney donations. Only for kidneys, however, was there a noticeable increase in actual donors.

Conclusions.—Strategies to increase the supply of transplantable organs from brain stem dead potential donors in intensive care units include reducing the number of relatives' refusals, avoiding nonprocurement of suitable organs and deterioration of initially suitable organs, converting restricted offers to unrestricted ones, and ensuring discussion with the patient's family. Early referral to the transplant team or coordinator is beneficial.

▶ An audit of 5,803 intensive care unit deaths in England was undertaken to identify impediments to organ donation (see Figure 1 in the original article). The reasons for a failure to procure organs for transplantation were carefully analyzed. Four broad categories were identified. During a period of intense publicity concerning transplantation, physicians were more vigilant about organ procurement and the rate of refusal by families to donate kidneys, but not other organs, decreased.—T. Strom, M.D.

The Effect of Race on Access and Outcome in Transplantation

Kasiske BL, Neyland JF III, Riggio RR, Danovitch GM, Kahana L, Alexander SR, White MG (Hennepin County Med Ctr, Minneapolis; Emory Univ, Atlanta; Cornell Med Ctr, New York; Univ of California, Los Angeles; Univ of South Florida, Tampa; et al)
N Engl J Med 324:302–307, 1991   7–3

Objective.—A study on racial inequality in transplantation was commissioned by the American Society of Transplant Physicians. The organization's Patient Care and Education Committee examined some of the reasons why radical minorities do not have the same access as whites to organ transplantation.

Findings.—Blacks in the United States have about a 4-fold higher relative risk than whites for end-stage renal disease. Blacks make up 12% of the US population but account for 27% of patients with end-stage renal disease. Native Americans are also at increased risk for renal failure. However, of patients undergoing dialysis, fewer nonwhites than whites subsequently undergo kidney transplantation.

Discussion.—Several reasons have been suggested why proportionately fewer blacks receive kidney transplants. Because only 8% of donors are black, the distribution of ABO blood groups and major histocompatibility complement (MHC) antigens may influence the matching of donors and recipients. More minority patients are socioeconomically disadvantaged, leading to poorer compliance and inadequate insurance coverage for a transplant procedure. Allograft survival is reduced in black recipients, even with cyclosporine. Blacks also undergo proportionately fewer pancreas and liver transplantations than whites.

Reevaluations.—the Committee recommended that the reasons for racial differences in transplantation be examined more fully. Members of racial minorities should be encouraged to become organ donors, and health care providers should assist minority patients in obtaining suitable treatment.

▶ The issues raised by this study are volatile. Are blacks offered kidney transplants less often than whites as a result of bigotry or as a result of valid considerations? Because whites are overrepresented in the donor pool, marked racial differences in expression of the blood group A and B substances must play a role in limiting kidneys available to blacks with blood B. Blacks, but not whites, are often B+.

Socioeconomic factors are closely linked to compliance. I believe that it is perfectly reasonable to deny noncompliant patients a kidney graft given the marked shortage of transplantable kidneys. Under no circumstances will I condone transplantation into an active drug abuser. They routinely and preferentially spend their funds on the "wrong" drug. On the other hand, are we sure that many physicians do not "unconsciously" assume that most uneducated white, blacks, or hispanics are noncompliant? Who knows?

Is the lower rate of long-term engraftment in blacks the result of biologic differences in immunosuppressive drug metabolism, immune vigor, noncompliance or because most blacks receive kidneys from whites? Because of racial differences in MHC expression, these kidneys may be more susceptible to more vigorous chronic rejection than well matched grafts.

It is obviously crucial to verify that the organ distribution network system allocates organs fairly and efficiently. This is a zero sum game. Allocation of a graft to one individual denies another individual, at least temporarily, of the opportunity to receive a graft. I'm not certain that further study will identify the precise reason for the lower rate of transplantation among black recipients, but I am gratified that the question has been raised.—T. Strom, M.D.

Organ Procurement in Patients with Fatal Head Injuries: The Fate of the Potential Donor

Mackersie RC, Bronsther OL, Shackford SR (Univ of California at San Diego)
Ann Surg 213:143–150, 1991   7–4

Introduction.—Organ transplantation continues to increase the survival of patients with end-stage cardiac, hepatic, and renal diseases. Traumatic head injury and other nonsurvivable CNS injury can contribute to the failure of a transplanted organ, however. The overall efficacy of organ procurement was evaluated in a level 1 trauma center, with emphasis on the donor organ availability, reasons for organ procurement failure, organ function outcome when procured from a victim of fatal head injury, and physiologic factors affecting organ function.

Methods—Using a standard protocol, the patients' demographic data, severity of injury, admission prognosis, donor eligibility status, brain death, and organ availability were recorded. The follow-up data on 47 of 48 renal transplant recipients spanned an average of 23 months.

Results.—During the course of the 46-month study, 190 patients died of major head injury, 64 of whom were excluded and 90 (71%) had nonsurvivable injuries at admission with an average of 2 hours from injury to death. Of the 108 initial survivors, 73 could donate 1 or more vascular organ. The 2 major reasons for failure to procure an organ from eligible patients were the denial of consent in 25 patients and failure of the physiologic support procedures used in 18. The mean survival time for all patients was 64 hours. the overall consent rate for organ procurement was 54%.

Conclusion.—The existing shortage of donor organs will increase. The organ procurement from patients with fatal head injury remains limited because cardiopulmonary function cannot be maintained for the appropriate length of time and because of the high rate of denial of consent by the patient's family.

▶ The proliferation or organ transplant centers has intensified the demand for organ donors, yet the number of actual cadaveric donors has not kept pace with recipient pools. This study from the University of California, San Diego, exemplifies the type of analysis done at the level of the hospital to delineate the pool of potential donors and the efficacy of the procurement process. There is increasing interest in assessing efficiency of organ procurement agencies, and these types of data will likely provide the basis for such analysis. If the government or the transplant community moves toward certification of organ procurement agencies, it will likely be based on an efficiency score determined by data similar to that collected by these authors.—N.L. Ascher, M.D., Ph.D.

The Pattern of Organ Donation in a Large Urban Center
Sumrani N, Delaney V, Butt KM, Hong JH (State Univ of New York Health Sciences Ctr, Brooklyn)
NY State J Med 90:396–399, 1990   7–5

Introduction.—Progress in immunosuppressive therapies, operative techniques, and management of complications has led to increased solid organ transplantation. These improvements produced a demand for organs. The results of organ procurement in 1983–1988 were reviewed.

Methods.—Data on solid organ donor referrals and actual procurement were obtained from medical records from 1983–1988 from a local organ procurement agency. Donor screening and initial discussions were usually conducted by the specially trained transplant coordinators.

Results.—Potential donors increased from 1983 to 1987 and peaked at 180 in 1987. The number of donors used remained relatively constant at 28–39 per year. Postoperative donors were excluded because of a high incidence of complications, such as sepsis, carrier state, life style, and/or

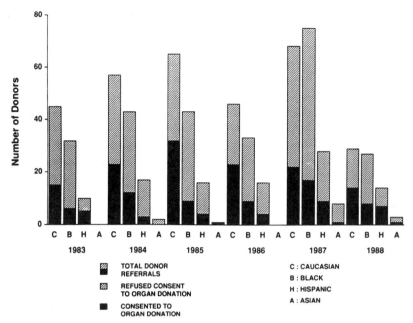

Fig 7–1.—Influence of race on organ donation, Gift of Life Program, New York City, 1983–1988. (Courtesy of Sumrani N, Delaney V, Butt KM, et al: *NY State J Med* 90:396–399, 1990.)

HIV disease. There were more potential donors who died before total brain death during 1983–1985, but this trend was reversed after 1986. Whites were the largest donor group at 50%, whereas 30% of blacks participated. Hispanics who agreed to organ donation increased from 17% in 1984 to 47% in 1988 (Fig 7–1). Asian donors formed a subgroup too small for analysis. Most of the organs used (50% to 75%) were obtained from whites, but the use of organs from blacks and Hispanics increased in the last 2 years of the study.

Conclusion.—Referrals for organ donations increased after passage of the Required Request Law in 1986. However, the number of actual donors did not change, although demand did increase. Organ procurement in the United States does not meet demand. Goal-oriented public education should be used to increase donations of transplant organs and physicians and hospital personnel should develop the appropriate amount of compassion and enthusiasm to encourage organ donation from grieving families.

▶ The transplant and legislative community had anticipated increased organ donation after institution of required request legislation. Unfortunately, the outcome of this legislation has been disappointing. Other measures under consideration to increase organ donation include presumed consent legislation, donor incentives, and the use of nonheart-beating donors. These sensitive measures require intensive study and a strong public mandate.—N.L. Ascher, M.D., Ph.D.

The Use of "Marginal" Donors for Organ Transplantation: The Influence of Donor Age on Outcome

Alexander JW, Vaughn WK (Univ of Cincinnati; United Network for Organ Sharing, Richmond, Va)
Transplantation 51:135–141, 1991   7–6

Background.—In the last 3 years, the number of solid organ donors has remained constant, whereas the recipient waiting list has grown by about 27% each year. Consequently, hundreds of people die each year for lack of a suitable transplantable organ. Because of the critical shortage, it is important to reevaluate the potential for use of organs from donors in older age groups.

Methods.—Investigators analyzed all kidney, heart, and liver transplantations performed from cadaveric donors during a 2-year period to determine the influence of donor age on the survival of the allografted organ. Follow-up data were available on 12,131 patients receiving renal allografts, 3,026 receiving heart transplants, and 2,913 receiving liver transplants. The oldest donor was 79 years old; 438 donors were <5 years old, 981 were 6–15 years old, 5,549 were 16–45 years old, 972 were 46–55 years old, 511 were 56–65 years old, and 68 were >65 years old.

Results.—Recipients of kidney transplants from donors aged 6 to 15 years had significantly better 1-year graft survival than did recipients from donors aged 56 to 65 years, but the difference was only 7%. Recipients of grafts from donors older than 65 years had better graft survival than did recipients from donors aged 56 to 65 years; organs from donors ≤5 years were less satisfactory. In patients with repeat transplants, diabetes, black race, age over 45 years, 0 HLA or 5 and 6 HLA matches, delayed graft function, shared kidneys, and panel reactive antibody (PRA) >50, kidneys from older donors survived as well as did kidneys from younger donors. Donor age was less important than the use of antilymphocyte globulin; donor race, diabetes, or peak PRA in ages 16 to 45 years; repeat transplant; delayed function; and HLA match. Recipients of heart transplants from donors aged 45 to 55 years had 8.4% reduced 1-year graft survival compared to that from heart recipients from donors aged 16 to 45 years. However, nearly 33% of heart patients died within the first year of listing without having received a transplant. Liver transplant recipients from donors aged 16 to 45 years had 10.8% better 1-year graft survival than liver recipients from donors >45 years, but a greater percentage of livers from older donors were transplanted to older and high-risk patients. Also, 24.3% of patients awaiting liver transplant died within 1 year before receiving the transplant.

Conclusions.—Older donors with normal organ function can provide transplants that will have satisfactory graft survival. Given the urgent need, age in itself should not be a barrier to organ donation.

▶ Expansion of the donor pool entails the use of organs previously considered "marginal." Although organs from older donors had slightly poorer outcome,

TABLE 1.—Summary of Data for Patients Who Were Seropositive for HIV Before Transplantation

Group and patient no.	Sex/age (y)	No. of CD4+ cells/mm³	CD4/CD8 ratio	Time to HIV disease posttransplantation (mo)	Immuno-suppression	Graft function	Follow-up posttransplantation (mo)	Outcome	Reference
Kidney recipients (n = 11)									
AIDS									
1	M/57	180	...	6	Reduced	Normal	24	Died	[27]
2	F/30	...	...	24	Normal	Normal	24	Died	[19]
3	.../...	...	...	9	...	...	9	Died	[26]
No HIV diseases									
4	.../...	...	...	...	...	...	2	Died	[26]
5	M/24	...	...	...	Discontinued	CRF, HD	60	Alive	[19]
6	M/13	...	...	...	Discontinued	CRF, HD	65	Alive	[10]
7	F/29	...	...	...	...	Normal	60	Alive	[10, 11]
8	F/29	...	...	...	Normal	Normal	36	Alive	[28]
9	F/48	...	...	...	Normal	Normal	24	Alive	[28]
10	M/...	...	...	...	...	...	22	Alive	[21]
11	.../64	...	...	...	Normal	Normal	12	Alive	[11]

Liver recipients (n = 10)

AIDS									
12	M/15	434	...	41	...	...	44	Died	[10, 11, 29]
13	M/36	...	0.27	14	Normal	Normal	27	Died	[29, 30]
14	./32	...	...	2.5	...	...	18	Died	[11]
15	M/48	285	...	...	...	...	4	Died	[10, 11, 29]
No HIV diseases									
16	./...	...	...	...	Normal	Normal	11	Died	[26]
17	F/0.5	...	...	...	...	...	9	Died	[10]
18	F/42	...	...	...	...	...	6	Died	[10]
19	F/47	...	...	...	...	...	5	Died	[10]
20	M/21	...	...	...	...	...	0	Died	[29, 31]
21	F/3	...	...	...	...	...	68	Alive	[10]
Heart recipient									
AIDS									
22	M/15	691	...	24	...	...	36	Alive	[11, 29]

Abbreviations: CRF, chronic renal failure; HD, hemodialysis.
(Courtesy of Erice A, Rhame FS, Heussner RC, et al: *Rev Infect Dis* 13:537–547, 1991.)

this factor alone was less significant than a number of recipient factors. Many transplant centers are reconsidering donor criteria, particularly in view of the significant number of potential heart and liver recipients who died awaiting transplants. The use of previously unused donors will require careful study to assure recipient safety.—N.L. Ascher, M.D., Ph.D.

Human Immunodeficiency Virus Infection in Patients With Solid-Organ Transplants: Report of Five Cases and Review
Erice A, Rhame FS, Heussner RC, Dunn DL, Balfour HH Jr (Univ of Minnesota, Minneapolis)
Rev Infect Dis 13:537–547, 1991   7–7

Background.—Although screening for HIV is now routine, patients undergoing organ transplantation were previously at risk of acquiring HIV infection from the transplant or blood transfusion. In addition, patients with unrecognized HIV infection might have undergone transplant operation. Five cases of solid organ transplantation patients who were infected with HIV are reported and compared with 83 such patients previously reported.

Methods.—The new patients were 3 women and 2 men who underwent transplant operations at 1 center in 1983 or 1984. There were 3 kidney, 1 heart, and 1 pancreas transplantations. The 83 patients from the literature were drawn from 29 reports appearing between 1985 and 1990. Data were collected and summarized for all patients. Sixty-six patients were seronegative for antibodies to HIV before transplantation and 22 were seropositive (Table 1).

Results.—Four kidney and 3 liver transplant recipients had their operations after routine HIV screening. In 28% of patients, AIDS developed. Of these, 80% died of related complications a mean of 37 months postoperatively. An additional 10% of patients developed HIV-related diseases. Overall, AIDS developed in a mean of 27.5 months, 32 months in patients who were seronegative before operation, and 17 months in patients who were seropositive before operation. Afebrile syndrome, attributed to HIV, developed in 17% of initially seronegative patients. Normal allograft function was maintained in 8 kidney and 2 liver recipients despite low-dose immunosuppressive therapy. Overall, 59% of patients died of AIDS-related causes (Table 2).

Conclusion.—The proportion of transplant recipients in whom AIDS develops does not appear to be greater than in other groups of HIV-infected patients, but AIDS may develop sooner in transplant recipients. Because transmission of HIV infection may still rarely occur in transplant patients, donors should be carefully investigated for HIV risk factors.

▶ The issue of transplantation outcome in the setting of an HIV-positive donor or recipient or in the setting of donor or recipient AIDS is an extremely important one. Patients with AIDs before transplant had uniformly fatal outcomes. Some HIV-positive kidney transplant recipients have survived 12–65 months.

TABLE 2.—Outcomes for HIV-Infected Recipients of Transplanted Organs

Type of patient and transplant	n	No. (%) of patients				
		HIV-related diseases	AIDS	Other HIV-related diseases	Deaths	AIDS-related deaths
All						
Kidney	59	36 (61)	16 (27)	7 (12)	17 (29)	14 (82)
Liver	22	13 (59)	7 (32)	2 (9)	13 (59)	5 (38)
Heart	6	4 (67)	2 (33)	. . .	3 (50)	1 (33)
Pancreas	1	1	. . .	. . .	1	. . .
Total	88	54 (61)	25 (28)	9 (10)	34 (39)	20 (59)
Seronegative at transplantation						
Kidney	48	28 (58)	13 (27)	7 (14.5)	13 (27)	11 (85)
Liver	12	7 (58)	3 (25)	2 (17)	4 (33)	1 (25)
Heart	5	4 (80)	1 (20)	. . .	3 (60)	1 (33)
Pancreas	1	1	. . .	. . .	1	. . .
Total	66	40 (61)	17 (26)	9 (14)	21 (32)	13 (62)
Seropositive at transplantation						
Kidney	11	8 (73)	3 (27)	. . .	4 (36)	3 (75)
Liver	10	6 (60)	4 (40)	. . .	9 (90)	4 (44)
Heart	1	. . .	1	. . .	. . .	. . .
Total	22	14 (64)	8 (36)		13 (59)	7 (54)

(Courtesy of Erice A, Rhame FS, Heussner RC, et al: *Rev Infect Dis* 13:537–547, 1991.)

Seronegative patients may also have substantial outcomes. The issue to relative risks must be assessed individually for transplantation from an HIV-positive donor. In particular, relative risks must be considered in potential recipients of a heart or liver who are certain to die without immediate transplant.—N.L. Ascher, M.D., Ph.D.

Medicine and Ethics: How to Allocate Transplantable Organs

Halasz NA (Univ of California, San Diego)
Transplantation 52:43–46, 1991

7–8

Introduction.—Organ transplantation has advanced greatly in recent years. The demand for organs exceeds the supply; waiting lists are growing longer, and patients are dying because of a lack of transplantable organs. Organ allocation policies have been based on medical and ethical considerations, but these policies have frequently grown by accretion. Medical and ethical aspects must be integrated to develop a coherent and fair means of allocating transplantable organs.

Ethical Aspects.—Rationing is based on maximizing the number of lives saved. An alternative approach, distributive justice, attempts to maximize the years of quality life that are saved. Organ allocation may also be viewed as a value-based system in which considerations of urgency, fairness, and the physician's loyalty to the patient are taken into account.

Medical Considerations.—The age limits for transplants have broadened steadily during the past decade. The risk of recurrent disease is an important medical consideration, and noncompliant behavior is a prominent cause of transplant loss after the first year. The value of seeking ever better-matched donor-recipient pairs has been questioned.

Synthesis.—Most relevant ethical and practical considerations are currently being applied, but there is no clear national policy ordering priorities for organ distribution. The libertarian approach of most physicians conflicts with the limit-setting function of regulatory agencies. A rational first step might be to allocate half or more of the organs recovered to low-risk individuals with long life expectancies. Perhaps another fourth of the organs could go to high-risk recipients, including those with urgent needs; the remainder could be allocated to other groups of potential recipients.

▶ The proposal to modify organ allocation is based on the principal of maximizing use of every organ. A portion of organs would be allocated to patients with the best anticipated outcome. This modification of distribution is vastly different from current distribution of hearts and livers based on severity of illness. The institution of a system like the one suggested should be analyzed on the basis of "fairness" to the recipient pool as well as on the basis of anticipated improvement in transplant results. An alternative may be the development of broader contraindications for transplantation.—N.L. Ascher, M.D., Ph.D.

8 Opportunistic Infections Following Transplantation

▶ ↓ Infectious disease complications continue to be a major application of clinical transplantation. Cytomegalovirus infection remains a particularly vexing problem. Several successful attempts at chemoprophylaxis for cytomegalovirus have been reported. In a recent report by Plotkin, the Towne attenuated cytomegalovirus strain was given safely to subjects who were awaiting a kidney transplant. The rate of patients experiencing severe infection was diminished when compared with a control population. The benefit was obtained entirely in the group of patients who were seronegative at the time of transplantation and who received a graft from a seronegative donor. The reports by Boland and Mast et al. deal with attempts to refine the precision of diagnostic tests aimed at identifying individuals with active cytomegalovirus. The report by Miller's group associates the use of OKT3 treatments with cytomegalovirus infection.

Many groups administer trimethaprim sulfamethoxazole to transplant patients for the purpose of preventing urosepsis and *Pneumocystis carinii* pneumonia. In a new analysis by Fox et al., the efficacy and cost efficiency of this practice are reviewed. Finally, Higgins et al. review the experience of the Oxford group with regard to mycobacterial infections in renal transplant recipients.—Terry Strom, M.D.

Effect of Towne Live Virus Vaccine on Cytomegalovirus Disease After Renal Transplant: A Controlled Trial
Plotkin SA, Starr SE, Friedman HM, Brayman K, Harris S, Jackson S, Tustin NB, Grossman R, Dafoe D, Barker C (Univ of Pennsylvania, Philadelphia)
Ann Intern Med 114:525–531, 1991   8–1

Background.—The most common infectious complication of kidney, liver, heart, and bone marrow transplantation is cytomegalovirus (CMV). An attenuated human CMV strain called Towne was developed and that has proven to be immunogenic and well tolerated in initial trials. A double-blind, randomized, placebo-controlled trial of the efficacy of vaccination with the Towne live virus vaccine in patients undergoing renal transplantation was studied.

Methods.—The subjects were 473 patients awaiting renal transplantation who were randomly assigned to receive subcutaneous inoculation with either vaccine or placebo. Of these, 237 patients underwent renal transplantation and were followed up for at least 6 months. For both recipients and donors, the CMV serologic status was determined; both se-

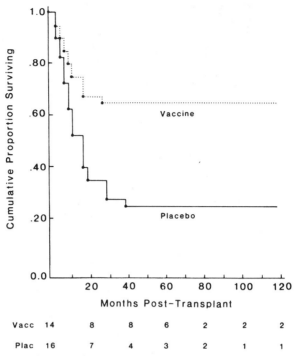

Fig 8–1.—Actuarial survival of the kidney graft in R − D + patients who received either vaccine *(Vacc)* or placebo *(Plac)* before transplant (*P* = .04 by Mantel-Cox test). Numbers of grafts surviving in patients who received either vaccine or placebo are shown at the bottom of the figure. R − D +, recipient seronegative for cytomegalovirus and donor seropositive. (Courtesy of Plotkin SA, Starr SE, Friedman HM, et al: *Ann Intern Med* 114:525–531, 1991.)

ronegative and seropositive patients were randomized. In the case of postoperative infection, the severity of disease was objectively scored by a prearranged system.

Results.—The patients who were vaccinated tolerated the vaccine well with no long-term adverse effects. There was no clear benefit in recipients who were originally seropositive. Recipients who were seronegative at the time of vaccination and whose donor was seropositive, considered to be at highest risk for CMV disease, were analyzed for protective efficacy of the vaccine. The patients who were vaccinated had significantly less severe CMV disease compared with patients who received placebo (Fig 8–1). The vaccinated group also had an 85% decrease in most severe disease, although the 2 groups showed similar infection rates. At 36 months, recipients of cadaver kidneys who were vaccinated showed better graft survival than recipients who were not vaccinated—50% vs. 25%.

Conclusions.—Administration of Towne live virus vaccine to seronegative renal transplant recipients appears to reduce the severity of CMV infection. It achieves this effect by mimicking the action of previous natural immunity. Studies are underway to confirm this effect.

▶ Active CMV disease has been a common and serious illness in renal transplant recipients. Seronegative recipients of kidneys from seropositive donors are at high risk to develop active CMV. Reactivation of latent virus can occur, especially after OKT3 or ALG antirejection therapy. Over the past several years, chemoprophylaxis and passive immunization have been proven to decrease the morbid complications of CMV disease in renal transplant recipients. Vaccination with attenuated Towne live CMV has now been tested, and this form of intervention has also been found beneficial in seronegative patients who eventually received a seropositive kidney. Vaccination resulted in a less morbid expression of CMV disease. Indeed, vaccination saved lives (see Fig 8–1). Should all seronegative potential kidney graft recipients at risk for developing active CMV receive passive immunization with anti-CMV globulin? Should all or certain patients receive chemoprophylaxis with acyclovir or gancyclovir? Are combinations of these interventions helpful and cost-effective? Control trial data are lacking. At present we administer chemoprophylaxis to all except seronegative recipients of seronegative kidneys. In addition, all seronegative recipients of seropositive grafts receive passive immunization. Until comparative control trials are available, we will continue this vigorous approach to prevent active CMV disease.—T. Strom, M.D.

Early Detection of Active Cytomegalovirus (CMV) Infection After Heart and Kidney Transplantation by Testing for Immediate Early Antigenemia and Influence of Cellular Immunity on the Occurrence of CMV Infection
Boland GJ, de Gast GC, Hené RJ, Jambroes G, Donckerwolcke R, The TH, Mudde GC (University Hospital, Wilhelmina Children's Hospital, Utrecht; University Hospital, Groningen, The Netherlands)
J Clin Microbiol 28:2069–2075, 1990   8–2

Background.—Active cytomegalovirus (CMV) infections, common after heart and kidney transplants, can cause serious disease. They develop only in immunocompromised hosts. The antigenemia test, along with quick cultures of urine, saliva, and buffy-coat cells, was assessed for the detection of active CMV infection in heart and kidney transplant recipients in relation to humoral and cellular immunity.

Methods.—Fifty-five renal and 14 cardiac transplant recipients were monitored closely for active CMV infection and immune parameters. The incidence of active CMV infection after organ transplantation and its relationship to the immune system were analyzed.

Findings.—All 19 CMV-seronegative recipients with seronegative donors remained seronegative. Thus, no CMV transmission occurred by leukocyte-depleted blood products. Primary CMV infection developed in 4 of 11, or 36%, of patients with positive donors. It was symptomatic in 1 patient. Active CMV infection was found in 29 of 39 seropositive patients, or 74%, being symptomatic in 8%. In all cases, CMV antigenemia was the first indication of active CMV infection. Cellular immunity, measured by lymphocyte proliferation (LPT), proved important in preventing active CMV infection. Fourteen of 15 patients with negative LPT had active CMV infections with antigenemia and positive cultures, whereas 1 of 10 with positive LPT had active infection.

Conclusions.—The antigenemia test provides an earlier indication of active CMV infection compared with cultures or a rise in IgG antibodies. Cellular immunity as measured by LPT appears to have an important part in preventing generalized and more serious CMV infections.

▶ The message is straightforward. Following infection with CMV, CMV antigen can be detected long before seroconversion occurs. Positive CMV cultures lag even longer following infection. A white blood cell "parasite," CMV produces an immunosuppressive effect in patients destined to develop active disease.—T. Strom, M.D.

Differentiation of Cytomegalovirus Infection From Acute Rejection Using Renal Allograft Fine Needle Aspirates

Nast CC, Wilkinson A, Rosenthal JT, Barba L, Bretan PN, Beaumont P, Danovitch GM (Harbor-UCLA Med Ctr, Torrance; UCLA Med Ctr, Los Angeles)
J Am Soc Nephrol 1:1204–1211, 1991   8–3

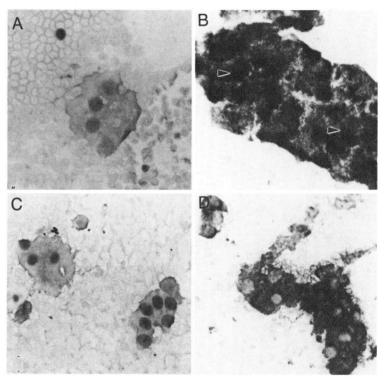

Fig 8–2.—Immunoalkaline phosphatase staining for CMV early nuclear protein (CMV-A) or HLA class II antigen (DR) of tubular cells from renal allograft fine-needle aspirates. **A,** a CMV-A-negative aspirate. No staining of tubular cell cytoplasm or nuclei is evident. **B,** a CMV-A-positive aspirate. There is marked CMV-A staining in the nuclei *(arrowheads)* with associated cytoplasmic staining; the cytoplasmic staining is possibly a cytospin artifact. **C,** a DR-negative aspirate. There is no staining present. **D,** a DR-positive aspirate. There is cytoplasmic staining without a nuclear component. Original magnification, ×325. (Courtesy of Nast CC, Wilkinson A, Rosenthal JT, et al: *J Am Soc Nephrol* 1:1204–1211, 1991.)

Introduction.—Because cytomegalovirus (CMV) infection may be difficult to distinguish from acute renal transplant rejection clinically and even histologically, immunohistochemical staining methods were used to assess aspirates from 27 transplant recipients. All the patients received cyclosporine and prednisone and some were given azathioprine as well.

Methods.—Of the 58 aspirates, 53 were stained with antibody against CMV early nuclear protein (CMV-A), and the same number were stained with antibody against leukocyte class II antigen (DR). A positive result consisted of 35% or more tubular cells staining for CMV-A and 30% or more for DR (Fig 8–2).

Results.—In 19 patients there was acute graft rejection and 5 had CMV infection; both were diagnosed in 1 patient. Of 9 positive CMV-A test results, 7 were associated with infection and there were no false negative results. Staining with DR never occurred in the absence of acute rejection, and all aspirates taken during acute rejection were DR-positive. Rejection was present 80% of the time when the aspirate was DR-positive.

Conclusion.—Immunohistochemical studies are a rapid and simple means of distinguishing between CMV infection of a renal graft and acute rejection.

▶ Graft dysfunction can occur during a bout of active CMV infection. At times, it may be difficult to discriminate between these entities. Occasionally, rejection and viremia may occur concurrently. Although latent CMV infection does not give rise to exuberant expression of viral proteins by the infected cell, such expression does occur during replicative infection. Hence, staining with monoclonal antibodies directed against certain viral proteins (e.g., early nuclear protein) are now routinely used to detect expression of viral proteins by mononuclear leukocytes that are actively infected. In this analysis of Nast et al., anti–CMV-A and anti-DR mAb were used to stain cells harvested from the graft by fine needle aspiration biopsy (FNAB). In other words, the allograft was examined as an alternative to peripheral blood white cells for expression of DR and CMV-A. Standards for staining of tubules by these antibodies were established using the immunoalkaline phosphatase method (see Fig 8–2).

The authors claim that aspirates from patients with rejection are never DR negative, and aspirates from patients with active CMV are never negative for CMV-A. Both DR and CMV-A were positive in 1 case where infection and rejection co-existed. While the results are fascinating, mononuclear leukocytes are a bit more readily accessible than renal tubular cells. The remarkable correlation of DR staining with rejection (and not infection) was blemished by only 3 potential false positive results. The authors correctly emphasize that elevations in host anti-CMV antibody titers lag behind active infection and are therefore a totally unreliable clinical tool. This study, if confirmed, suggests that FNAB is a grossly underused clinical tool. Can the diagnosis of rejection truly be established on the basis of anti-DR staining? It sounds too easy.—T. Strom, M.D.

Evidence That Antibodies to Cytomegalovirus and the T Cell Receptor (TCR)/CD3 Complex May Have Common Ligands

Yang W-C, Carreno M, Esquenazi V, Fuller L, Ranjan D, Burke G, Roth D, Miller J (Miami VA Hosp; Univ of Miami School of Medicine, Fla)
Transplantation 51:490–498, 1991   8–4

Background.—Human cytomegalovirus (CMV) often occurs in a carrier state without symptoms in nonimmunosuppressed individuals. Previous research has shown that about 25% of renal transplant recipients undergo a long immunosuppressive phase after OKT3 monoclonal antibody (MAb) therapy. The immunosuppression leads to decreased CD3 expression on peripheral blood T cells, and CMV infection. A study was undertaken to analyze the potential for an autoinduced immunosuppressive state in patients receiving OKT3 treatment.

Methods.—Sera were tested from renal allograft recipients who were treated with mouse monoclonal antibody OKT3 during rejection and who later developed a decrease in CD3 expression on peripheral blood lymphocytes (PBLs). Serum immunoglobulins were fractionated and measured. The CMV serology was assayed using enzyme-linked immunoassay techniques. An analysis was made of lymphocyte responsiveness to OKT3 stimulation, and on the binding to T cells of WT31, an MAb against a monomorphic epitope of the T cell receptor (TCR) αβ chain in flow cytometry. Other MAbs associated with immunosuppression were assayed, including αF1 (generated against the TCRα chain) and an MAb against the CMV late nuclear antigen.

Findings.—Immunoglobulins from sera from renal transplant patients receiving OKT3 MAb therapy bind to several bands of T cell membrane lysates, indicating molecular weights ranging from 40 to 55 KD. A significant decrease in the binding of WT31 in flow cytometry was observed during the second immunosuppressive phase (phase III) in which CD3 expression on PBL decreased, which did not occur during Phase II. The sera from patients during Phase II (the early interim phase with normal CD3 expression) did not affect the expression of CD2, CD4, and CD8. These derived immunoglobulins also suppressed the activation of normal PLBs generally induced by OKT3. Seven of 32 patients who developed the anti-antiidiotypic antibody (Ab2) had culture-proven CMV infections. From immunoblot analyses, αF1 MAb demonstrated binding to protein bands of the CMV lysate derived from virus-infected embryonic fibroblasts and to several ligands in the membrane lysate of CMV-infected cells. An anti-CMV MAb binding to the late nuclear antigen (LAb) strongly bound to a band of T cell membrane lysates and several bands of H33HJAJ1, a human T leukemia cell lysate. Sera containing Ab2 blocked αF1 binding to acetone-fixed cytofuged PBL slide preparations. Both LAb and αF1 inhibited the mitogen-stimulated lymphocyte activation in vitro.

Conclusion.—These findings add support to the concept that T cell functional abnormalities associated with CMV infection in renal transplant recipients with anti-T cell antibodies may result from the binding to T cell ligands by crossreacting regulatory human immunoglobulins.

▶ These investigators have discovered a common pathway linking treatment of the host with OKT3 antibody and the development of cytomegalovirus infection. They found common epitomes shared by antibody to CMV and antiidiotypic antibody induced by OKT3 treatment. This discovery may explain the frequent association made between rejection therapy and viral infection.—N.L. Ascher, M.D., Ph.D.

A Prospective, Randomized, Double-Blind Study of Trimethoprim-Sulfamethoxazole for Prophylaxis of Infection in Renal Transplantation: Clinical Efficacy, Absorption of Trimethoprim-Sulfamethoxazole, Effects on the Microflora, and the Cost-Benefit of Prophylaxis
Fox BC, Sollinger HW, Belzer FO, Maki DG (Univ of Wisconsin, Madison)
Am J Med 89:255–274, 1990   8–5

Introduction.—Infection continues to be a cause of significant morbidity and mortality in patients undergoing renal transplantation. The efficacy of long-term prophylaxis with trimethoprim-sulfamethoxazole (TMP-SMZ) for preventing bacterial infection in such patients was examined and the absorption of TMP-SMZ in transplant recipients, the effects of prophylaxis on the microflora, and the cost-benefit of prophylaxis were determined.

Observations.—One hundred thirty-two adults were enrolled in the randomized, double-blind, placebo-controlled trial. Those receiving TMP-SMZ had fewer hospital days with fever and significantly fewer bacterial infections after removal of a urethral catheter and after hospital discharge. A daily dose of 320/1,600 mg of TMP-SMZ was highly effective during hospitalization. A daily dose of 160/800 mg produced unexpectedly low blood levels and effectively prevented only urinary tract infections after catheter removal. Prophylaxis was most effective in preventing urinary tract and bloodstream infections and infections caused by enteric gram-negative bacilli, enterococci, or *Staphylococcus aureus*. In the early posttransplant period, prophylaxis did not prevent urinary tract infections associated with urethral catheters. After catheter removal, however, it reduced the risk of urinary tract infection 3-fold. There were no significant between-group differences in colonization by TMP-SMZ–resistant gram-negative bacilli. Paradoxically, patients given TMP-SMZ were less likely to become colonized by *Candida,* probably because of less exposure to antibiotics for treatment of infection. The prophylaxis group did not have a higher rate of infections caused by TMP-SMZ–resistant bacteria or Candida. However, their infections were more likely to be caused by resistant bacteria than were infections in patients given placebo (table).

Discussion.—Prophylaxis with TMP-SMZ is well tolerated and significantly decreases the incidence of bacterial infection after renal transplantation, especially infection of the urinary tract and bloodstream. It also protects against *Pneumocystis carinii* pneumonia. It is cost-beneficial. Subnormal absorption of TMP-SMZ in the early posttransplant period

Microbial Profile of Infection in the 2 Treatment Groups

Organisms	Placebo (n = 66)	TMP-SMZ (n = 66)	p Value
Gram-positive bacteria (TMP-SMZ–resistant)	47 (11)	25 (12)	0.05
Coagulase-negative staphylococci	11 (7)	17 (11)	NS†
Staphylococcus aureus	9 (1)	1 (0)	0.01
Enterococci	22 (3)	6 (1)	0.006
Gram-negative bacilli (TMP-SMZ–resistant)	48 (5)	10 (9)	<0.000
Enterobacteriaceae	46 (4)	4 (3)	<0.001
Escherichia coli	33 (2)	3 (3)	<0.001
Proteus mirabilis	4 (0)	0 (...)	NS
Klebsiella pneumoniae	3 (0)	0 (...)	NS
Citrobacter freundii	3 (1)	0 (...)	NS
Enterobacter cloacae	0 (...)	1 (0)	
Other enterobacteriaceae	3 (1)	0 (...)	NS
Pseudomonas aeruginosa	0 (...)	3 (3)	NS
Other	2 (1)	3 (3)	NS
Fungi	9	8	NS
Candida species	9	8	NS
Filamentous fungi	0	0	NS
Pneumocystis carinii	1	0	NS
Viruses	17*	12	NS
Herpes simplex virus	5	6	NS
Cytomegalovirus	10	5	NS
Varicella-zoster	2	1	NS
Epstein-Barr virus	1	0	NS

*Includes 1 patient with simultaneous infection of herpes simplex virus and varicella zoster virus.
†Not significant at p < .05.
(Courtesy of Fox BC, Sollinger HW, Belzer FO, et al: *Am J Med* 89:255–274, 1990.)

indicates that 320/1,600 mg daily is the best dose. This prophylaxis appears to have little effect on the microflora.

▶ For some years, many hospitals, including our own, have used TMP-SMX prophylaxis. Because urosepsis and *Pneumocystis carinii* pneumonia (PCP) are common and horrifying complications after transplantation, it seemed reasonable to use this agent. Nonetheless, several questions remained unanswered, because prospective, randomized studies had not been completed. Thanks to this study we can now be reassured of the following: (1) TMP-SMX prophylaxis does help prevent urosepsis, PCP, and other infections; (2) there is little discernable effect on the gut microflora; and (3) prophylaxis is cost-effective. Although the numbers are small, the benefit of TMP-SMX in OKT3-treated patients was of special interest. It was also noteworthy that whereas infection in SMP-TMX–treated patients was often caused by TMP-SMX–resistant organisms, a discernable increase in *Candida* or other candidate serious infections was not detected.—T. Strom, M.D.

Mycobacterial Infections After Renal Transplantation

Higgins RM, Cahn AP, Porter D, Richardson AJ, Mitchell RG, Hopkin JM, Morris PJ (University of Oxford, England)
Quart J Med 78:145–153, 1991   8–6

Introduction.—Tuberculosis occurs more often during dialysis and after renal transplantation than in the general population because of immunosuppression, which itself is secondary to both uremia and the use of drugs to prevent rejection. The occurrence of mycobacterial infection was examined in 633 patients successfully given renal transplants between 1975 and May 1989. All had cadaveric grafts that functioned for longer than 3 months.

Findings.—Three patients had localized pulmonary tuberculosis and recovered uneventfully when placed on chemotherapy for 11 to 16 months. Three other patients had extrapulmonary tuberculosis, 4 had miliary infection, and 7 had a *Mycobacterium kansasii* infection. One of the patients with miliary tuberculosis died of liver failure that might have been related to toxicity from antituberculosis treatment. Two others lost their grafts from rejection after withdrawal of cyclosporine because of rifampicin therapy and withdrawal of azathioprine because of neutropenia. Tuberculosis occurred in 22% of the 27 patients not given chemoprophylaxis but who were at risk because they lived in an endemic region or had been exposed. None of the 12 patients given chemoprophylaxis, usually because of a history of disease, had tuberculosis.

Recommendation.—The chief morbidity in these cases was allograft rejection secondary to reduced immunosuppressive therapy. Treatment with rifampicin and isoniazid for 9 months, with ethambutol added for the first 2 months, probably is adequate.

▶ OK, I'll faithfully promise to give isoniazide prophylaxis to patients at high risk of developing a mycobacterial infection. Because about one fourth of such patients not given antimicrobial prophylaxis develop an active infection, this is a necessary approach. Whereas the infections were controlled with appropriate treatment, the active infection required cessation of immunosuppression and thereby led to frequent rejection episodes.—T. Strom, M.D.

Use of Indium 111-Labeled White Blood Cell Scan in the Diagnosis of Cytomegalovirus Pneumonia in a Renal Transplant Recipient With a Normal Chest Roentgenogram

Chinsky K, Goodenberger DM (Washington Univ School of Medicine
Chest 99:761–763, 1991   8–7

Introduction.—Cytomegalovirus (CMV) infection is an important cause of morbidity and death in renal transplant recipients. Cytomegalovirus pneumonia has been described in transplant recipients whose chest radiographs are normal, but histologic confirmation generally is lacking.

Case Report.—Man, 33, underwent living-related-donor kidney transplantation for end-stage pyelonephritis disease. A second graft was transplanted after several rejection episodes. The donor was seropositive for CMV and, despite treatment with acyclovir and CMV immune globulin, the patient became febrile and had CMV-positive buffy coat and urine cultures. Fever recurred after ganciclovir treatment. The chest roentgenogram remained normal, but a ^{111}In-white blood cell scan showed diffuse uptake in both lungs, and bronchial washings were CMV-positive. Transbronchial biopsy specimens showed inclusions diagnostic of CMV infection. The patient responded to intravenous ganciclovir therapy. Radiographs transiently showed mild infiltration.

Implications.—A normal chest roentgenogram should not preclude a search for a pulmonary origin of fever in renal transplant recipients. The ^{111}In-white blood cell scan can help diagnose CMV pneumonia in this setting.

▶ I have no experience with this method, but it certainly worked in this case (see Figures 2 and 3 of the original article). The usefulness of gallium scan in detection of *Pneumocystis carinii* pneumonia is well established. Gallium scans have also been used to detect CMV in a transplant recipient.—T. Strom, M.D.

Reference

1. Hamed IA, Wenzl JE, Leonard JC, et al: *Arch Intern Med* 139:286–288, 1979.

The Effect of the Graft-Versus-Host Reaction on B Lymphocyte Production in Bone Marrow of Mice: Depressed Genesis of Early Progenitors Prior to μ Heavy Chain Expression
Xenocostas A, Osmond DG, Lapp WS (McGill University, Montreal)
Transplantation 51:1089–1096, 1991   8–8

Introduction.—The systemic graft-vs.-host (GVH) reactions caused by parental-strain lymphoid cell injection into F_1 hybrid recipients can lead to severe immunodeficiencies. Various suppressor cells mediate the early phase GVH, whereas the later phase occurs without any suppressor cell activity. The effects of GVH reactions on the size of early precursor cell populations that contribute to primary B-lymphocyte genesis were studied in mice.

Methods.—Experiments were conducted in female inbred A strain mice and female C57BL/6×A F_1 (B6AF$_1$) hybrid mice. The lymphoid cells from the A-strain mice were injected into the bone marrow of the C57BL/6×A F_1 mice. Three possible early B cell progenitors were quantitated using double immunofluorescence labeling methods for terminal deoxynucleotidyl transferase (TdT), the intranuclear enzyme, for the B220 cell surface glycoprotein detection by the 14.8 monoclonal antibody, and for the surface or cytoplasmic μ chains of the IgM molecule.

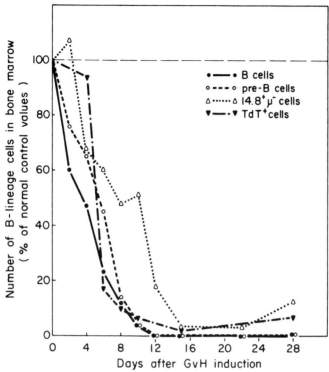

Fig 8–3.—The number of B-lineage precursor cells in the bone marrow during GVH reactions. (Courtesy of Xenocostas A, Osmond DG, Lapp WS: *Transplantation* 51:1089–1096, 1991.)

Cells were pooled from 3 mice to obtain samples necessary for immunofluorescence analysis.

Results.—On inducing the GVH reactions, the early B-precursor cells, the pre-B cells, and the B lymphocytes decreased rapidly in the bone marrow. After 10–15 days, these cells had almost completely disappeared and remained so for the rest of the 30 days of the experiment. Of the 35 total GVH-reactive mice, 3 died. Hypocellularity developed in the femoral bone marrow of the GVH-reactive mice at 6 days, achieving minimum numbers by day 15. The double immunofluorescence labeling with mAb 14.8 and the anti-μ antibodies demonstrated 2 groups of cells in the bone marrow: 1 expressed the B220 surface antigen and the μ chains (sμ ± cμ) and the other expressed the B220 antigen but no μ chains. The onset of depletion of the terminally differentiated B lymphocytes and the pre-B cells preceded the total reduction of the earlier $14.8^+\mu^-$ and the TdT^+ progenitor cells, both of which decreased after 2 and 4 days, respectively (Fig 8–3).

Conclusions.—There is a marked reduction of B-lineage progenitor cells in the bone marrow of GVH-reactive mice, which relates to humoral immunodeficiency. This appears to lead to the failure of B-cell genesis and ultimately to an absolute deficiency in the primary humoral immune response. These findings suggest a mechanism for the development of the immunodeficiencies related to GVH syndrome in human beings.

▶ Graft-vs.-host disease is associated with susceptibility to infection. These investigators demonstrate a failure of B-cell genesis and subsequent antibody production in a mouse model of GVH disease. Understanding the specific defective pathway is essential for effective therapy of GVH disease.—N.L. Ascher, M.D., Ph.D.

9 Lymphoma After Transplantation

▶ ↓ Epstein-Barr virus–associated lymphoma is an important complication after solid and bone marrow organ transplantation. These articles address mechanism of induction and treatment of lymphoma.—Nancy L. Ascher, M.D., Ph.D.

Anti-B-Cell Monoclonal Antibodies in the Treatment of Severe B-Cell Lymphoproliferative Syndrome Following Bond Marrow and Organ Transplantation

Fischer A, Blanche S, Le Bidois J, Bordigoni P, Garnier JL, Niaudet P, Morinet F, Le Deist F, Fischer A-M, Griscelli C, Hirn M (Hôpital des Enfants-Malades, Paris; Hôpital E Herriot, Lyons; Hôpital Sainte-Louis, Paris; Immunotech, Marseilles)

N Engl J Med 324:1451–1456, 1991   9–1

Introduction.—The B-cell lymphoproliferative syndrome is a rare life-threatening complication of marrow or organ transplantation that results from immunosuppression. The results of an open, multicenter, prospective trial of CD12 and CD24 monoclonal antibodies in the treatment of 26 patients with this syndrome after organ or marrow transplantation were reviewed.

Methods.—The B-cell–specific antibodies, including those with anti-immunoglobulin heavy-chain and light-chain isotype antibodies, were used to characterize the B cells in the blood and biopsy samples of the patients. Monoclonal antibodies included the ALB9, a mouse IgG1 specific for CD24, .2 mg/kg, which was infused for 4–6 hours every day for 10 days.

Results.—In 3 patients there was grade 2 fever, 2 had pain, and 1 had vomiting, diarrhea and thrombocytopenia from the monoclonal antibody infusion. No patient produced antibodies against the mouse immunoglobulins. The B cells were not detectable in the serum of the 18 patients analyzed. Some patients received antiviral drugs during the study. The anti–B-cell antibodies produced a complete remission in 16 patients who received treatment in 15–45 days (median, 21 days) (table). The complete remission occurred only in patients with oligoclonal B-cell lymphoproliferative syndrome, whereas patients with the monoclonal B-cell lymphoproliferative syndrome died within 38 days of beginning therapy. Of the 15 patients in complete remission evaluated, there was CD21 and CD24 expression on the proliferative B cells in 10 patients and CD21 or CD24 expression in 5 patients. Of the 16 patients in complete remission, 2 marrow-transplant recipients had a relapse.

Outcome of Treatment of Oligoclonal and Monoclonal B-Cell
Lymphoproliferative Syndrome With Anti-B-Cell Antibodies

TYPE OF SYNDROME	No. of PATIENTS	COMPLETE REMISSION	PARTIAL REMISSION	No RESPONSE
Oligoclonal				
Marrow transplantation	10	9	1*	0
Organ transplantation	8	7	1*	0
Total	18	16	2	0
Monoclonal				
Marrow transplantation	4	0	0	4
Organ transplantation	3	0	0	3
Total	7	0	0	7
Unknown	1	—	—	1†

*Progression of CNS disease.
†The clonality of the disease was unknown in 1 patient who underwent organ transplantation and died early in the course of the study.
(Courtesy of Fischer A, Blanche S, Le Bidois J, et al: *N Engl J Med* 324:1451–1456, 1991.)

Conclusion.—Intravenous infusion of the anti–B-cell antibodies can control the oligoclonal B-cell proliferation of cells, as long as the CNS is not involved. A randomized, controlled trial is recommended to evaluate this monoclonal antibody as a treatment for B-cell lymphoproliferative syndrome.

▶ Epstein-Barr virus–induced B-cell lymphoma is a significant source of mortality in solid organ and bone marrow transplant recipients. These investigators used 2 murine monoclonal antibodies directed against B cells to treat lymphoma in 14 marrow and 11 organ transplant recipients. Sixteen of 18 patients with oligoclonal disease had complete response; in contrast, none of the patients with monoclonal disease responded to the antibody. This therapy will need to be compared to antiviral agents, surgical excision, and decreased immunosuppression, which are the current mainstays of therapy in solid organ transplant recipients. It is likely that monoclonal antibodies will prove useful in combination with these modalities.—N.L. Ascher, M.D., Ph.D.

Promotion of B Cell Stimulation in Graft Recipients Through a Mechanism Distinct from Interleukin-6 Gene Superinduction
Kunzendorf U, Brockmöller J, Bickel U, Jochimsen F, Walz G, Roots I, Offermann G (Freie Universität of Berlin, Germany)
Transplantation 51:1312–1315, 1991   9–2

Background.—The risk of B cell-derived non-Hodgkin's lymphoma appears to be increased in graft recipients given cyclosporine (CsA). This treatment is associated with B cell activation and increased immunoglobulin production. Lymphoproliferative responses are reversed by cessation or reduction of CsA therapy. Because enhanced interleukin-6 (IL-6) gene expression results from CsA in cell culture, overproduction of this interleukin might lead to B-cell stimulation and lymphoproliferative disorders in CsA-treated patients.

Study Design.—A group of 91 patients was studied. All patients had undergone a kidney graft within a 6-year period and had stable graft function. Of the 91 patients, 11 received CsA alone; 30 received CsA and low-dose methylprednisolone; 30 were given CsA, azathioprine, and steroid; and 20 received azathioprine and steroid.

Observations.—Serum immunoglobulin levels were highest in those patients who were given monotherapy with CsA. The plasma IL-6 levels were similar in all groups, including a control group; they did not correlate with the immunoglobulin levels in any of the treatment groups.

Implications.—Renal graft recipients who are given CsA exhibit increased B cell stimulation; however, they retain normal plasma IL-6 levels. It appears that CsA may increase the risk of lymphoproliferative disease through a mechanism distinct from overexpression of IL-6.

▶ These authors attempt to explain the increased incidence of lymphoproliferative disease in patients treated with cyclosporine after organ transplantation through B cell stimulation by IL-6. Although cyclosporine enhances IL-6 gene expression and IL-6 production in vitro, these investigators could not find increased IL-6 levels in the plasma of renal transplant recipients. These investigators may be examining the wrong site for IL-6 levels. There may be a subset of patients in whom there is increased IL-6 gene expression in select lymphoid depots with local stimulation of B lymphocytes.—N.L. Ascher, M.D., Ph.D.

Orthotopic Liver Transplantation, Epstein-Barr Virus, Cyclosporine, and Lymphoproliferative Disease: A Growing Concern

Malatack JJ, Gartner JC Jr, Urbach AH, Zitelli BJ (Univ of Pittsburgh Health Science Ctr)
J Pediatr 118:667–675, 1991   9–3

Introduction.—Liver transplantation with cyclosporine immunosuppression has become increasingly effective, but at the cost of adverse effects of cyclosporine such as renal dysfunction. Long-term immunosuppression carries a risk of lymphoproliferative disease, presumably secondary to Epstein-Barr virus infection.

Methods.—Data were reviewed on 12 of 132 pediatric patients given orthotopic liver transplants in whom lymphoproliferative disease developed. Of the patients, 5 died of progressive lymphoproliferative disease or its complications, and 7 patients survived.

Results.—In 4 patients who were otherwise well, there was hyperplastic lymphatic tissue, usually in the form of tonsillar enlargement with mild upper airway obstruction. Examination of the excised tonsils (or axillary nodes) showed polymorphic polyclonal disease. After the cyclosporine dose was halved, 3 patients did well. Disseminated disease with lymphomatous clinical manifestations developed in the remaining patient, who died. In 3 patients, there were systemic symptoms with fever, vomiting, progressive encephalopathy, and/or respiratory distress; 1 improved spontaneously, but the other 2 died. In 5 patients, there was a lymphomatous condition resembling non-Hodgkin's lymphoma; only 1 of these patients lived without disease.

Conclusion.—Early recognition of lymphoproliferative disease in liver transplant recipients may improve the outcome. Disease should be resected and immunosuppression reduced. The new agent FK506 appears to be an even more potent immunosuppressive agent than cyclosporine and to have fewer adverse effects.

▶ Epstein-Barr virus–associated lymphoproliferative disease has long been a concern of the transplant community. A multidirectional approach using tumor excision and decreased immunosuppressor and antiviral agents has been the mainstay of therapy. Any immunosuppressant that interferes with the development of Epstein-Barr virus–specific cytotoxic T cells will inhibit the normal host response to virus infection. Although the article relates to patients immunosuppressed with cyclosporine, it is likely that newer, more potent immunosuppressants will also be associated with Epstein-Barr virus–associated lymphoma.— N.L. Ascher, M.D., Ph.D.

Increased Incidence of Lymphoproliferative Disorder After Immunosuppression With the Monoclonal Antibody OKT3 in Cardiac-Transplant Recipients
Swinnen LJ, Costanzo-Nordin MR, Fisher SG, O'Sullivan EJ, Johnson MR, Heroux AL, Dizikes GJ, Pifarre R, Fisher RI (Loyola Univ of Chicago, Maywood, IL; Hines VA Hosp, Hines IL)
N Engl J Med 323:1723–1728, 1990   9–4

Introduction.—A sharp increase in incidence of posttransplantation lymphoproliferative disorder was noted in heart transplantation patients in association with the monoclonal antibody OKT3. Heart transplantation patients at 1 institution were reviewed to identify factors that predict the development of this disorder.

Patients and Methods.—The study sample was comprised of 154 patients who received cardiac transplants during a 6-year period. Of these, 79 received OKT3 prophylactically or for treatment of rejection and 86 received prophylaxis with antithymocyte globulin. All patients received methylprednisolone, azathioprine, prednisone, and cyclosporine. Statistical analysis of the results included univariate analyses and multivariate analysis by logistic regression.

Results.—Posttransplantation lymphoproliferative disorder occurred in 1 of 75 patients who did not receive OKT3, a rate of 1.3%, compared to 11.4% of patients who did receive OKT3. The OKT3-treated group was 9 times more likely to develop the disorder. Use of OKT3 was shown by multivariate analysis to be the only factor having a significant association with development of the disorder. Increasing doses of this agent significantly increased risk; of 65 patients whose overall dose was 75 mg or less, only 4 developed the disorder, compared to 5 of 14 patients who received more than 75 mg. Seven deaths were attributed to the disorder.

Conclusion.—The use of OKT3 increases the incidence of posttransplantation lymphoproliferative disorder in heart transplant patients, especially those who have had cumulative doses of more than 75 mg. The use of prophylactic OKT3 should be reassessed, particularly since the value of prophylactic immunotherapy is yet to be firmly established. All patients who have received OKT3 should be monitored closely for signs of posttransplantation lymphoproliferative disorder.

▶ On a background of potent immunosuppressive therapy, patients receiving at least a 14-day course of OKT3 are at increased risk to develop lymphoproliferative disease. Indeed, longer courses of 5 μg/day therapy appeared to lead to more rapid onset of lymphoproliferative disease. Insofar as OKT3 is a potent and often useful antirejection therapeutic, it is important to discern whether OKT3 is a unique menace to incite lymphoproliferative disease and whether OKT3 treatment at any dose/duration is dangerous.

A burgeoning literature links expression of EBV with posttransplant lymphoproliferative disease. In vitro infection of B cells with EBV "immortalizes" the infected B cell. In the current report and in other reports, Epstein-Barr virus DNA was detected in malignant B cells. Another line of evidence links T cell-dependent immune mechanisms with resistance to emergence of EBV driven lymphoid neoplasia. Hence, it seems reasonable that the intense long-lasting immunodeficiency facilitates development of posttransplant lymphoproliferative disease. A 14-day (or more) course of OKT3 that targets all T cells for immunosuppression carries an inherent risk to patients receiving other immunosuppressive agents. Kidney transplant patients, by convention, often receive 10-day, not 14-day, courses of OKT3. Is this regimen safer? Because repeat courses of OKT3 carry a risk of reactivating cytomegalovirus and other viruses, many have limited their course of OKT3 to no more than 10 days.

This report should also serve to warn about the double-edged sword of long-lasting pan-T cell immunosuppression. Further studies are needed to evaluate the safety of briefer courses of therapy. More precise targets for immunosuppression than CD3 proteins are needed to improve the safety of monoclonal antibody treatment.—T. Strom, M.D.

10 Induction of Donor-Specific Unresponsiveness

▶ ↓ As a community, we are still looking for a reliable means to induce donor-specific hyporesponsiveness or unresponsiveness. The following group of articles add insight about the mechanism underlying donor-specific unresponsiveness. Mixed chimerism is a new model that holds great promise for clinical applicability.—Terry Strom, M.D., Nancy L. Ascher, M.D., Ph.D.

Induction of Donor-Specific Unresponsiveness to Cardiac Allografts in Rats by Pretransplant Anti-CD4 Monoclonal Antibody Therapy
Shizuru JA, Seydel KB, Flavin TF, Wu AP, Kong CC, Hoyt EG, Fujimoto N, Billingham ME, Starnes VA, Fathman CG (Stanford Univ)
Transplantation 50:366–373, 1990   10–1

Background.—Previous research has shown that monoclonal antibodies directed against the CD4 surface molecule can generate profound immunosuppression in mice. A monoclonal antibody designated OX-38 di-

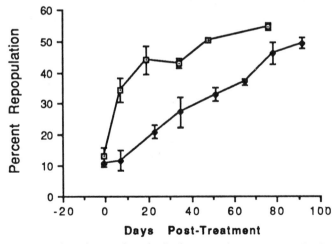

Fig 10–1.—Repopulation kinetics of CD4⁺ cells after OX-38 therapy. Rats treated with OX-38 and transplanted with heterotopic heart allografts were monitored for return of CD4⁺ cell levels in peripheral blood by fluorescence-activated cell-sorter analysis. Y-axis is percentage of CD4⁺ cells relative to untreated controls. Treatment group A levels *(filled diamonds)* initially lagged behind group B *(open boxes)*; however, both stabilized at approximately 60% control levels at 3 months posttreatment. (Courtesy of Shizuru JA, Seydel KB, Flavin TF, et al: *Transplantation* 50:366–373, 1990.)

TABLE 1.—Cardiac Allograft Survival With Anti-CD4
Monoclonal Antibody Treatment

Treatment group	Strain combination	Graft survival (days)
Control	Lewis-to-ACI	8, 8, 9, 10, 11, 12
(A) − 4 weeks	Lewis-to-ACI	8,*>28,†>200, >200, >250, >250
(B) − 4 days	Lewis-to-ACI	14, >176, >200, >200, >250, >250

*Showed CD4⁺ cell-depletion levels and enzyme-linked immunosorbent assay response significantly different from all other treated rats.
†Rat died of causes unrelated to allograft.
(Courtesy of Shizuru JA, Seydel KB, Flavin TF, et al: *Transplantation* 50:366–373, 1990.)

rected against the rat CD4 molecule was tested for its capacity to prolong the survival of heterotopic vascularized rat heart allografts transplanted across major histocompatibility barriers.

Methods and Results.—Adult male ACI rats were used as recipients, and adult male Lewis and Brown-Norway rats were used as heart donors. Fluorescence-activated cell-sorter analysis demonstrated that OX-38 administration selectively depleted 80% to 95% of CD4⁺ cells from peripheral blood of treated rats. The in vivo immunosuppressive effects of OX-38 were verified by suppression of an antibody response against OX-38 as a heterologous protein immunogen. Recipients were given OX-38 antibody as a single agent in pretransplant regimens. Nine of 12 treated rats maintained heterotopic abdominal heart allografts for more than 175 days, whereas rats not given antibody therapy rejected their grafts within 14 days. Rats maintaining heart allografts for more than 100 days did not reject second donor strain hearts but did reject third party heart grafts transplanted into the femoral space. Anti-CD4– induced allograft unresponsiveness persisted for 90 days or more after donor tissue was surgically removed and the second donor-matched heart was retransplanted (Tables 1 and 2; Fig 10–1).

TABLE 2.—Survival of Femoral Cardiac Allografts: Anti-CD4
Monoclonal Antibody Induces Donor-Specific Unresponsiveness

Treatment group	Strain combination	Graft survival (days)
Control	Lewis-to-ACI	8, 8, 9, 10, 10, 13
Control	BN-to-ACI	5, 5, 6, 7, 7, 7
Long-term graft survivor	Lewis-to-ACI	>16,*>49,* >50,* >100, >100
Long-term graft survivor	BN-to-ACI	>12,†>13,†>17,†>32

*Grafts removed for histologic evaluation, all functionally 4⁺ at time of excision.
†Grafts removed for histologic evaluation, all functionally 2⁺ at time of excision.
(Courtesy of Shizuru JA, Seydel KB, Flavin TF, et al: *Transplantation* 50:366–373, 1990.)

Conclusions.—Transient, pretransplant treatment with monoclonal antibodies directed against the CD4$^+$ lymphocyte induced specific, long-lasting unresponsiveness to wholly major histocompatibility complex-mismatched cardiac allografts in rats without additional immunosuppression. Of course, the findings from rodent studies cannot be directly extrapolated to human beings. The properties of the monoclonal antibodies that yield optimal immunosuppression must be further explored.

▶ Pretransplant treatment with high doses of an anti-CD4 monoclonal antibody that causes massive in vivo lysis of CD4 cells (Fig 10–1) creates a state of donor-specific graft tolerance (see Tables 1, 2). Indeed, the treated host also fails to mount a response against the anti-CD4 monoclonal antibody, which is a foreign protein. This powerful treatment does not, however, erase immunologic memory. Until most recently, only first generation monoclonal antibodies have been available for use in the clinic. These first generation anti-CD4 monoclonal antibodies activate human complement or antibody-dependent cell-mediated cytotoxicity mechanisms. Hence, they lacked the ability to clear CD4$^+$ cells. Will the fully humanized monoclonal antibodies (anti-CD4 and other monoclonal antibodies such as anti-CD3 and anti-CD25) have a profound impact on human subjects? Will it be necessary to search for monoclonal antibodies that react with special CD4 epitopes? In preclinical models some, but not all, nonlytic anti-CD4 monoclonal antibodies are also tolerogenic. This may be important because it is uncertain how well patients will tolerate AIDS-like CD4 counts.—T. Strom, M.D.

Influence of Antiidiotypic Antibody Activity on Renal Transplant Outcome
Al-Muzairai IA, Dolhain R, Taylor Y, Stewart KN, MacMillan M, Catto GRD, Mac-Leod AM (University of Aberdeen; Western Infirmary, Glasgow, Scotland)
Kidney Int 40:80–85, 1991   10–2

Background.—The presence of cytotoxic histocompatibility leukocyte antigen (HLA) antibodies (Ab1) against donor lymphocytes in sera before transplantation is almost always associated with rapid renal transplant rejection. The possibility that anti-idiotypic antibodies (Ab2) to cytotoxic HLA antibodies may modulate the immune response and favorably affect renal allograft outcome was investigated.

Methods and Findings.—Sera were obtained from 63 patients before transplantation and tested for inhibitory or potentiating activity in the short anti-idiotypic assay. Thirty patients had inhibitory activity. In 28 of those patients, the transplant survived more than 1 year. Of the patients without antibody activity, 11 of 17 had grafts that survived more than 1 year. Of those showing potentiating activity, 11 of 16 were functioning at 1 year. Transplant survival in the first group was significantly different from that in the other 2 groups. No significant difference in survival rates was seen in the latter 2 groups.

Conclusions.—Antibodies of the idiotypic/anti-idiotypic network may be present before transplantation in patients not previously showing cytotoxic activity to donor lymphocytes. The presence of inhibitory activity correlates with improved allograft survival. Potentiating activity is not an indicator of poor transplant outcome. The rapid short anti-idiotypic assay done before transplantation may be used to select patients for successful transplantation.

▶ Although Jerne won a Nobel prize for his "network theory," I and many others are basically agnostic about the truth of this dogma. This report suggests, but does not prove, that patients elaborating anti-idiotypic antibodies (Ab2) against donor-specific anti-HLA antibodies have a very high rate of engraftment (see Table 6 in the original article). The detection system used to screen for anti-idiotypic antibodies does not definitively prove that the antibodies are indeed anti-idiotypic. Nonetheless, the correlation between a positive assay and engraftment is impressive. This interesting report warrants thorough follow-up analysis to determine the precise nature of the substance that scores as a positive in the screening assay. The presence of anti-anti-idiotypic (Ab3) antibodies that should neutralize the anti-idiotypic (Ab2) antibodies, did *not* influence the rate of engraftment. Whew! I'm exhausted just thinking about anti-antibodies and anti-anti-antibodies.—T. Strom, M.D.

Specific Unresponsiveness in Rats With Prolonged Cardiac Allograft Survival After Treatment With Cyclosporine. IV. Examination of T Cell Subsets in Graft-Versus-Host Assays

Pearce NW, Dorsch SE, Hall BM (Stanford Univ, Stanford, Calif; University of Sydney, Sydney, Australia)
Transplantation 50:493–497, 1990   10–3

Background.—Short-term cyclosporine treatment induces a specific unresponsiveness in DA rats that receive PVG heart allografts. If the graft survives for more than 75 days, the W3/25$^+$ (CD4$^+$) subset becomes unable to mediate rejection of PVG, but not third-party, grafts when they are placed into irradiated DA hosts. Experiments were performed using this model to ascertain whether there was a related change in the ability of peripheral lymphoid T cell subsets from unresponsive animals to induce graft-vs.-host (GVH) reactivity.

Findings.—Naive CD4$^+$ and CD8$^+$ cells demonstrated synergy in the popliteal lymph node (PLN) assay; however, alone, only CD4$^+$ cells proliferated. Similar PLN enlargement was seen in both donor-specific (DA×PVG)F$_1$ hosts and third-party (W/F×DA)F$_1$ hosts with unfractionated and CD4$^+$ cells from unresponsive animals. No PLN enlargement was produced by MRC OX8$^+$ cells from unresponsive and naive hosts, unless large numbers of cells were injected. With small numbers of MRC OX8$^+$ cells, specific PLN enlargement was seen. In an in vivo assay adapted from the host-vs.-graft (HVG) PLN assay, CD4$^+$ cells from DA rats treated with cyclosporine showed no response to DA anti-PVG idiotype. A lethal GVH assay was used to test cells from cyclosporine-treated DA rats because the PLN assay does not test the capacity of cells to cause tissue damage. They proved to have the same ability to induce lethal GVH in irradiated $(DA \times PVG)F_1$ and $(DA \times W/F)F_1$ hosts.

Conclusions.—Cells from unresponsive animals have a normal response in both proliferative and effector GVH assays. This suggests that cells, which could respond to PVG alloantigen and mediate tissue damage, exist in unresponsive animals but cannot mediate rejection. This may be because of the relatively weak immune stimulus of organ grafting. Clinically, it is possible that tolerance to a graft can exist without clonal deletion.

▶ My laboratory may have been the first to point out that short courses of CsA in allografted rats result in emergence or unopposed activity of donor specific T cell–dependent immune phenomena. This current work carefully catalogues such effects in a rat cardiac transplant model. These effects have been noted by many workers, although the molecular basis of these effects have remained mysterious. Since the publication of this current work, Suthanthiran's laboratory has determined that while CsA blocks expression of multiple pro-inflammatory cytokines, CsA amplifies expression of TGF-β, a powerfully immunosuppressive cytokine. Hence, CsA-mediated immunosuppression just might result from skewing the program of T cell activation. This deviated activation profile may render potentially alloaggressive cells into cells that home to the graft but secrete immunosuppressive, not immunostimulatory, molecules.—T. Strom, M.D.

Kidney Allograft Tolerance in Primates Without Chronic Immunosuppression—The Role of Veto Cells
Thomas JM, Carver FM, Cunningham PRG, Olson LC, Thomas FT (East Carolina Univ, Greenville, NC)
Transplantation 51:198–207, 1991   10–4

Background.—Infusion of specific donor bone marrow cells after transplant into antithymocyte globulin (ATG)-treated recipients promotes long allograft survival in the absence of immunosuppressive drug treatment. Infusion of donor bone marrow cells also inhibits antidonor cytotoxic T lymphocyte (CTL) activation in allograft recipients. This trend is analogous to the veto phenomenon. The hypothesis that veto activity in donor bone marrow cells is involved in the induction of donor-specific unresponsiveness was tested in rhesus monkey kidney transplant recipients treated with ATG and donor bone marrow.

Methods.—Normal monkey bone marrow cells were fractionated into subpopulations through depletion with monoclonal antibodies and immunomagnetic beads. Unfractionated bone marrow cells and subsets were assessed for veto activity in in vitro mixed lymphocyte reaction (MLR)-induced CTL and for in vivo tolerance-promoting activity in ATG-treated monkey kidney transplant recipients.

Results.—Bone marrow cells specifically suppressed CTL activity to peripheral blood lymphocytes from the bone marrow cell donor in MLR-induced CTL assays. A small population of bone marrow cells mediated the suppression. This population expressed a $CD2^+$, $CD8^+$, $CD16^+$, DR^-, $CD3^-$, $CD38^-$ phenotype. The in vivo study results were highly correlated with the in vitro results. The ATG-treated recipients given DR^- or DR^- $CD3^-$ bone marrow cell infusions had significantly longer graft survival and a 40% to 50% rate of long-term survivors over 150 days. The tolerance-promoting effect of donor bone marrow cell infusions was absent in recipients given $CD2^-$ or DR^- $DC16^-$ donor bone marrow cell infusions. There were no long-term survivors in this group. Long survival was associated with suppressed in vivo antidonor CTL activity.

Conclusions.—A minor donor bone marrow cell subpopulation with similar phenotypic markers suppressed acute rejection and in vivo and in vitro antidonor CTL responses. A veto mechanism may control the induction phase of allograft tolerance in this model, providing a critical period of CTL silence so that host immunoregulatory mechanisms needed to maintain graft tolerance can develop.

▶ There is absolutely no evidence that allograft tolerance is associated with permanent deletion of alloreactive clones. In some models, T cells that have the appropriate T cell receptor molecules to recognize and attack the graft have been rendered anergic. These anergic cells are immunologically paralyzed and do not proliferate in response to donor antigen. In the total lymphoid irradiation model, the cells that re-populate the irradiated nodes do not often secrete IL-2; they use IL-4 as their growth factor. This and other investigations suggest that T cells in the tolerant host may express a skewed pattern of cytokine secretion. In this study, Thomas et al. demonstrate defective antidonor CTL activation takes place. In some models, this failure to normally activate CTLs has been attributed to a so-called veto cell mechanism. Veto cells are maladroit antigen-presenting cells that inactivate rather than activate CTLs. Thomas et al. point to a veto cell mechanism in this model. As I read this paper, I wonder whether the veto cell mechanism and T cell clonal anergy are the opposite sides of the same coin.—T. Strom, M.D.

Downregulation of Antidonor Cytotoxic Lymphocyte Responses in Recipients of Donor-Specific Transfusions

Hadley GA, Kenyon N, Anderson CB, Mohanakumar T (Washington Univ School of Med, St. Louis; Diabetes Research Inst, Miami)
Transplantation 50:1064–1066, 1990   10–5

Background.—Research results have demonstrated that donor-specific blood transfusions (DST) lengthen the survival of histocompatibility leukocyte antigen (HLA)-disparate allografts to a level similar to that of HLA-identical transplants. The types of changes in cellular immunity that occur in human DST recipients were tested using a limiting dilution assay for cytotoxic T lymphocyte precursors (CTLp) in 7 patients before and after they underwent DST conditioning.

Methods.—The DST patients had 3 transfusions of 200 mL donor blood spaced 2 weeks apart while taking azathioprine continuously for immunosuppression. Pre-DST blood samples were taken 1–2 weeks before the initial transfusion, and post-DST samples were taken 2 weeks after the final infusion. The lymphocyte-dependent antibody assay was used to assay antidonor CTL responses.

Findings.—After the DST procedures, the 7 patients demonstrated 2 different kinds of antidonor LDA plots. Four patients had post-DST antidonor plots with single-hit kinetics; in the other 3, biphasic post-DST plots to donor antigens were produced (Fig 10–2). Six of the 7 patients receiving transfusions demonstrated no significant change in reactivity to any third-party antigens after DST ($P = .05$). One patient had a significant increase in the third-party reactivity after DST ($P = .05$), while another patient demonstrated a significant decrease.

Comment.—These findings are consistent with the hypothesis that the DST conditioning procedure increases an immunoregulatory cell population that downregulates production of antidonor CTL responses in a subset group of DST recipients. This type of mechanism could partially explain the beneficial effects of DST conditioning on renal allograft survival.

▶ The limiting dilution analysis is an interesting assay that allows one to differentiate between clonal deletion and the presence of a suppressor phenomenon. It is to be anticipated that the beneficial effects offered by donor-specific transfusions will represent a number of different mechanisms that are operative to varying degrees.—N.L. Ascher, M.D., Ph.D.

Cross-Species Bone Marrow Transplantation: Evidence for Tolerance Induction, Stem Cell Engraftment, and Maturation of T Lymphocytes in a Xenogeneic Stromal Environment (Rat → Mouse)
Ildstad ST, Wren SM, Boggs SS, Hronakes ML, Vecchini F, Van den Brink MRM (Univ of Pittsburgh; Childrens Hosp of Pittsburgh)
J Exp Med 174:467–478, 1991   10–6

Introduction.—Limitations to xenogeneic transplantation might be overcome by induction of tolerance through transplantation of bone marrow between species to produce fully xenogeneic chimeras. Few studies have addressed the question of whether marrow from the donor species can survive for long periods and function normally in the stromal environment of the recipient species. Experiments were conducted in which untreated rat bone marrow was transplanted into irradiated mice to produce fully xenogeneic chimeras.

Methods.—Fully xenogeneically reconstituted animals were prepared by transplanting non-T-cell-depleted (TCD) F344 or Wistar Furth rat bone marrow into irradiated B10 mouse recipients. Mixed xenogeneically reconstituted animals were prepared by transplantation of TCD mouse

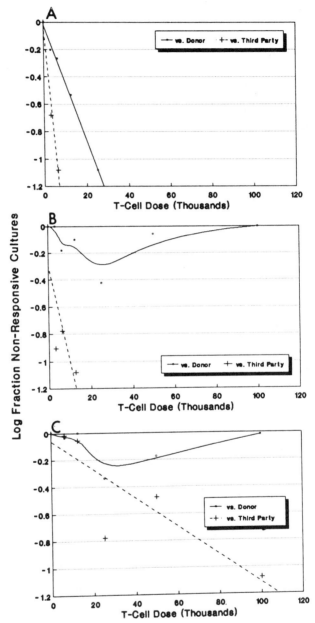

Fig 10–2.—Limiting dilution analysis of cytolitic T lymphocyte precursors directed to donor *(solid line)* and third-party antigens *(dashed line)* for recipient GB: **A,** pre-DST; **B,** post-DST, pretransplant; and **C,** post-DST, posttransplant. (Courtesy of Hadley GA, Kenyon N, Anderson CB, et al: *Transplantation* 50:1064–1066, 1990.)

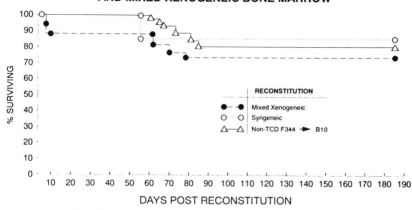

Fig 10–3.—Life-table survival of fully xenogeneic chimeras (non-TCD F344 rat → B10 mouse) (n = 36). Syngeneically reconstituted mice (B10 → B10) (n = 10) and mixed xenogeneic chimeras (B10 + non-TCD F344 → B10) (n = 10) which received a mixture of syngeneic B10 plus untreated F344 rat bone marrow were prepared as controls. Minimum follow-up was 77 days. Experimental animals prepared for lineage-specific analysis by flow cytometry were not included in survival analyses because killing of the animals was required. (Courtesy of Ildstad ST, Wren SM, Boggs SS, et al: *J Exp Med* 174:467–478, 1991.)

bone marrow cells plus non-TCD F344 rat bone marrow cells. Radiation controls were also prepared.

Results.—Stable xenogeneic lymphoid chimerism was produced in fully xenogeneically reconstituted animals, ranging from 82% to 97% rat derivation. All of these animals survived for at least 50 days without evidence of graft-vs.-host disease, whereas all unreconstituted radiation controls died within 10 days (Fig 10–3). Highly donor-specific tolerance was achieved, with major histocompatibility complex (MHC) disparate third-party mouse and rat skin grafts being promptly rejected, but donor-specific F344 grafts surviving greater than 130 days. Up to 7 months after transplantation, the fully xenogeneic chimeras had multi-lineage rat stem cell-derived progeny, including T and B lymphocytes, myeloid cells, erythrocytes, platelets, and natural killer cells. Rat T lymphocytes matured and acquired the α/β T-cell receptor in the thymus of chimeras in a way similar to that seen in normal rat controls, suggesting that normal maturation and differentiation could occur by interaction of immature T lymphocytes of rat origin with murine xenogeneic thymic stroma.

Conclusion.—Stable rat pluripotent stem-cell engraftment and maturation of rat T lymphocytes can occur in the stromal environment of irradiated B10 mice after transplantation of untreated rat bone marrow. The mechanisms of induction and maintenance of donor-specific transplantation tolerance across a species barrier can be studied by this model.

▶ The work of Ildstad and Sachs using mixed syngeneic and allogeneic marrow to induce mixed chimerism offers promise for transplantation tolerance. In these experiments, Ildstad et al. produced stable xenogeneic lymphoid chimerism without graft vs. host disease. The implications for the field of xenotransplantation are obvious.—N.L. Ascher, M.D., Ph.D.

Mixed Chimerism to Induce Tolerance for Solid Organ Transplantation
Wren SM, Nalesnik M, Hronakes ML, Oh E, Ildstad ST (Univ of Pittsburgh; Children's Hosp of Pittsburgh)
J Pediatr Surg 26:439–443, 1991   10–7

Introduction.—Chimerism in which tissue elements from more than 1 genetically diverse strain or species coexists in another organism can induce donor-specific transplantation tolerance. Mixed allogeneic chimeras can result from the transplantation of a mixture of T cell-depleted (TCD) syngeneic (host-type) plus TCD allogeneic (donor) bone marrow. The outcome of allogeneic donor-specific skin grafts inserted specifically at the time of mixed bone marrow reconstitution were reviewed.

Methods.—Several strains of mice were used. Mixed allogeneic reconstitutions were produced. Syngeneically reconstituted control animals received the bone marrow cells. Skin grafts of full-thickness tail skin tissue measuring 1 cm × 1 cm were used, with representative samples from 3 animals analyzed using hematoxylin-eosin staining.

Results.—Permanent survival of the B10.BR skin grafts were observed in all chimeras, even if the graft was inserted at the mixed allogeneic reconstitution time. However, normal B10 controls rejected the skin grafts early with a median survival time of about 11 days. Third-party grafts were quickly rejected, but the donor-specific B10.BR grafts remained patent. Histologic evaluation of grafts from mixed chimeras showed all grafts to be healthy and viable. Even the graft sampled at 62 days postimplantation demonstrated no signs of rejection. In the 2 samples from animals that had skin grafts inserted at marrow transplant at 90 days, some small increases in the number of mononuclear cells, basophils, and neutrophils occurred. Mild edema and slight inflammation were also observed.

Conclusion.—Mixed chimerism can be accomplished with nonlethal preparative techniques using monoclonal antibodies in conjunction with cytoreductive drugs or low-dose irradiation. This model could ultimately have clinical application, and both living and related donor tissue could be used, as well as cadaver bone marrow and solid organ grafts.

▶ Ilstad et al. have developed an important model, which holds promise for clinical application to induce tolerance in transplantation. Mixed T cell-depleted syngeneic and allogeneic bone marrow transplantation into a lethally irradiated host results in stable mixed chimerism and tolerance to donor skin. This group has also shown tolerance induction in this model tested in a solid organ allograft. Modification of this technique for human beings will likely substitute the use of antilymphocyte preparations for high-dose irradiation. Concern regarding graft vs. host disease is the major limitation in clinical application.—N.L. Ascher, M.D., Ph.D.

Induction of Kidney Transplantation Tolerance Across Major Histocompatibility Complex Barriers By Bone Marrow Transplantation in Miniature Swine

Guzzetta PC, Sundt TM, Suzuki T, Mixon A, Rosengard BR, Sachs DH (National Cancer Inst, Bethesda, Md)
Transplantation 51:862–866, 1991   10–8

Background.—Marrow transplantation across major histocompatibility complex (MHC) barriers can induce donor-specific tolerance in mice, preserving immunocompetence against third-party antigens. Permanent lymphohemopoietic chimerism can be induced in MHC-disparate miniature swine by transplanting bone marrow after lethal whole-body radiation. Whether such chimerism allows permanent tolerance of a vascularized allograft without the need for exogenous immune suppression was investigated.

Methods.—Renal transplantation was carried out in miniature swine given MHC-mismatched marrow transplants more than 5 months previously. Kidneys from both MHC-matched and mismatched donors (relative to the marrow donor) were transplanted.

Results.—All the animals regained in vitro responsiveness to third-party MHC antigens but remained unresponsive to MHC antigens of the marrow donor and of self. Mismatched kidneys were promptly rejected, but most animals given kidneys matched for marrow-donor MHC showed no evidence of rejection and functioned for longer than 200 days (table).

Conclusions.—It appears that marrow transplantation is an effective means of inducing tolerance to an MHC-mismatched kidney transplant in this large animal model. If the results are replicated in studies using a nonlethal preparative regimen, they may be applicable clinically to patients requiring poor-prognosis transplants, such as intestinal transplants.

▶ This work builds on that of Ilstad et al.—transplantation of allogeneic bone marrow after host lethal whole-body irradiation. Sach's group shows that chimerism can be induced in a large animal model (the miniature swine) using this

Results of Kidney Transplants in Bone-marrow-transplanted Miniature Swine

	Animal No.	BMT combination haplotypes	KTX donor haplotype	Results
A. BMT and KTX donors MHC mismatched	2009	dd → cd	ac	Died day 6 KTX rejection
	2420	cd → dd	ad	Died day 8 KTX rejection
	2408	ad → cd	Yucatan	Died day 7 KTX rejection
B. BMT and KTX donors MHC matched	2246	ac → ad	ac	CREAT 1.8 at 14 months
	2256	ac → ad	ac	Died day 75 KTX rejection
	2308	ag → gg	ag(2)[a]	CREAT 1.5 at 11 months
	2396	ac → ad	ac	CREAT 1.4 at 9 months
	2409	ad → cd	ad	CREAT 1.7 at 8 months

[a]First KTX was a technical failure, replaced at day 6 with the other kidney from the same donor.
(Courtesy of Guzzetta PC, Sundt TM, Suzuki T, et al: *Transplantation* 51:862–866, 1991.)

technique. Further, the level of chimerism achieved induces tolerance to a kidney transplant from the bone marrow donor. Although cadaveric bone marrow infusion with kidney transplantation has been applied clinically by the University of Alabama group, these experiments support the deliberate institution of the chimeric state.—N.L. Ascher, M.D., Ph.D.

Evidence for Involvement of Clonal Anergy in MHC Class I and Class II Disparate Skin Allograft Tolerance After the Termination of Intrathymic Clonal Deletion

Tomita Y, Nishimura Y, Harada N, Eto M, Ayukawa K, Yoshikai Y, Nomoto K (Kyushu University, Fukuoka, Japan)
J Immunol 145:4026–4036, 1990   10–9

Background.—Recent studies of mice suggest that self-tolerance to major histocompatibility complex (MHC) molecules involves intrathymic clonal deletion. The presence of extrathymic mechanisms of tolerance to both class I and class II antigens has also been demonstrated. A method of inducing tolerance by administering cyclophosphamide after an injection of allogeneic spleen cells and/or bone marrow cells resulted in long-lasting skin allograft tolerance with minimal mixed chimerism in most H2-identical combinations.

Study Plan.—This model of tolerance was used to examine mechanisms of cyclophosphamide-induced tolerance to class I (D) and class II (IE) alloantigens in mice.

Findings.—In the tolerant mice, intrathymic clonal deletion of T cells reactive to IE-encoded antigens was seen in association with intrathymic mixed chimerism. Skin grafts continued to survive after the clonal deletion was terminated 6 months after tolerance induction. The T cells that reappeared in the periphery of graft-bearing mice were incapable of proliferating in response to receptor cross-linking with specific monoclonal antibody. The cytotoxic T lymphocyte activity against class I alloantigens of spleen cells from tolerant mice was restored by adding interleukin-2 to the mixed lymphocyte cultures.

Implications.—These findings provide direct evidence that tolerance to both class I and class II alloantigens by clonal allergy develops during the termination of intrathymic clonal deletion. The major mechanisms of such tolerance include the destruction of antigen-stimulated T cells in the periphery, intrathymic clonal deletion associated with mixed chimerism, and clonal anergy.

▶ Tomita et al. have induced low level chimerism and tolerance to class I and class II murine antigens using antigen challenge and cyclophosphamide injection. Their studies indicate that intrathymic clonal deletion is not the mechanism by which skin grafts are maintained over the long term. Although precursor cytolytic cells can be identified in the periphery, local lack of differentiation factors prevent the presence of mature cytolytic cells. This clonal anergy involved lack of maturation of precursor cells.—N.L. Ascher, M.D., Ph.D.

Induction of Donor-Specific Unresponsiveness by Intrathymic Islet Transplantation

Posselt AM, Barker CF, Tomaszewski JE, Markmann JF, Choti MA, Naji A (Univ of Pennsylvania, Philadelphia)
Science 249:1293–1295, 1990   10–10

Induction.—The most specific therapy for insulin-dependent diabetes mellitus is isolated pancreatic islet transplantation; however, its applicability has been hampered by the vulnerability of allografts to immunologic rejections. Whether the thymus might be an immunologically privileged site for such transplantation was investigated.

Methods.—Islets were taken from rat donors and transplanted into major histocompatibility complex incompatible rats in which diabetes had been induced. Islets were inoculated into conventional transplant sites into the testicle which is known to be a privileged site and into the thymus. Some islets were fresh and others were cultured before transplantation. Some recipients had a single injection of rabbit antiserum to rat lymphocytes.

Results.—All thymus allografts in recipients who received antilymphocyte serum survived indefinitely (table). Survival of a second donor strain islet allograft was permitted by a state of donor-specific unresponsiveness. This state may have been induced by maturation of T-cell precursors in a thymic microenvironment that was harboring foreign alloantigen.

Condition.—Pancreatic islet allografts transplanted into the thymus survive indefinitely and can induce donor-specific unresponsiveness. This model provides a method for successful pancreatic islet transplantation and may offer new information on the development of tolerance.

▶ This group has made the important observation that education of those cells in thymic microenvironment with allogeneic cells results in tolerance to donor alloantigen. Decreased precursor cytolytic cells were identified in these hosts. These experiments are consistent with the presumed role of the thymus in induction of self-tolerance.—N.L. Ascher, M.D., Ph.D.

Survival of Fresh Lewis Islet Allografts in Wistar Furth Recipients		
Site of islet transplantation	Individual graft survival (days)	
	Without ALS	1 ml of ALS*
Liver (intraportal)	5, 8, 8, 9 (8)†	6, 22, 29, 35, 36 (29)
Renal subcapsule	9, 9, 10, 13 (9.5)	27, 33, 38, 47, 61, >200 × 2 (47)
Thymus	13, 13, 16, 17, 17, 18, >200 (17)	28, 33, 57, >200 × 10 (>200)‡
Testicle		50, 50, 76, 110, >200 × 2 (76)

*Accurate Chemical & Scientific C., Westbury, NY.
†Median survival times.
‡Three recipients of intrathymic islets that were not used for further transplantation experiments remained normoglycemic after 17 months.
(Courtesy of Posselt AM, Barker CFR, Tomaszewski JE, et al: *Science* 249:1293–1295, 1990.)

Termination of Immune Privilege in the Anterior Chamber of the Eye When Tumor-Infiltrating Lymphocytes Acquire Cytolytic Function

Ksander BR, Mammolenti MM, Streilein JW (Univ of Miami, Fla; Bascom Palmer Eye Inst, Miami, Fla)
Transplantation 52:128–133, 1991   10–11

Introduction.—Progressively growing intraocular tumors form when minor H incompatible P815 tumor cells are injected into the anterior chamber of eyes of BALB/c mice, which is an immunologically privileged site. However, the cells are rejected in the subconjunctival space. Fully functional T cells (Tc) emerge only at the subconjunctival site at the time the tumor graft is rejected.

Methods.—Whether precursor cytotoxic T cells (pTc) can differentiate into Tc in the anterior chamber was invested. Previous studies had shown that P815 tumor cells grew transiently in the anterior chamber after injection into the eyes of MHC-incompatible C57BL/6 mice but were eventually rejected. In the present study, the intraocular T-cell response was analyzed before, during, and after rejection of P815 tumors injected into the anterior chambers of C57BL/6 mice.

Results.—Tumor-specific pTc-infiltrated eyes containing MHC-incompatible tumors in a way similar to that seen in eyes containing minor H-incompatible tumors. Tumor-specific, directly cytotoxic Tc were present during and after rejection of major histocompatibility complex-incompatible intraocular tumor allografts. The tumor implant was rejected and the intraocular tumor cell count decreased, indicating that the immune privilege had ended at the same time that fully functional Tc were detected in the eye. The pTc that infiltrated the tumors during the phase of progressive growth appeared to differentiate into Tc.

Conclusion.—The anterior chamber of the eye appears to have an immune privilege in which terminal differentiation of pTc is suppressed. This privilege ends if pTc are converted to Tc. Emergence of delayed hypersensitivity may account for the delivery of "help" to tumor-specific pTc.

▶ This work serves to elucidate the mechanism by which an anterior chamber of the eye transplant is a privileged transplantation site. The failure of differentiation of precursor cytolytic cells to antigen-specific cytolytic cells accounts for the privileged status. Once the signals and growth factors necessary to differentiate with cytolytic cells is understood, therapy such as antibody to growth factors could be designed.—N.L. Ascher, M.D., Ph.D.

11 Immunosuppression Agents in Transplantation

▶ ↓ Cyclosporine is the immunosuppressive drug of the present. Is FK 506 the drug of the future? The in vivo effects of FK 506 continue to receive a great deal of attention, particularly from the Pittsburgh group. The initial reports regarding the effects of FK 506 in clinical transplantation have now been issued.—Terry Strom, M.D.

Kidney Transplantation Under FK 506

Starzl TE, Fung J, Jordan M, Shapiro R, Tzakis A, McCauley J, Johnston J, Iwaki Y, Jain A, Alessiani M, Todo S (Univ Health Ctr of Pittsburgh; VA Med Ctr, Pittsburgh)
JAMA 264:63–67, 1990   11–1

Introduction.—The immunosuppressive agent FK 506 has yielded encouraging results in liver transplantation trials. The drug, which is produced by the fungus *Streptomyces tsukubaensis*, has an effect on the immune system similar to that of cyclosporine. The results of a trial of FK 506 in 36 kidney recipients were evaluated.

Patients.—Most of the patients had complex clinical problems or were at high risk because of adverse medical or immunologic factors (table). Ten patients were undergoing kidney retransplantation. Ten also had liver transplantation at an earlier time or concomitantly. Two received a third organ in addition to a liver and kidney. The patients were followed for 4–13 months. All but 2 of the 36 patients were alive at last follow-up.

Results.—Eighty-one percent of the patients became dialysis free, and most had good renal function. Twenty of the 29 dialysis-free patients were receiving no or low-dose prednisone treatment. Only 1 kidney was lost because of cellular rejection. Patients who had antidonor cytotoxic antibodies in current or past serum samples, however, had a high rate of irreversible humoral rejection. There was a low incidence of posttransplant hypertension. No hirsutism or gingival hyperplasia developed. Patients who took FK 506 had unexpectedly low serum levels of cholesterol. The effect on uric acid levels was minimal. Adverse effects included nephrotoxicity, neurotoxicity, and the potential induction of a diabetic state. These side effects are similar to those associated with cyclosporine but are probably less severe.

Conclusions.—The efficacy and safety of FK 506 in this difficult group

Clinical Features of 36 Kidney Recipients

	No. of Organs	No. of Recipients
Complexity Factors		
Primary kidney transplant only	...	16
Previous kidney transplant		
Patients	...	10
Kidneys	12	...
Previous liver transplant		
Patients	...	6
Livers	9	...
Simultaneous liver transplant	...	4
Liver only	2	...
Liver–pancreas	1	...
Liver–heart	1	...
Total	...	36
Causes of Renal Failure		
Glomerulonephritis	...	8
Cyclosporine toxicity	...	7
Diabetes mellitus	...	7
Chronic renal rejection and cyclosporine toxicity	...	4
Hypertension	...	3
Polycystic disease	...	2
Hemolytic uremia syndrome	...	2
Focal glomerulosclerosis	...	1
Lupus nephritis	...	1
Sickle-cell disease	...	1
Total	...	36

Note: The median age was 40 years (range, 10–67 years). The group included 16 males and 20 females. (Courtesy of Starzl TE, Fung J, Jordan M, et al: *JAMA* 264:63–67, 1990.)

of patients were impressive. This treatment appears to be relatively free of side effects. Further trials in kidney transplant recipients are warranted.

▶ This preliminary communication is interesting but does not provide enough information to reach firm conclusions about the eventual place of FK 506 in the immunosuppressive firmament. In vitro studies indicate that FK 506 produces immunosuppression through a mechanism that appears startlingly similar to cyclosporine's effects. Both drugs block transcription of an identical select subset of T-cell activation genes (including the interleukin-2 gene) that are induced through the calcium-dependent signaling pathway that is stimulated on activation of the T-cell receptor for antigen. Both cyclosporine and FK 506 bind to and inhibit enzymes that are involved in folding proteins (isomerase) at proline residues. However, the isomerases targeted by FK 506 and cyclosporine are not identical, and recent evidence suggests that inhibition of isomerases is not the mechanism by which these drugs block T-cell activation.

This article provides results of a pilot study and is not a comprehensive, randomized, prospective study. The pilot study indicates that FK 506 is a promising agent, but FK 506 does not appear to be a panacea. Immunologic graft failure did occur; the list of side effects closely matches the problems associated with cyclosporine. Perhaps FK 506 has less potential for causing hypertension. The results of this pilot study certainly justify continuing interest in FK 506. To date, the rate of 1-year kidney transplant engraftment at Pittsburgh using FK

506 therapy is not superior to the results obtained with cyclosporine. Indeed, the rate of engraftment obtained with cyclosporine is slightly superior to the results obtained with FK 506 treatment. This may reflect the vast experience with cyclosporine and the meager experience accrued to date with FK 506. A controlled, comparative analysis of FK 506 and cyclosporine is eagerly awaited.—T. Strom, M.D.

Effect of FK506 Treatment on Allocytolytic T Lymphocyte Induction In Vivo: Differential Effects of FK506 on L3T4$^+$ and Ly2$^+$ T Cells

Maruyama M, Suzuki H, Yamashita N, Yano S (Toyama Medical and Pharmaceutical University, Toyama, Japan)
Transplantation 50:272–277, 1990   11–2

Background.—The antibiotic FK 506 has been widely researched as a potent suppressor of organ allograft rejection in animals. However, little is known about its effect on T-cell responses to allografts in vivo.

Methods and Results.—The effect of FK 506 on the induction of allocytolytic T lymphocyte was studied using mice primed with alloantigens and treated with FK 506. In a dose-dependent fashion, FK 506 suppressed the cytotoxic T lymphocyte (CTL) induction of spleen cells and peritoneal exudate cells (PEC). Time-course kinetic studies showed that CTL activity depended greatly on the time of administration of FK 506 to the mice. Lymphocytes from the FK 506-treated animals were reactivated on exposure to the same alloantigens in a secondary mixed lymphocyte culture (MLC). The FK 506 also had a differential effect on the activation of helper (L3T4$^+$) and cytotoxic (Ly2$^+$) T cell subpopulations. The L3T4$^+$ T cells from the mice primed with alloantigens and treated with FK 506 had normal helper activity in CTL generation in MLC. However, Ly2$^+$ T cells from those mice had profoundly suppressed CTL activity on reexposure to the same alloantigens in a secondary MLC. Exogenous IL-2 or L3T4$^+$ T cells were able to overcome the immunosuppressive effect of FK 506 on CTL induction of Ly2$^+$ T cells in a secondary MLC. That FK 506 effect was apparently antigen-nonspecific, because Ly2$^+$ T cells from alloprimed FK 506-treated mice did not induce CTL against the third-party alloantigens or the same alloantigens in a secondary MLC.

Conclusions.—The findings raise major questions about the mechanism of action of FK 506 in vivo. Its mechanism in vivo may be unrelated to its mechanism in vitro. Metabolites of FK 506 formed in vivo may have immunosuppressive effects unrelated to the ability of the native drug to inhibit in vitro.

▶ There is no doubt that FK 506 is a potent immunosuppressive that shares many properties with CsA. This in vivo analysis shows that FK 506 powerfully induces broad immunosuppression that is not confined to a dampening of anti-donor responses. The immunosuppressive effects appear to be targeted primarily against helper T-cell effects. Because FK 506 and CsA block expression

of multiple "helper cell released" lymphokines, these results might be anticipated. Indeed, exogenous IL-2 can resurrect some CTL activity.—T. Strom,
M.D.

Kidney Transplantation Under FK 506 Immunosuppression
Shapiro R, Jordan M, Fung J, McCauley J, Johnston J, Iwaki Y, Tzakis A,
Hakala T, Todo S, Starzl TE (Univ Health Ctr of Pittsburgh; VA Med Center,
Pittsburgh)
Transplant Proc 23:920–923, 1991   11–3

Background.—Experience with FK 506 in 36 patients undergoing renal transplantation was previously reported. The outcomes in 26 patients
from that experience who were pure kidney recipients, plus 19 additional
patients treated more recently, were assessed after 2.5 to 11 months.
   Methods.—The 65 patients received 66 grafts, all but 2 cadaveric. All
were given FK 506 and corticosteroids. The initial FK 506 dose—.075 or
.15 mg/kg—was usually begun intravenously 2 hours after transplantation and given for 2 to 4 hours. Further intravenous doses of .075 mg/kg
were delivered every 12 hours until the patient could tolerate FK 506
orally. The oral dose was begun at .15 mg/kg twice a day.
   Outcomes.—Sixty-two percent of the kidneys functioned immediately,
whereas 38% had some form of delayed graft function. Eighty percent of
the patients are free of dialysis. The most frequent cause of graft loss was
rejection. The infectious profile was similar to that associated with past
immunosuppressive regimens. However, there was no lethal systemic sepsis, possibly because of the limited use of steroids.
   Conclusions.—Kidney transplantation trials have added to the impression that FK 506 is a safe drug to the extent that any powerful immunosuppressant is safe. In this series, mortality was only 1.5%. The freedom
from historical posttransplant morbidity was impressive, resulting mainly
from the ability to minimize or stop steroid treatment within the first 2
months in 75% of the cases.

▶ In this update of an ongoing study of FK 506 immunosuppression, 65 FK
506-treated patients receiving a total of 66 transplants were analyzed. This uncontrolled study shows good, but not extraordinary, graft survival (see Table 3
in the original article). The benefits and side effects of FK 506 therapy appear
comparable to cyclosporine. Randomized controlled trials will be required to
precisely evaluate the relative merits of these 2 agents. Of course, the clinical
experience with FK 506 is meager in comparison to that with CsA. As a consequence, it may be difficult to fully appreciate the full merits or problems associated with FK 506 treatment until a greater clinical experience accrues. Remember that the rate of engraftment of CsA-treated patients steadily increased
for several years after introduction of the drug. The "learning curve" for FK 506
administration may well follow a similar several year long path.—T. Strom,
M.D.

▶ ↓ For the present, cyclosporine-based immunosuppression regimens remain the linchpin of immunosuppressive therapy. These regimens have been in place for a long time, and it is not surprising that many groups are now taking a careful look at the individual components of these multidrug regimens. These attempts to improve cyclosporine-based immunosuppressive regimens also include efforts to more accurately profile drug levels or pharmacologically offset the nephrotoxic properties of cyclosporine with use of dietary fish oil or the administration of inhibition of thromboxane synthesis. In addition, the relationship of cyclosporine administration to various other clinical problems in the transplant recipient continues to receive attention.—T. Strom, M.D.

A Randomized Trial Comparing Double-Drug and Triple-Drug Therapy in Primary Cadaveric Renal Transplants

Brinker KR, Dickerman RM, Gonwa TA, Hull AR, Langley JW, Long DL, Nesser DA, Trevino G, Velez RL, Vergne-Marini PJ (Methodist Med Ctr, Dallas)
Transplantation 50:43–49, 1990   11–4

Introduction.—A prospective, randomized, controlled trial was carried out to compare the effects of a double-drug immunosuppression regimen with that of a triple-drug regimen in primary cadaveric renal transplantation.

Methods.—Of 209 patients undergoing renal transplantation, 99 were treated with the double-drug regimen consisting of cyclosporine and prednisone, and 110 received the triple-drug regimen, consisting of cyclosporine at a lower initial dose, azathioprine, and prednisone.

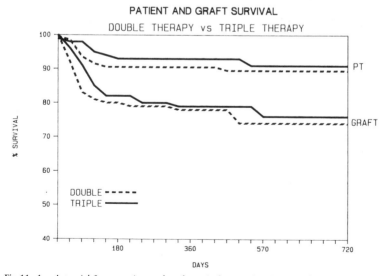

Fig 11–1.—Actuarial 2-year patient and graft survival curves in primary cadaver kidney recipients assigned to double or triple therapy. (Courtesy of Brinker KR, Dickerman RM, Gonwa TA, et al: *Transplantation* 50:43–49, 1990.)

Results.—Actuarial 2-year graft survival and 2-year patient survival were similar in both groups (Fig 11–1). There were no differences between the 2 groups in iothalamate clearance at any time. The duration of the initial hospitalization, the frequency of rehospitalization, and the rejection frequency were also similar. Triple-therapy patients had a higher frequency of hypertension in the first 6 months posttransplantation.

Conclusion.—Double-drug therapy and triple-drug therapy for primary cadaveric renal transplantation are equally effective.

▶ I am a devout prescriber of triple therapy. Inherently, it makes good sense to use a combination of agents that block T-cell alloactivation at various steps of the process that leads to rejection. The use of multiple agents to interrupt a given process is a successful and time-honored tactic in pharmacology. Triple therapy offers other theoretic advantages. I like the luxury of the reduced CsA dosages that are used in triple therapy for these ATN-prone patients in the early posttransplant period. I also like the flexibility of drug dosing that is provided in the 3 drug program to avoid toxicity. If a given drug causes a problem, the other 2 agents can be used in full doses. These are the theoretic advantages for triple therapy. Nonetheless, Brinker et al. have conducted a study that indicates equivalence for double and triple therapy, as indicated through analysis of a variety of indices in primary cadaveric donor kidney allograft recipients. While longer term studies are underway, it is apparent that triple therapy does not provide a major advantage over double therapy in primary cadaver donor recipients. On the other hand, this study by no means excludes the possibility that in the more troublesome situation of retransplantation triple therapy is most useful.—T. Strom, M.D.

Effects of Steroid Withdrawal on Posttransplant Diabetes Mellitus in Cyclosporine-Treated Renal Transplant Recipients
Hricik DE, Bartucci MR, Moir EJ, Mayes JT, Schulak JA (Univ Hosps of Cleveland; Case Western Reserve Univ, Cleveland)
Transplantation 51:374–377, 1991   11–5

Background.—Posttransplant diabetes mellitus (PTDM) has traditionally been attributed to steroid treatment. However, cyclosporine may also be diabetogenic. The effects of steroid withdrawal on PTDM in renal transplant recipients treated with cyclosporine (CsA) were studied.

Methods.—The records of all patients without diabetes receiving kidney transplants from January 1987 to July 1989 were reviewed retrospectively. Posttransplant diabetes mellitus was defined as hyperglycemia requiring treatment with oral hypoglycemic agents or insulin.

Findings.—Posttransplant diabetes mellitus developed in 9 of 70 patients receiving prednisone, azathioprine, and CsA and in 8 of 83 receiving azathioprine and prednisone alone at an earlier time, for incidences of 12.9% and 9.6%, respectively. The difference between these groups was not significant. Among those receiving triple-drug therapy, complete prednisone withdrawal was tried in 7 renal transplant recipients with

PTDM and 1 recipient of a combined kidney-pancreas transplant who showed signs of type II diabetes mellitus. Seven of the patients were able to stop taking insulin or oral hypoglycemic agents within 4 months of discontinuing the steroids. Mean glycohemoglobin levels dropped from 10.6% before steroid withdrawal to 6% within a month of stopping steroids. Mean CsA dose and trough CsA blood levels remained the same. Mild rejection episodes in 2 patients prompted a return to steroid treatment.

Conclusions.—The possibility that CsA is diabetogenic has not been excluded. However, withdrawing steroid treatment is a safe, effective way to manage PTDM in patients subsequently given maintenance therapy of CsA and azathioprine.

▶ This is a useful study. Posttransplant diabetes mellitus is not uncommon. In the past, 2 components of the standard triple-therapy regimen have been implicated. Corticosteroids have long been known to cause insulin-resistant diabetes. Cyclosporine has a clearly diabetogenic effect in several species, and it impairs insulin release by cultured human islet cells. Reports indicating that CsA withdrawal can alleviate posttransplant diabetes in humans have also been published. This study implicates corticosteroids as the major culprit in this syndrome. It would be interesting to randomize posttransplant diabetic subjects into control, steroid withdrawal, and CsA withdrawal arms, but I bet that corticosteroid withdrawal will prove to be the "way to go."—T. Strom, M.D.

A Prospective Randomized Trial of Prednisone Versus No Prednisone Maintenance Therapy in Cyclosporine-Treated and Azathioprine-Treated Renal Transplant Patients
Schulak JA, Mayes JT, Moritz CE, Hricik DE (Univ Hosps of Cleveland; Case Western Reserve Univ, Cleveland)
Transplantation 49:327–332, 1990   11–6

Background.—Cyclosporine is the single most important agent for maintaining immunosuppression after renal transplantation. In an attempt to reduce the toxicity of this agent, low doses have been used with steroids and azathioprine. Although this 3-drug regimen is effective, the problem of steroid-associated morbidity persists. The use of cyclosporine and azathioprine without steroids in the early posttransplantation period has not been widely studied. The early withdrawal of prednisone from renal transplant recipients treated with cyclosporine and azathioprine was attempted.

Methods.—The series included 8 recipients of living-related donor kidneys and 59 recipients of cadaver donor kidneys. The patients were randomized prospectively to receive or not receive prednisone in addition to antilymphocyte globulin, cyclosporine, and azathioprine. Rejection episodes were treated initially with methylprednisolone pulses, and the OKT3 monoclonal antibody was used to treat biopsy-verified steroid-resistant rejection.

Findings.—Patient survival and graft survival for those receiving living-related donor kidneys were 100% in both treatment groups at 12 months. These rates in cadaver kidney recipients at 1 year were 94% and 83%, respectively, in those given prednisone. For those not given prednisone, the rates were 88% and 77%, respectively. Rejection episodes occurred more often and earlier in patients not given maintenance steroids. The severity of rejection was also greater in the group not given prednisone. The incidence of serious infection in both groups was similar. The protocol failed in 40% of living-related donor kidney recipients and in 59% of cadaver kidney recipients.

Conclusions.—Initiating maintenance treatment without prednisone in renal transplantation patients is safe, but it is associated with a higher risk of rejection developing. Because of the greater incidence and severity of early rejection episodes in patients not given prednisone in this series, the use of this immunosuppressive strategy in renal transplantation is not recommended.

▶ If this article and the preceding article (Abstract 11–4) are to be taken at face value, all double-drug protocols are not created equal. Corticosteroids appear to remain useful in our armentarium despite the litany of side effects caused by this class of drugs.—T. Strom, M.D.

A Randomized Prospective Trial Comparing Cyclosporine Monotherapy With Triple-Drug Therapy in Renal Transplantation
Tarantino A, Aroldi A, Stucchi L, Montagnino G, Mascaretti L, Vegeto A, Ponticelli C (Maggiore Hospital, Milan, Italy)
Transplantation 52:53–57, 1991   11–7

Background.—Cyclosporine immunosuppression has improved the results of renal allotransplantation, but the best treatment regimen remains uncertain. Some have suggested that cyclosporine be used without steroid to avoid steroid toxicity, but cyclosporine itself can produce dose-dependent nephrotoxicity that can limit graft function.

Study Design.—Seventy-four new renal transplant recipients aged 14–60 years were randomized to receive cyclosporine monotherapy, intravenously and then orally in a maintenance dose of about 5 mg/kg daily. The goal was a trough blood level of 200–600 ng/mL. Another 77 patients received cyclosporine in a final maintenance dose of 3 mg/kg daily along with azathioprine and steroid. The maintenance dose of methylprednisolone was 8 mg daily.

Results.—Patient survival at 2 years exceeded 95% in both groups. The 2-year graft survival rate was 84% on cyclosporine monotherapy and 90% on triple therapy, not a significant difference. Acute renal failure was more frequent in the monotherapy group and was irreversible only in these patients. Rejection was comparably frequent in the 2 treatment groups. Early cyclosporine-related nephrotoxicity was more frequent with monotherapy. Infectious episodes were equally frequent in the 2 groups, and renal function was similar at most intervals.

Conclusions.—Both these regimens can be effective. Cyclosporine monotherapy may be recommended for those who are at particular risk of steroid toxicity, but many patients will not tolerate treatment without steroids. Combined treatment provides good graft survival over the long term without increasing the risk of complications.

Therapeutic Cyclosporine Monitoring: Comparison of Radioimmunoassay and High-Performance Liquid Chromatography Methods in Organ Transplant Recipients

Hirvisalo E-L, Kivistö KT, Neuvonen PJ (University of Helsinki; University of Turku, Finland)

Ther Drug Monit 12:353–358, 1990   11–8

Background.—Recently many laboratories monitoring cyclosporine (CsA) have started using more specific analytical techniques. The relative contribution of parent CsA to the total amount of drug and metabolites in blood varies markedly among patients and sometimes within the same patient. Results obtained with different methods have therefore produced some confusion in the interpretation of CsA levels in different groups of organ transplant recipients. Results of 3 different methods for therapeutic monitoring of blood CsA levels were compared.

Methods.—A specific (SRIA) and nonspecific (RIA) radioimmunoassay method and a high-performance liquid chromatography (HPLC) method were used in 212 blood samples from heart, liver, kidney, and bone marrow transplant recipients. The ratios of whole-blood CsA concentrations were recorded.

Results.—With the nonspecific antibody, mean RIA/HPLC ratios in different patient groups ranged from 2.3 to 5.5. The variability in this ratio was large in all groups. With the specific antibody, mean SRIA/HPLC ratios in different groups ranged from 1.1 to 1.5. Variability was smaller with this method.

Conclusions.—Radioimmunoassay using a specific monoclonal antibody is well suited for therapeutically monitoring blood CsA levels. However, even with this method CsA levels can be overestimated in some cases.

▶ The precision of HPLC to individually identify native cyclosporine and its multiple metabolites is not challenged by RIA methods. As expected, a polyclonal-based analysis is far less exacting than a monoclonal antibody-based system. Nonetheless, the monoclonal antibody was not specific for native cyclosporine because substantial overestimates of cyclosporine levels were routinely encountered with this method. The imprecision of these assay kits must aid to the vagaries of CsA monitoring.—T. Strom, M.D.

Improved Survival of Heterotopic Cardiac Allografts in Rats With Dietary n-3 Polyunsaturated Fatty Acids

Otto DA, Kahn DR, Hamm MW, Forrest DE, Wooten JT (Baptist Med Ctrs Princeton, Birmingham, Ala; Rutgers Univ, New Brunswick, NJ)
Transplantation 50:193–198, 1990   11–9

Background.—Acute rejection is still a major problem in cardiac transplantation. The effect of dietary n-3 polyunsaturated fatty acids on acute rejection was investigated in a heterotopic cardiac transplant model.

Methods.—The model was designed with male Fischer 344 rats as donors and Long Evans rats as recipients. Donor and recipient rats were fed purified diets high in n-3 polyunsaturated fatty acids from concentrated n-3 ethyl esters (EE) or fish oil or n-6 polyunsaturated fatty acids from corn oil for 2 to 3 weeks or 3 to 4 weeks before transplantation. Recipients continued their diets until rejection occurred.

Results.—Compared with the group fed the corn oil diet, recipient rats fed EE had an allograft survival significantly increased by 45%, regardless of the donors' diet. When only donor rats were fed the EE diet 2 to 3 weeks before transplant, there was a slight but significant increase in allograft survival. With the fish oil diet, only the group in which fish oil was fed to both recipient and donor 2 to 3 weeks before transplantation had a significant increase in allograft survival compared with the corn oil diet group. When fish oil diets were fed for 3 to 4 weeks before transplantation, survival was increased in groups in which fish oil was fed to either the donor or recipient alone. In this case, allograft survival with fish oil feeding to both recipient and donor did not differ from recipient feeding alone. Allograft survival was significantly and directly correlated with the donor heart phospholipid n-3/n-6 fatty acid ratio and n-3 fatty acid content at rejection. Its relationship with the n-6 fatty acid content was indirect. No detectable 20:3 (n-9) was found in the cardiac phospholipids, which indicated the absence of essential fatty acid deficiency.

Conclusions.—The strongest determinant of the fatty acid composition of the transplanted donor heart was recipient diet. Providing dietary n-3 polyunsaturated fatty acids before and after cardiac transplant to recipient animals significantly protects against acute rejection.

▶ Fish oil possesses at least modest immunosuppressive properties. It is useful in treatment of murine lupus and humans with rheumatoid arthritis. We have previously shown additive-synergistic effects with CsA in a mouse allograft model. Fish oil itself did not have a big effect. In this study, fish oil administration as a monotherapy improves survival of rat heart allografts; however, pretreatment was required.—T. Strom, M.D.

The Effects of Dietary Supplementation With Fish Oil on Renal Function in Cyclosporine-Treated Renal Transplant Recipients

Homan van der Heide JJ, Bilo HJG, Tegzess AM, Donker AJM (University Hospital Groningen, The Netherlands; Free University Hospital, Amsterdam)
Transplantation 49:523–527, 1990   11–10

Introduction.—Cyclosporine has become indispensible in transplantation medicine. However, it has been associated with considerable side effects such as nephrotoxicity. A study recently demonstrated that fish oil reduces CsA-induced renal dysfunction in rats. The effect of daily fish oil supplementation on renal function and blood pressure in CsA-treated renal transplant recipients was explored in a prospective, randomized, double-blind study.

Methods.—Stable CsA-treated transplant recipients were studied at least 9 months after grafting. Eleven patients were given fish oil, 6 g, and 10 were given placebo. Glomerular filtration rate and effective renal plasma flow (ERPF) were measured before and after 3 months of oil ingestion.

Findings.—There were no changes in the placebo group. In the fish oil-treated group, glomerular filtration rate increased by 20.3% and ERPF by 16.4%. Mean arterial pressure and calculated total renal vascular resistance (TRVR) did not change in the placebo group but fell by 8.6% and 21.1%, respectively, in the fish oil group.

Conclusions.—Renal dysfunction in CsA-treated renal transplant recipients can at least partly be reversed for about 1 year with dietary fish oil supplementation. The increases in glomerular filtration rate, ERPF, and creatinine clearance were remarkable in patients receiving fish oil supplementation.

► Several preclinical studies have demonstrated that fish oil administration produces modest immunosuppressive effects, as deduced by the effects of therapy in transplant and autoimmune preclinical models. Patients with cyclosporine acute nephrotoxicity excrete large amounts of thromboxane, a potent vasoconstrictor. It is likely, but not certain, that this abnormality is directly linked to the causation of drug toxicity. Certainly, early reversible cyclosporine toxicity is characterized by diminished renal ischemia. The nature of alterations in eicosanoid metabolism in hosts that receive fish oil, (i.e., elaboration of inactive forms of thromboxane but active forms of prostaglandin E and prostaglandin I) suggested that cyclosporine nephrotoxicity might also be obviated by fish oil. Indeed, in rodents, fish oil administration attenuates CsA-induced nephrotoxicity but enhances CsA-induced immunosuppression. Are these salubrious effects sustained in humans? This study suggests that administration of fish oils may produce a needed respite from cyclosporine nephrotoxicity. because drug-induced nephrotoxicity has prevented widespread application of this drug in autoimmune disease, despite a favorable effect on the autoimmune process, this study may provide insight about how to circumvent nephrotoxicity for many patients.—T. Strom, M.D.

Modulation of Experimental Cyclosporine Nephrotoxicity by Inhibition of Thromboxane Synthesis
Petric R, Freeman D, Wallace C, McDonald J, Stiller C, Keown P (University Hospital, London, Ontario, Canada)
Transplantation 50:558–563, 1990 11–11

Background.—The intrinsic nephrotoxicity of cyclosporine (CsA) constrains its clinical usefulness. One possible mechanism of CsA-mediated renal injury could involve changes in the prostaglandin-thromboxane cascade. The effects of nonselective and selective inhibition of thromboxane-mediated vasoconstrictor limb on the nephrotoxicity of CsA and the production of these mediators were studied.

Methods.—The prostaglandin-thromboxane system in normal and nephrotoxic Sprague Dawley rats was manipulated by means of the specific thromboxane synthetase inhibitor U63,557A and the cyclooxygenase inhibitor indomethacin. Nephrotoxicity was induced by giving CsA, 50 mg/kg/day for 7 days, whereas control rats received vehicle alone.

Results.—The nephrotoxic rats had a 99% increase in urinary thromboxane B_2 excretion compared with the control rats. The nephrotoxic animals also had a 48% decrease in creatinine clearance and a 25% reduction in fractional excretion of sodium (FeNa). On histologic examination, the rats were found to have cortical tubular vacuolization and necrosis. Prostanoid excretion was significantly reduced in both normal and nephrotoxic rats by indomethacin, 8 mg/kg/day. This treatment did not worsen glomerular function, but there was an exaggerated decrease in renal function when indomethacin was given with CsA. These animals had a further 27% reduction in creatinine clearance and a 76% decrease in FeNa, along with increased histologic injury. Animals that received U63,557A with CsA had no increase in urinary thromboxane excretion, a 20% improvement in creatinine clearance, and restoration of FeNa. They also had diminished vacuolization.

Conclusions.—The clinical nephrotoxic effects of CsA might be curbed by selective inhibition of thromboxane production. The nephrotoxicity appears to result from linked but separate mechanisms, including renal prostanoids. Caution is needed when combining prostaglandin inhibitors and CsA.

▶ Activation of membrane fatty acids can result in synthesis of vasodilating, antithrombolic prostaglandin E and prostaglandin I prostanoid molecules as well as vasoconstrictor, prothrombotic thromboxanes. It is of considerable interest that cyclooxygenase inhibitors (indomethacin) that block prostaglandin E and thromboxane synthesis in a balanced manner do not protect from CsA toxicity, while selective blockade of thromboxane synthesis is indeed protective. These data support my personal bias that CsA toxicity is an ischemic lesion.

It is interesting to recall that administration of fish oils also block CsA toxicity. Fish oils cause synthesis of biologically inactive trienoic thromboxane but biologically active prostaglandin E/prostaglandin I. Fish oil is also a modest immunosuppressive. Hence, we are currently testing the hypothesis that the balance of vasodilating and vasoconstricting eicosanoids is of great importance in CsA nephrotoxicity by administrating fish oil to human renal allograft recipients. We believe that fish oil also blocks CsA toxicity by preventing ischemic injury.—T. Strom, M.D.

Arteriolosclerosis of the Human Renal Allograft: Morphology, Origin, Life History, and Relationship to Cyclosporine Therapy

Rossmann P, Jirka J, Chadimová M, Reneltová I, Saudek F (Czechoslovak Academy of Sciences; Institute of Clinical and Experimental Medicine, Prague)

Virchows Archiv Pathol Anat 418[A]:129–141, 1991   11–12

Objective.—Vascular rejection is the chief cause of renal allograft failure in both its early (obliterative arterio-arteriolopathy) and late (rejection endarteritis) forms. There were 658 biopsies from 568 cadaveric renal allografts reviewed for the occurrence of vascular pathology. Immunosuppression was based on azathioprine or, after 1982, on cyclosporine.

Observations.—In 118 grafts the afferent vessels exhibited nonproliferative changes that included fibrinoid and hyaline masses of varying extent, transmural "knobs," intimal edema with metachromasia, and microthrombosis. The prevalence and extent of these changes increased in the later years of the review period when cyclosporine immunosuppression was used. Grafts from patients given cyclosporine exhibited early edema and hypergranulation of endothelial cells on ultrastructural study. Microfibrils in smooth muscle cells were disrupted. The changes were progressive only in cyclosporine-treated patients. Endarteritis predominated in nephrectomy specimens. Graft survival rates were not significantly dependent on the presence or degree of vasculopathy.

Conclusions.—Even apparently optimal cyclosporine therapy can produce a nonproliferative vasculopathy, which, however, does not seem to markedly influence the posttransplantation course. It is possible that longer posttransplantation follow-up will alter this conclusion.

▶ Early immunologic graft failure is usually associated with an insidious progressive vascular lesion that is called rejection end arteritis by these authors. By any name, the lesion is distinct from the obliterative lesion that the authors claim is more common in cyclosporine-treated hosts than in patients not given CsA. This lesion is characterized by transmural "insudative" lesions. These authors maintain that many biopsies reveal this lesion; however, progressive disease is seen in CsA-treated hosts, but not in azathioprine-treated hosts. This comparison is based on analysis of biopsies of patients who underwent transplantation before 1983 or after CsA became available. Hence, this is a retrospective study. The original CsA protocol (1983) used high cyclosporine doses. Because high cyclosporine can clearly cause a hemolytic uremic syndrome-like vascular lesion, the importance of this more subtle lesion arising in CsA-treated patients requires examination. Data from the large transplant registries in Heidelberg, Germany, and Los Angeles show that CsA treatment results in an increase of early graft survival, but the tempo of insidious chronic graft loss is identical in the CsA and azathioprine eras. If CsA causes a nasty chronic vasculopathy, this form of renal disease is not evident in these large data bases.—T. Strom, M.D.

Renal Handling of Urate and the Incidence of Gouty Arthritis During Cyclosporine and Diuretic Use

Noordzij TC, Leunissen KML, Van Hooff JP (University Hospital, Maastricht, The Netherlands)
Transplantation 52:64–67, 1991   11–13

Introduction.—Hyperuricemia is found in renal transplant recipients given cyclosporine for immunosuppression. The occurrence of gout was studied in a group of 85 patients having a functioning cadaver graft for at least 2 years. Fifty-five patients were maintained on cyclosporine, and 23 used azathioprine as baseline immunosuppression. Seven others changed from cyclosporine to azathioprine because of toxicity caused by cyclosporine.

Dosages.—Cyclosporine was given intravenously and then orally in a dose needed to produce trough blood levels of 0.1–0.15 mg/L. Prednisolone was given in a final dose of 5 mg daily but was withdrawn in patients having a first graft. Azathioprine was used in a dose of 2–3 mg/kg daily along with 10 mg of prednisolone daily.

Observations.—One fourth of the patients on cyclosporine developed gouty arthritis within 2 years after transplantation. These patients had higher serum urate levels than those without gout but not lower glomerular filtration rates. Apart from the serum urate, gouty arthritis correlated with the creatinine clearance, fractional urate clearance, and furosemide use. Urate clearance remained abnormal after conversion to azathioprine.

Conclusions.—Urate handling is impaired in renal transplant recipients given cyclosporine. Those also given furosemide are at particular risk of developing gouty arthritis.

▶ What? One quarter of CsA-treated transplant recipients develop gout. It is interesting to me that I have rarely diagnosed acute gout in transplant recipients. Meticulous methods of diagnosis were used in this analysis, and the authors claim that 25% of CsA-treated recipients, especially those on furosemide, experienced acute gout. I'm most surprised, but I'll take a more careful look at my patients. The cause of these episodes apparently relates to impaired renal tubular handling of urate. Are Dutch patients more gout prone than Bostonians or do the Dutch patients just have better diagnosticians than I as their physicians? I'll bet the answer turns out to be a bit of both—a higher incidence and alert physicians!—T. Strom, M.D.

12 Mechanisms of Action of Immunosuppressive Drugs

▶ ↓ A detailed analysis of the immunosuppressive effects of cyclosporine, FK 506, 15-deoxyspergualin, rapamycin, and RS-61443 have proven both exciting and highly informative. An analysis of the mechanism by which these agents block T-cell activation has given insight into the molecular means of T-cell activation. It is now clear that FK 506 and cyclosporine have identical calcium dependent pathways in the activated T-cell. Rapamycin, in spite of some superficial similarities to FK506, blocks an entirely different pathway from that blocked by cyclosporine and FK 506. Genistein 15-deoxyspergualin, and RS-61443 each block unique components of the T-cell activation pathway. New techniques have also enabled us to reexamine drugs that have been the mainstay of immunosuppression.—Terry Strom, M.D.

Evidence That the Immunosuppressive Effects of FK506 and Cyclosporine Are Identical

Johansson A, Möller E (Huddinge Hospital, Karolinska Institute, Huddinge, Sweden)
Transplantation 50:1001–1007, 1990   12–1

Background.—The immunosuppressive agent FK 506, classified as a fungal metabolite, can inhibit the production of interleukin-2-receptor (Il-2R) in vitro. In mice, FK 506 suppresses the humoral response to foreign erythrocytes. The agent FK 506 has many similarities with cyclosporine A (CsA), another immunosuppressive fungal metabolite.

Study Design.—The in vitro immunosuppressive properties of FK 506 alone and when combined with CsA were analyzed. Studies with CsA and FK 506 were performed in cell cultures of human lymphocytes (PBLs) and monocytes. Human lymphocytes without monocytes were combined with allogeneic irradiated PBLs and subjected to mitogens. The Il-2 activity on this in vitro system was also assessed.

Findings.—The mean FK 506 and CsA concentrations that achieved 50% inhibition of the mixed lymphocyte reaction induced proliferation were .38 ng/mL and 44 ng/mL, respectively. The 2 drugs stopped the cell-mediated lympholysis response when present from the experiment's beginning, but did not inhibit the response when either drug was added to the effector phase of the procedure. The FK 506 activity occurred at 1-100th the concentration of CsA required for the same blocking action. Neither drug affected the $CD3^+$ cells, and both CsA and FK 506 affected the Il-2R-alpha expression on the Con A lymphoblasts only a minor amount. Both drugs block transcription of several T-cell activation genes. Various amounts of FK 506 and CsA were combined to assess any possible additive or synergistic effect; the inhibition obtained by .1 ng/mL FK 506 and 10 ng/mL CsA was similar to the suppression achieved by doubling the CsA concentration.

Implications.—The effects of FK 506 and CsA are similar, producing an inhibition response from human PBLs to various mitogenic and alloantigenic stimulants. Thus, both fungal agents may share the same mechanism of action in vivo.

▶ Well, let's say the activities of the 2 drugs are similar, but they are not identical. Both drugs do, however, block transcription of a strikingly similar series of T-cell activation genes. These pretranscriptional events are Ca^{2+} dependent. The drug FK 506 and CsA are not structurally related—CsA is a peptide, and FK 506 is a macrolide. Both drugs bind to and inactivate peptidyl-prolyl isomerase (see Abstract 12–2) in low concentrations. The target peptidyl-prolyl isomerases, however, are not identical.

One clear functional distinction is the noted ability of FK 506—not CsA—to block rapamycin-mediated suppression (2). The irony here is that both rapamycin and FK 506 bind to and inactivate the same peptidyl-prolyl isomerase. Hence, inactivation of the peptidyl-prolyl isomerase is not the mechanism of FK 506-mediated immunosuppression. As previously noted (1) CsA's mechanism of action is not mediated by its ability to inactivate the peptidyl-prolyl isomerase cyclophillin.—T. Strom, M.D.

Reference

1. Wicker LS, et al: *Eur J Immul* 20:2277–2283, 1990.

Is Cyclophilin Involved in the Immunosuppressive and Nephrotoxic Mechanism of Action of Cyclosporin A?
Sigal NH, Dumont F, Durette P, Siekierka JJ, Peterson L, Rich DH, Dunlap BE, Staruch MJ, Melino MR, Koprak SL, Williams D, Witzel B, Pisano JM (Merck, Sharp, and Dohme Research Labs, Rahway, NJ; Univ of Wisconsin-Madison)
J Exp Med 173:619–628, 1991   12–2

Introduction.—Some questions remain about the mechanism of action of cyclosporin A (CsA). It is not known whether the major cytosolic protein for CsA, cyclophilin, is directly involved in mediating the immunosuppressive activity of the drug, particularly whether inhibition of this protein's peptidyl-prolyl *cis-trans* isomerase (PPIase) activity inhibits murine T-cell activation. Also, it is not known whether the nephrotoxicity associated with CsA is related to the inhibition of PPIase-dependent pathways in cells other than lymphocytes.

	Summary of the Correlation Between Cyclophilin Binding and Immunosuppressive Activity		
Class	Cyclophilin binding	Immunosuppression	No. of compounds
I	+	+	37
II	−	−	10
III	−	+	1
IV	+	−	13

*Analogues are designated as showing agreement between the 2 assays (class I or II) if they show less than a fivefold difference between cyclophilin binding and immunosuppression.

(Courtesy of Sigal NH, Dumont F, Durette P, et al: *J Exp Med* 173:619–628, 1991.)

Observations.—A series of 61 cyclosporin analogues was used. Generally, there was a good correlation between cyclophilin binding and immunosuppressive activity for most analogues analyzed. There were a number of compounds of distinct structural classes that could interact with cyclophilin but that were much less immunosuppressive than expected. The inability of these analogues to inhibit lymphocyte activation could not be explained by their failure to enter the cell and bind to cyclophilin under the conditions used in the cellular assays. A nonimmunosuppressive analogue, MeAla-6, bound well to cyclophilin and was active as a PPIase inhibitor, but did not induce renal pathology in vivo. In addition, another analogue, MeBm$_2$t, was immunosuppressive in vitro but had little or no activity as a PPIase inhibitor (table).

Conclusion.—These observations raise serious questions about a direct role of cyclosporin in mediating immunosuppressive and nephrotoxic activities of CsA. They also cast doubt on whether PPIase has a direct function in lymphocyte signal transduction.

▶ A tidy story crashes! Like cyclophilin, PPI'ases are enzymes that fold proteins at proline residues. Proline residues are of extreme architectural importance in 3-D protein structure. Because CsA (and FK 506) bind to and inactivate PPI'ases, it seemed reasonable that inactivation of PPI'ases would be the mechanism by which these immunosuppressive agents block T-cell activation. This thorough analysis of the properties of CsA structural analogues reveals that most, but not all, PPI'ase inhibitors are immunosuppressive. Yet some CsA analogues that fail to block PPI'ases are potent immunosuppressives. So much for theory! PPI'ases are not the target molecules for CsA's immunosuppressive action. It seems likely that CsA targets a close structural analogue of PPI'ase, but not PPI'ase itself. It all seemed so reasonable. Unfortunately, this analysis also reveals that immunosuppressive and nephrotoxic activities are closely linked. It may be difficult to construct a non-nephrotoxic, immunosuppressive CsA analogue.—T. Strom, M.D.

Complementary DNA Encoding the Human T-Cell FK506-Binding Protein, a Peptidylprolyl *cis-trans* Isomerase Distinct From Cyclophilin

Maki N, Sekiguchi F, Nishimaki J, Miwa K, Hayano T, Takahashi N, Suzuki M (Tonen K K, Saitama, Japan)

Proc Natl Acad Sci USA 87:5440–5443, 1990

12–3

Background.—The drug FK 506 is a newly detected macrolide with potent immunosuppressive activity at concentrations 100 times lower than cyclosporin A. The cyclosporin A binding protein cyclophilin is identical to peptidyl-prolyl *cis-trans* isomerase. The cellular binding protein for FK 506 is distinct from cyclophilin but has the same enzymatic activity. Little is known about the structure of this FK 506 binding protein (FKBP). A cDNA coding for FKBP was isolated and its nucleotide sequence was examined.

Findings.—Coding was isolated from human peripheral blood T cells using mixed 20-mer oligonucleotide probes synthesized according to the sequence Glu-Asp-Gly-Lys-Lys-Phe-Asp that was previously reported for bovine FKBP. This DNA consisted of an open reading frame encoding 108 amino acid residues, the first 40 of which were identical to those of the amino-terminal sequence for bovine KFBP. This finding suggested that the sequence represented gene coding for FKBP. The deduced amino acid sequence was analyzed with computer assistance that indicated no internal homology and no significant sequence similarity to any other known amino acid sequences, including cyclophilin. Messenger ribonucleic acid species of 1.8 kilobases, which hybridized with human FKBP cDNA, were found in poly(A)$^+$ RNAs from brain, lung, liver, and placental cells and leukocytes according to Northern blot analysis. Level of FKBP mRNA was unaffected by induction of Jurkat leukemic T cells with phorbol 12-myristate 13-acetate and ionomycin. Southern blot analysis suggested that there were only a few copies of the DNA sequence encoding FKBP, whereas the mammalian genome may encode up to 20 copies of the cyclophilin gene and possible pseudogenes.

Conclusions.—The nucleotide sequence of human FKBP was studied. Cyclophilin genes appear to have diverged extensively in the course of evolution, but the FKBP has not. This difference in genomic complexity may indicate that FKBP exhibits much less functional diversity than cyclophilin. More study is needed to clarify the induction of cyclophilin and FKBP in normal lymphoid cells.

▶ After the discovery that the intracellular target protein for CsA binding is cyclophilin, a peptidyl-prolyl *cis-trans* isomerase, (rotamase or foldase), it was remarkable to learn that FK 506 also binds to a rotomase. Although the agents are not structurally related, CsA and FK 506 both block a set of Ca^{2+} dependent events that are crucial to T-cell activation. Hence, the fact that both agents bind to rotamases is absolutely fascinating. The FK 506 target protein is called FK 506 binding protein (FKBP).

A structural understanding of the FKBP protein will certainly be enhanced by analysis of cDNA encoding human FKBP. Maki et al. sequenced and isolated

FKBP cDNA. It is interesting that this analysis shows that cyclophilin and FKBP are not structurally related. At the time this report was published, many believed that the immunosuppressive effects of CsA and FK 506 resulted from their ability to block the enzymatic function of their target rotamases. This assumption has proven incorrect. Inhibition of rotamase function is not at the heart of the immunosuppressive activity. The drug/target protein complex targets other cellular proteins including a vital phosphatase. Nonetheless, the structure of CsA/cyclophilin and FK 506/FKBP complexes must hold the key to their target protein specificity and ultimate immunosuppressive properties.—T. Strom, M.D.

15-Deoxyspergualin for Induction of Graft Nonreactivity After Cardiac and Renal Allotransplantation in Primates
Reichenspurner H, Hildebrandt A, Human PA, Boehm DH, Rose AG, Odell JA, Reichart B, Schorlemmer HU (University of Cape Town, Republic of South Africa)
Transplantation 50:181–185, 1990   12–4

Background.—The drug 15-deoxyspergualin (15-DS) is a spegualine derivative with antitumor activity. Its immunosuppressive action is not completely understood, but it has prolonged graft survival in several organ transplant models in rats. There have been few studies of its efficacy in larger animals. Its immunosuppressive potential was evaluated in a preclinical experiment in baboons that received cardiac and renal allografts.

Methods.—The study animals were 52 Chacma baboons. Twenty-seven animals, comprising group 1, received heterotopic cardiac allotransplantation, and 25, comprising group 2, received classic renal allotransplantation. Groups 1A and 2A received no immunosuppressive treatment. Groups 1B and 2B received 15-DS alone, in a dose of 4 mg/kg/day for 9 days. Groups 1C and 2C received cyclosporine A 10 to 40 mg/kg/day for 30 days. Groups 1D and 2D received both treatments. Animals underwent noninvasive cytoimmunologic monitoring and weekly transmyocardial or renal core biopsy.

Results.—Mean graft survivals were 11 days for group 1A, 28.2 days for group 1B, 32.4 days for group 1C, and 43.1 days for group 1D. Survivals were 12.3 days for group 2A, 8.5 days for group 2B, 30.4 days for group 2C, and 148.9 days for group 2D (Fig 12–1). The most common cause of graft failure was acute rejection. Serious treatment-related adverse effects, especially gastrointestinal complications, occurred only in animals that received 15-DS alone. No permanent state of graft nonreactivity was achieved in the heart transplant group, but within a mean of 21.8 days after immunosuppression was stopped, there was a delayed reaction. Likewise, graft nonreactivity was not achieved in groups 2B and 2C, but 50% of animals in group 2D were graft tolerant up to 340 days after discontinuation of treatment.

Conclusions.—Combined 15-DS and cyclosporine A treatment signifi-

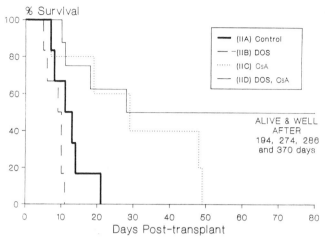

Fig 12−1.—Survival rates after renal transplantation. Only group IID (15-DS and CsA) showed a significant increase in survival time when compared with the controls, IIA. Three primates are still alive 370, 286, and 274 days after surgery. One baboon died 194 days after transplantation. (Courtesy of Reichenspurner H, Hildebrandt A, Human PA, et al: *Transplantation* 50:181−185, 1990.)

cantly prolongs graft survival in baboon models of cardiac and renal allotransplantation. Some animals that receive this treatment achieve renal graft nonreactivity. More research, both in vitro and in vivo, with 15-DS is needed; it has much promise as an adjunct immunosuppressive treatment.

▶ Whereas 15-DS did not produce potent immunosuppression when given alone, a 15-DS plus CsA regimen successfully prolonged engraftment of heart and kidney allografts in subhuman primate models. Indeed, 4 of 8 renal allograft recipients (Fig 12−1) experienced continuing engraftment that persisted after drug cessation. The mechanism of action of 15-DS is poorly understood. Use of 15-DS with azathioprine has proven toxic, yet the agent may prove to be a useful adjunct to CsA therapy. This agent is a guanidine-like derivative of spergualine with antitumor effects.—T. Strom, M.D.

Evidence That Deoxyspergualin Prevents Sensitization and First-Set Cardiac Xenograft Rejection in Rats by Suppression of Antibody Formation
Valdivia LA, Monden M, Gotoh M, Nakano Y, Tono T, Mori T (Osaka Univ, Fukushimaku, Osaka)
Transplantation 50:132−136, 1990   12−5

Background.—A major problem in the control of xenograft rejection is the lack of understanding of the immunologic mechanisms underlying it. A study was done to try to confirm that humoral antibodies have an important role in rejecting hamster-to-rat cardiac xenografts by simple transfer of serum from animals that rejected xenografts. The effects of 15-deoxyspergualin (DSG) on antibody-mediated cardiac xenograft rejec-

		Survival of Cardiac Xenografts		
Group	n	Survival (days)	MST *	P†(vs. group)
1. Untreated	10	3, 3, 3, 3, 3, 3, 4, 4, 4, 4	3.4±0.5	
2. Spx	8	5, 5, 5, 5, 5, 5, 6, 6	5.2±0.4	<.01 (vs. 1)
3. DSG, 2.5 mg/kg/day	8	7, 7, 8, 9, 9, 10, 11, 15	9.5±2.6	<.01 (vs. 1, 2)
4. DSG, 2.5 mg/kg/day + Spx	10	(15),‡(15), 18, 20, 20, 22, 24, 28, 28, 31	22.1±5.5	<.01 (vs. 1, 3)
5. DSG, 5 mg/kg/day	7	(7), (11), (14), (18), (21), (22), (22)	16.4±5.9	

*MST indicates mean survival time ± 1 SD.
†Student's *t* test.
‡Days in parentheses indicate death of a recipient with a functioning graft.
(Courtesy of Valdivia LA, Monden M, Gotoh M, et al: *Transplantation* 50:132–136, 1990.)

tion were also tested, as were the effects of recipient splenectomy as an adjunct to DSG in controlling first-set xenograft rejection.

Methods and Results.—Hyperimmune serum was obtained from control recipients at the time of rejection and injected intravenously into new recipients of cardiac xenografts. Hyperacute graft rejection resulted. Survival dependent on the amount of serum injected. It ranged from 14.7 minutes with 3 mL of serum to 233.3 minutes with .5 mL. Experiments on first-set xenograft rejection showed that DSG, 2.5 mg/kg/day, could prolong xenograft survival from 3.4 days in untreated control animals to 9.5 days. A DSG dose of 5 mg/kg/day increased graft survival to 16.4 days but was toxic to the recipients. Splenectomy alone prolonged xenograft survival to 5.2 days. When combined with 2.5 mg/kg/day of DSG, it prolonged graft survival to 22.1 days. Cytotoxic antibody appearance was delayed. Titers dropped from 1:256 in untreated controls to 1:16 to 1:64 in the group that had splenectomy only and in the group receiving 2.5 mg/kg/day of DSG. Combined therapy suppressed antibody response for more than 2 weeks. Experiments on hyperacute rejection induced by sensitization showed that 1 mL of hamster whole blood transfused into prospective heart recipients a week before transplantation led to graft loss in a mean 18.2 minutes. Hyperacute rejection was prevented and graft survival prolonged to 7 days after pretransplant transfusion and concomitant daily administration of DSG, 5 mg/kg, until 1 day after grafting. The survival associated with this treatment was significantly longer than that associated with DSG alone (table).

Conclusions.—An important mechanism in graft destruction in hamster-to-rat cardiac xenograft transplantation is antibody-mediated injury. Suppressing this branch of the immunologic response by DSG becomes the key to preventing first-set xenograft rejection and hyperacute rejection induced by sensitization. Even later cellular rejection is controlled to some degree with this agent. Splenectomy as an adjunct enhances xenograft survival.

▶ In xenografts undertaken with a recipient species harboring preformed antibodies against donor cell surface determinants (discordant species), hyperacute rejection occurs. Xenografts in so-called discordant species are doomed to hyperacute rejection. Although the hamster-to-rat combination has been termed concordant, it appears that antibodies play a prominent role in rejection of hamster-to-rat xenografts. There was a modest effect on rejection with 15-DSG or splenectomy alone, but the combination was more potent (table). The effect on xenograft rejection correlated with, but was not necessarily the result of, suppression of synthesis of antigraft antibodies. Although the precise mode of action of 15-DSG is enigmatic, the agent clearly possesses interesting immunosuppressive effects.—T. Strom, M.D.

RS-61443–A New, Potent Immunosuppressive Agent
Platz KP, Sollinger HW, Hullett DA, Eckhoff DE, Eugui EM, Allison AC (Univ of Wisconsin, Madison; Syntex Research, Palo Alto, Calif)
Transplantation 51:27–31, 1991   12–6

Background.—The semisynthetic mycophenolic acid derivative RS-61443 demonstrated powerful immunosuppressive action in initial in vitro and in vivo animal studies. The immunosuppressive effect of RS-61443 was evaluated in renal allografts in dogs.

Methods.—The study animals were unrelated female mongrel dogs. Five animals received no immunosuppressive treatment, 6 received cyclosporin A, 5 mg/kg/day, and methylprednisolone, .1 mg/kg/day; 6 received RS-61443, 40/mg/kg/day; and 16 received RS-61443, 20 mg/kg/day, cyclosporin A, 5 mg/kg/day, and methyl prednisolone, .1 mg/kg/day.

Results.—Median survival times were 8.1 days in the nontreatment group, 8.5 days in the treatment control group, 36 days in the RS-61443 monotherapy group, and 122.4 days in the triple-therapy group (Fig 12–2). Graft survival was significantly prolonged with triple therapy. Six of the animals in this group survived more than 150 days, and none

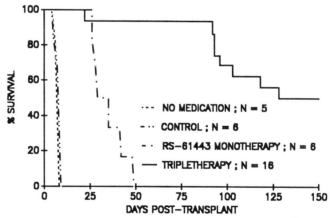

Fig 12–2.—Comparative dog survival of the 4 experimental groups under different treatment schedules. (Courtesy of Platz KP, Sollinger HW, Hullett DA, et al: *Transplantation* 51:27–31, 1991.)

showed any major adverse effects. There was a slight elevation of alkaline phosphatase levels, but there was no nephrotoxicity, hematotoxicity, or hepatotoxicity. There were some gastrointestinal symptoms, (e.g., gastritis, diarrhea, and anorexia), particularly in the monotherapy group. These effects appeared to be dose-related. There was no increased susceptibility to bacterial or viral infection. On examination, the kidneys showed slight interstitial cell infiltration but no vascular or glomerular damage.

Conclusions.—In dogs, RS-61443 is shown to have potent immunosuppressive effects and prolongation of graft survival. This agent appears to have significant promise as an adjunct agent for use in combination with current immunosuppressive agents. A clinical trial in cadaver renal allograft recipients is underway.

▶ The agent RS-61443 is an ester derivative of mycophenolic acid (MPA), which causes a selective cellular depletion of quanine nucleotides and selective depression of the de novo purine synthetic pathways, based on theoretical considerations. Derivatives of MPA were predicted to be effective and safe immunosuppressive agents; MPA also exhibits modest antimicrobial effects.

In this analysis, RS-61443 was tested as an antirejection agent in "large" animals—mongrel dogs. Monotherapy with RS-61443 is modestly effective in preventing rejection of renal allografts (Fig 12–2). Triple therapy (RS-61443 + CsA + steroids) was very effective; however, in preclinical and early clinical studies, RS-61443 appears to be very nicely tolerated and is a beneficial agent. It can be used as a maintenance or antirejection agent. This is a lovely result since RS-61443 was actually designed as an immunosuppressive. This is a rationally designed, not an empirically discovered, agent. Bravo.—T. Strom, M.D.

Production of Synergistic But Nonidentical Mechanisms of Immunosuppression by Rapamycin and Cyclosporine

Kimball PM, Kerman RH, Kahan BD (Univ of Texas Med School, Houston)
Transplantation 51:486–490, 1991   12–7

Background.—Kidney transplant recipients usually receive cyclosporine (CsA) along with several other drugs to produce the greatest degree of immunosuppression with the least side effects. Rapamycin RAP), a fungal metabolite of *Streptomyces hygroscopieus*, appears to work cooperatively with CsA to enhance immunosuppression.

Objective.—The possible synergistic relations between RAP and CsA were investigated by measuring the comparative effects of the 2 agents on peripheral blood lymphocytes.

Methods.—The in vitro methods used to study how RAP and CsA work together include culture of peripheral blood lymphocytes and extracts from the cells' cytoplasm. The activator of DNA replication (ADR) activity was measured in cultured resting nuclei. Rapamycin and CsA were each dissolved at 1 mg/mL in 80% ethanol/20% Tween 80 buffer and diluted in the RPMI culture medium.

Findings.—Results of the in vitro experiments demonstrate that RAP

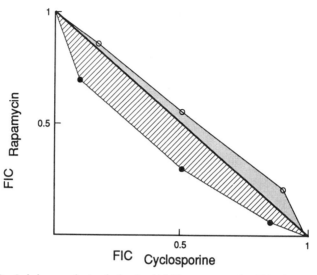

Fig 12–3.—Isobolograms plotting the fractional inhibitory concentration (FIC) of rapamycin and cyclosporine when 3 concentrations of drugs near their respective 50% inhibitory concentration were mixed. The *line of unity* indicates the concentration that reduces proliferation by 50% for each drug. Drug combinations below the line of unity indicate synergy; those above the line indicate antagonism. Rapamycin/CsA combinations were synergistic in suppressing proliferation (area below the line of unity), whereas their effect on ADR generation was additive (area slightly above the line of unity). (Courtesy of Kimball PM, Kerman RH, Kahan BD: *Transplantation* 51:486–490, 1991.)

inhibited the proliferation of T cells after application of mitogen (phytohemagglutinin antigen) and/or after alloantigen (mixed lymphocyte reaction) stimulation. The RAP doses of 100, 33, 11, and 3.6 ng/mL lowered proliferation by 81%, 84%, 81%, and 83%, respectively. The activation of the alloantigen showed the same type of individual variability in sensitivity to RAP. The RAP inhibitory effects occurred during all phases of the cell cycle, but CsA blockage of inhibition was effective only in the G_0 phase of the cell cycle. The addition of RAP to pokeweed mitogen-stimulated B lymphocytes produced cell cycle-restricted proliferation. Cyclosporine produced an equal degree of inhibition of the generation of the ADR whereas RAP caused a linear, indirect reduction in proliferation versus ADR synthesis (Fig 12–3).

Conclusions.—Rapamycin, but not CsA, blocks B cell activation. Rapamycin inhibited the activator of DNA replication apparently through a different mechanism of action. Rapamycin and CsA given together worked synergistically to inhibit proliferation of T cells in vitro and additively to block cytoplasmic activation of signal ADR.

▶ Rapamycin, CsA, and FK 506 all inhibit certain PPI'ases. Rapamycin and FK 506 bind to the same PPI'ase. It is interesting that rapamycin and CsA are synergistic in vitro. As noted in Abstract 12–1, FK 506 actually antagonizes rapamycin. All of this is interesting and highly confusing. The basic mechanism of action of these drugs remains mysterious.—T. Strom, M.D.

Evidence That Genistein, a Protein-Tyrosine Kinase Inhibitor, Inhibits CD$_{28}$ Monoclonal-Antibody-Stimulated Human T Cell Proliferation

Atluru S, Atluru D (Kansas State Univ, Manhattan)

Transplantation 51:448–450, 1991   12–8

Background.—The isoflavinoid compound genistein, which was previously shown to inhibit both protein tyrosine kinase and topoisomerase enzyme specifically, has recently been shown to inhibit the anti-CD$_{28}$ stimulated T cell proliferation via interleukin-2 (IL-2) dependent pathway. The immunosuppressive action of genistein was measured on anti-CD$_{28}$ stimulated T cell proliferation, IL-2 production, and IL-2R expression from cell cultures.

Methods.—T lymphocytes were isolated from the peripheral blood of healthy volunteers and cell cultures were prepared for proliferation studies. Interleukin-2 production was measured by using CTLL-2 cells, and IL-2R expression was measured by flow cytometry.

Results.—T cell proliferation stimulated by phorbol-12-myristate-13-acetate (PMA) plus anti-CD$_{28}$ was inhibited by genistein, but the same proliferative activity resisted the inhibitory effect of cyclosporin A (Fig 12–4). Interleukin-2 synthesis induced by PHA plus anti-CD$_{28}$ or PMA plus anti-CD$_{28}$ was also inhibited by genistein. Interleukin-2 synthesis induced by PHA plus PMA was inhibited by cyclosporin A, but that induced by PMA plus anti-CD$_{28}$ was unaffected by cyclosporin A. At the concentration, which inhibited T cell proliferation and IL-2 synthesis, genistein also significantly inhibited IL-2R expression stimulated by PMA plus anti-CD$_{28}$. Interleukin-2R expression stimulated by the same cultures was unaffected by cyclosporin A.

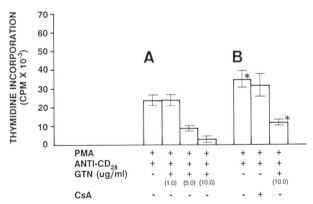

Fig 12–4.—A, dose-response inhibition of phorbol-12-myristate-13-acetate (PMA) plus anti-CD28 stimulated T-cell proliferation. T cells were cultured with culture additives for 3 days to measure ^{3}H-thymidine incorporation. Genistein (1, 5, and 10 μg/mL) was added at time 0 hour. Data represent mean ± SD of 2 experiments using different donors. **B**, inhibitory effects of CsA or genistein on PMA plus anti-CD$_{28}$ induced T-cell proliferation. Culture conditions are the same as described in **A**. Data represent mean ± SEM from 3 experiments using different donors. Culture additives are used as follows: PMA, 10 ng/mL; anti-CD$_{28}$, .5 μg/mL; CsA, 250 ng/mL; genistein 10 μg/mL. (*) Cultures stimulated with PMA plus anti-CD$_{28}$ and genistein are significantly different ($P < .05$) from PMA plus anti-CD$_{28}$ cultures. (Courtesy of Atluru S, Atluru D: *Transplantation* 51:448–450, 1991.)

Conclusions.—Genistein appears to be a potent immunosuppressive compound that has no toxic effects on T cells and might be useful in prevention and treatment of allograft rejection. Genistein and cyclosporin A could be used in combination to produce a better immunosuppressive effect with less cyclosporin A-induced nephrotoxicity because genistein blocks the cyclosporin A-resistant pathway of T cell proliferation.

▶ Activation of the T-cell receptor complex by antigen is required but not sufficient for T-cell proliferation. A second co-stimulatory signal is derived from certain cytokines or ligan specific T-cell to APC protein interaction is required for T-cell proliferation. A lengthy list of co-stimulatory signals that are effective in vitro includes various cytokines IL-1, IL-6, IL-7, and interaction of CD2 to LFA-3 and CD28 to B7 molecules of T-cells and antigen-presenting cells. It is fascinating that only the CD28 driven signal is insensitive to CsA and FK 506. Could blockade of this signal be the missing pharmacologic link to vastly reduced immunologic graft failure and elusive goal of tolerance? I personally believe that this pathway will prove to be of great importance in vivo. Cross-linking of surface T-cell CD28 molecule can be accomplished in a test tube with anti-CD28 mAbs. Genistein blocked T-cell proliferation in this "drug resistant" system (Fig 12–4). The authors suggest that therapy with genistein may prove beneficial.

Whereas the effects of genistein are clear cut, they are hardly specific for the CD28 pathway. Genistein inhibits protein tyrosine kinases (enzymes that phosphorylate proteins at tyrosine residues). Protein tyrosine kinases are crucial for proliferation of a myriad of cell types. Thus, protein tyrosine kinase blockers inhibit proliferation of many (most?) cell types. Genistein also blocks both the T-cell receptor and IL-2 receptor signaling pathways. Indeed, the authors provide no evidence that the effects of genistein were specific for blocking the CD28 signal in this experimental set up since this agent inhibits the PHA and IL-2 derived signals. I'm sure that in vivo administration of genistein would lead to immunosuppression, but I'm not certain that this drug can be safely administered. Can life go on in the face of genistein?—T. Strom, M.D.

Evidence That Glucocorticosteroid-Mediated Immunosuppressive Effects Do Not Involve Altering Second Messenger Function
Almawi WY, Hadro ET, Strom TB (Harvard Med School, Boston)
Transplantation 52:133–140, 1991   12–9

Introduction.—Several immune disorders have been treated using glucocorticosteroids as immunosuppressive agents, although the exact mechanism remains unknown. Glucocorticosteroids block transcription of interleukin (IL)-1 and IL-6 genes in a concentration-dependent manner. The way in which glucocorticosteroids suppress proliferation of human peripheral blood mononuclear leukocytes (PBML) was investigated.

Results.—Dexamethasone and 6α-methylprednisolone inhibited PBML in a concentration-dependent manner, as shown by proliferative responses to immobilized anti-CD3 mAb or mitogens. Dexamethasone did not block the entry of Ca^{2+} into cells stimulated by anti-CD3$^+$ phorbal-

12β-myristate-13a-acetate (PMA), and dexamethasone-mediated suppression was not circumvented by Ca^{2+} ionopheres; these findings indicated that the glucocorticosteroid mechanism did not involve interference with Ca^{2+} fluxes. Protein kinase C (PKC) inhibitors and stimulators did not prevent dexamethasone-mediated suppression. Dexamethasone did not affect upregulation of CD4 and CD8 expression, which is an indirect index of PKC activity, nor did it change translocation of PKC from cytosolic to membrane-bound compartments; thus, dexamethasone had no effect on PKC activity.

Conclusion.—Given the previous findings that glucocorticosteroids inhibit cytokine gene transcription, and the rIL-1 plus rIL-6 plus rIFNγ completely abrogate the suppressive effects of glucocorticosteroids, these findings suggest that the immunosuppressive effects of glucocorticosteroids result from inhibition of cytokine gene expression. Glucocorticosteroids may enter the cytoplasm of T and accessory cells and bind to the glucocorticosteroid receptor, which becomes a DNA-binding protein.

▶ Although glucocorticosteroids have been the mainstay of solid organ transplantation, the mechanism of action of these drugs is unknown. These experiments indicate that steroids do not affect calcium fluxes but instead inhibit cytokine gene expression. To plan combination agents to take advantage of the synergetic effects, it is important to understand specific mechanisms of action.—N.L. Ascher, M.D., Ph.D.

Soluble Suppressive Molecule Released by Human T Lymphocytes Induced by Heat-Inactivated Allostimulator Cells in the Presence of Cyclosporine
Nelson PA, Tam AW, Sukiennicki T, Wong-Lee J, Brenner CA, Larrick JW (Genelabs Inc, Redwood City, Calif)
Transplantation 50:286–293, 1990   12–10

Introduction.—Human suppressor cells can be selectively activated by incubation of lymphocytes with heat-inactivated allogeneic cells. A soluble suppressive factor was produced from CD4+ cells, which were derived from the peripheral blood lymphocytes (PBLs) that were incubated with heat-inactivated allogeneic Epstein-Barr virus (EBV) in the presence of cyclosporine (CsA). The soluble suppressive factor is capable of inhibiting a primary MLR.

Methods.—The PBLs were obtained from buffy coat cells of randomly selected normal blood donors. These cells were stimulated with allogeneic heat-inactivated (HI) EBV-transformed lymphoblastoid cells. The T-suppressor cell lines were derived from cells after 1–2 weeks of culture with the HI-EBV stimulator cells. Cell viability, bioactivity, cytotoxicity, and mRNA were assessed.

Results.—Culturing of fresh E-rosette-positive PBLs with irradiated allogeneic stimulator cells for 7 days produced an MLR. With the addition of irradiated CsA/HI-treated sheep red blood cell-rosetted T lymphocytes

(E+ cells), this proliferation response ceased. The attempts to generate CD8+ T-suppressor cells that would work in a syngeneic manner was not successful. When the CsA/HI-activated cells were added directly to allogeneic ^{51}Cr-labeled EBV-transformed B-lymphoblastoid target cells, no cytotoxicity was found. Kinetic studies showed that suppression occurs only if the supernatant is added during the first 3 days of culture. The E+ PBL cells produced a soluble molecule, concentrated in greater than 1,000 units of suppressive activity per milliliter. This suppressor factor has an apparent molecular weight of 90 kd and is sensitive to change in pH and to boiling. Neutralization with anti-TGF-β antibody and tests for mRNA expression demonstrated that this factor is not the suppressive cytokine TGFβ.

Conclusion.—The findings of this study support earlier reports that CsA/HI-activated T cells do produce a new cytokine that is not antigen-specific or MHC-restricted.

▶ Lymphocytes stimulated by heat-inactivated EBV-transformed cells in the presence of cyclosporine secrete a suppressor factor that suppresses MLR nonspecifically but not mitogen responses. This cytokine proved not to be TGF-β and will need to be characterized to determine whether it represents a novel suppressor molecule. This molecule may represent an important mechanism by which cyclosporine exerts its immunosuppressive effect.—N.L. Ascher, M.D., Ph.D.

13 Role of Monoclonal Antibody in Clinical and Experimental Transplant

▶ ↓ Therapeutic administration of anti-CD3 pan T-cell monoclonal antibodies (mAbs) continues to be a lively topic in preclinical and clinical transplantation. Anti-CD3 mAb can render unsensitized T cells prone to receive tolerogenic signals. Administration of OKT3, an anti-CD3 mAb, appears beneficial in several rather difficult circumstances, such as vascular rejection and in patients with positive antiglobulin crossmatch. The powerful immunosuppressive effect of anti-CD3 mAbs does not require donor cell lysis. In the sensitized host, anti-CD4 antibody may be effective if administered before grafting. These mAbs probably prevent the T-cell receptor complex from binding antigen, and they can be highly tolerogenic in several preclinical models.

Progress has been made in dealing with 2 problems that plague anti-CD3 mAb therapy: (1) elaboration of neutralizing anti-mAb antibodies by the treated host; and (2) the OKT3 induced cytokine syndrome. The vexing association of high, repeated doses of OKT3 with lymphoma formation has been emphasized. Modification of antibody may prevent the formation of antibodies to neutralize it.—Terry Strom, M.D.

Induction of Specific Nonresponsiveness in Unprimed Human T Cells by Anti-CD3 Antibody and Alloantigen

Anasetti C, Tan P, Hansen JA, Martin PJ (Fred Hutchinson Cancer Research Ctr, Seattle; Univ of Washington, Seattle)
J Exp Med 172:1691–1700, 1990
13–1

Background.—Human T cell antigen recognition is mediated by the α and β polymorphic chains of the TCR, noncovalently associated on the cell surface with 5 invariant polypeptides that collectively represent the CD3 complex responsible for signal transduction. Co-stimulation of unprimed human T cells with soluble anti-CD3 antibody and allogeneic MHC was demonstrated to induce a sustained state of antigen-specific nonresponsiveness.

Methods and Results.—Fresh peripheral blood mononuclear cells were exposed to alloantigen for 3 to 8 days in the presence of anti-CD3 antibodies. Although these cells showed no response after restimulation with cells from the original donor, they were still able to respond to third-party donors. Both nonmitogenic and mitogenic anti-CD3 antibodies induced antigen-specific nonresponsiveness, but antibodies against CD2, CD4, CD5, CD8, CD18, and CD28 did not. Anti-CD3 antibody-induced nonresponsiveness in mixed leukocyte culture was sustained for at least 34 days from culture initiation and 26 days after antibody removal. In addition, anti-CD3 antibody induced antigen-specific nonresponsiveness in cytotoxic T cell generation assays. Anti-CD3 antibody did not induce nonresponsiveness in cells that were previously primed. The anti-CD3-induced nonresponsiveness was apparently not associated with suppressor cell activation.

Conclusions.—Co-stimulation of the T cell receptor-CD3 complex on unprimed T cells with a fluid phase anti-CD3 antibody and allogeneic major histocompatability complex antigens may induce either clonal anergy or deletion. These findings suggest novel approaches for attaining transplantation tolerance.

▶ Creation of a state of specific tolerance to the graft remains the unfilfilled aspiration of clinical transplanters. How can this elusive goal be achieved? A series of proteins that includes members of T-cell receptor/CD3 complex as well as T-cell proteins that foster T cell to antigen-presenting cell co-mitogenic signals (e.g., CD2, CD4, CD5, CD8, C18, and CD28) are obvious potential therapeutic targets. The impact of mAbs directed against these proteins was analyzed in a MLC system. In a primary mixed lymphocyte culture system, anti-CD3, but not anti-CD2, anti-CD4, anti-CD5, anti-CD8, anti-CD18, or anti-CD28, produced a lingering state of antigen-specific unresponsiveness. A state of anergy was achieved with a nonlytic anti-CD3 mAb. Because development of anergy requires antigen recognition (see Figure 1 in the original article), I would guess that partial capping of TCR/CD3 proteins with anti-CD3 produces suboptimal T-cell activation and thereby produces anergy. Anergy was not evident when pre-activated T cells were tested in this mixed lymphocyte culture system. These results suggest an experimental preclinical protocol in which pre-activated T cells are selectively destroyed before exposure to alloantigen (IL-2 toxin, anti-IL-2R mAb) and anti-CD3 mAb is used to produce anergy.— T. Strom, M.D.

The Efficacy of OKT3 in Vascular Rejection
Schroeder TJ, Weiss MA, Smith RD, Stephens GW, First MR (Univ of Cincinnati Med Ctr)
Transplantation 51:312–315, 1991   13–2

Introduction.—The murine-derived monoclonal antibody OKT3 is directed against the CD3 receptor on human T lymphocytes. It is effective in the treatment of acute cellular rejection in kidney, liver, heart, and pancreas transplant recipients. However, there has been only 1 report of patients with acute vascular rejection treated successfully with OKT3.

Methods.—Sixty-six consecutive biopsies of renal allograft recipients treated with OKT3 monoclonal antibody were divided into 2 groups.

The 29 patients in group 1 had evidence of acute vascular and cellular rejection. The 32 in group 2 had only cellular rejection. Samples were inadequate to determine the presence or absence of vascular rejection in 5 cases. Cellular rejection severity was graded as mild, moderate, or severe histologically.

Findings.—Severity of rejection was comparable in the 2 groups and there was no difference in the rejection reversal rate. At 6 and 12 months, however, graft loss was higher in the group with vascular rejection. Patients with both severe acute cellular rejection and acute vascular rejection had the worst outcomes. Serum creatinine levels were higher both before and after OKT3 treatment at 1, 6, and 12 months in group 1.

Summary.—Treatment with OKT3 was equally successful in reversing acute cellular rejection and acute vascular rejection. Patients with vascular rejection, however, had increased graft loss at 6 and 12 months.

▶ The ability of OKT3 to reverse acute cellular and or acute vascular rejection was studied. Vascular rejection was defined as endothelial swelling and intimal mononuclear cell infiltrates plus or minus IgM/C3 deposits. The results of this descriptive analysis indicate that while both cellular and "vascular" rejection episodes respond to OKT3 with similar frequency, the long-term outcome was inferior in patients with vascular rejection—especially in those with both cellular and vascular rejection. The results are not surprising. Rejection is a T-cell–dependent process that spreads throughout the kidney in a fairly reproducible manner. Intense infiltration of the intima and/or endothelium is often a late event. In the event that this process is not aborted, endothelial-intimal damage can eventually lead to ischemia of the organ. Therefore, cellular infiltration of these structures is worrisome but not inevitably devastating. The process causing vascular rejection is merely an extension of the T-cell–dependent process that we call cellular rejection. Why give a special name—vascular rejection—to these forms of vascular rejection that remain T-cell dependent? When T-cell–dependent B-cell and macrophage activation goes unchecked, the process eventually becomes T-cell independent. For T-cell–dependent processes such as DTH-like processes, OKT3 is a useful treatment. Responsiveness to OKT3 does not, as often implied, mean that the injury is necessarily directly mediated (as opposed to dependent on) by T cells. I would have liked to have seen an analysis of all patients with the diagnosis of vascular rejection broken down into categories where Ab/complement was present versus those lacking such deposition. Perhaps it would be of greater value to analyze biopsies and therapeutic outcome with attempts to integrate the molecular basis of the immune attacks. At a certain point Ab production becomes a T-cell–independent process. The broad descriptive category of vascular rejection used in this analysis is almost useless. For example, cellular infiltration of the intima (not so bad) and microthrombi in the capillary (a disaster) are both covered by this near meaningless term.—T. Strom, M.D.

Renal Transplantation Despite a Positive Antiglobulin Crossmatch With and Without Prophylactic OKT3

Dafoe DC, Bromberg JS, Grossman RA, Tomaszewski JE, Zmijewski CM, Perloff LJ, Naji A, Asplund MW, Alfrey EJ, Sack M, Zellers L, Kearns J, Barker CF (Hosp of the Univ of Pennsylvania, Philadelphia)

Transplantation 51:762–768, 1991   13–3

Introduction.—Many transplant centers use the antiglobulin crossmatch (AGXM) to enhance detection of preformed antibody-to-donor antigens that may cause hyperacute rejection. However, positive AGXM sometimes detects irrelevant or very low titers of anti-HLA antibody, which precludes transplantation in suitable recipients.

Methods.—To determine the significance of a positive AGXM, cadaveric renal transplantation was performed in 48 patients despite a weakly positive AGXM, defined as cell killing above background but not greater than 20%.

Results.—In an initial group of 10 patients treated with cyclosporine, azathioprine, and prednisone, accelerated rejection occurred in 4 patients and graft loss in 3. In 38 patients who were treated with a prophylactic course of OKT3 followed by triple therapy, there were no episodes of accelerated acute rejection, although clinical hyperacute rejection occurred in 1 patient. The incidence of delayed graft function was high (75%). Patients treated prophylactically with OKT3 had a decreased incidence of acute rejection per recipient and a delayed onset of first episodes. The 1-year actuarial primary graft survival was 88% in the group treated with OKT3 and 50% in the initial group. Overall, the outcome in patients with the weakly positive AGXM was similar to that in a comparison group of 32 patients with a negative AGXM and immediate graft function. However, a subset of positive AGXM regraft recipients treated prophylactically with OKT3 did not do well, with a 36% incidence of primary nonfunction.

Conclusion.—A positive AGXM is not a contraindication to primary renal transplantation. The use of the AGXM can identify transplant recipients who would benefit from prophylaxis with OKT3.

▶ Clinical decision making would be far easier if there were more black or white, yes or no prognostic categories. Does a positive in the sensitive antiglobulin donor-specific crossmatch uniformly predict hyperacute rejection? Does prophylactic OKT3 benefit patients receiving primary grafts or retransplants despite the presence of low titer antidonor T-cell–specific antibodies detected by this sensitive crossmatch? In primary kidney graft recipients treated with triple therapy bearing low titer antidonor T-cell–specific antibodies, the rate of 1-year engraftment was 50%. Thus, the presence of the sensitive antiglobulin crossmatch places patients in a high risk group, but the test does not accurately predict graft failure. Half the patients experience immunologic failure; half obtain successful engraftment. A subsequent group of similar patients were subsequently given prophylactic OKT3 (5 mg/day intravenously for 10–14 days). Prophylactic therapy with OKT3 appears useful in these primary graft recipients, although the trial was not prospective, randomized, etc. Of course, the rate of engraftment in a retransplant, especially in the sensitized population, is compromised. It was of interest, therefore, to study the impact of OKT3 in patients with low titer antidonor T-cell–specific antibodies. They fared very poorly! Bottom line: these data suggest that sequential immunotherapy may be valuable in patients receiving primary grafts but not in retransplants with low titer antidonor antibodies. A "correct" randomized, prospective trial should be undertaken.—T. Strom, M.D.

Dose-Related Mechanisms of Immunosuppression Mediated by Murine Anti-CD3 Monoclonal Antibody in Pancreatic Islet Cell Transplantation and Delayed-Type Hypersensitivity
Mackie JD, Pankewycz OG, Bastos MG, Kelley VE, Strom TB (Charles A Dana Research Inst; Brigham and Women's Hosp, Boston)
Transplantation 49:1150–1154, 1990   13–4

Background.—The mouse antihuman CD3 monoclonal antibody OKT3 blocks human allograft rejection, but the exact mechanisms of this immunosuppressive effect have not been defined. The results of antibody dosage on these immunosuppressive properties in murine models of allograft transplantation and delayed-type hypersensitivity were studied.

Methods.—Mice were subjected to either pancreatic islet cell allograft or delayed-type hypersensitivity reaction models of T-cell–dependent immunity. In the pancreatic islet allograft model, varying doses of anti-CD3 mAB 145-2C11—50, 5, or .5 µg/day was given for 15 days. In the delayed-type hypersensitivity model, mAb treatment began on day 0 and continued through the day of antigen challenge—day 6—except in animals that received a single intravenous dose of 400 µg on day 0 or day 6.

Results.—Clinical immunosuppression was superficially equal and effective in animals receiving low-dose anti-CD3 therapy and those receiving a single high-dose injection. There was no response to in vitro restimulation in T cells from animals that received high-dose anti-CD3. On the other hand, T cells from the low-dose group continued to demonstrate in vitro proliferative capacity on stimulation with polyvalent anti-CD3 mAb. Administration of anti-CD3 mAb caused immunosuppression in C5-deficient mice, demonstrating that the terminal complement components were not needed to support in vivo immunosuppression mediated by the antibody. Some of the allograft recipients attained permanent engraftment but not tolerance. In recipients with long-term, well-accepted grafts, replacement of donor leukocytes induced acute rejection.

Conclusions.—A study in mice demonstrates that anti-CD3 mAb therapy can suppress delayed-type hypersensitivity without complement-mediated cell lysis to confer immunosuppression. In vivo T-cell activation results from MAb administration, but changes in T-cell reactivity vary with dose and time after administration. If treatment is prolonged, this may allow time for replacement or inactivation of donor leukocytes.

▶ Gosh, who authored this great article? The hamster antimurine CD3 145–2C11 mAb has many of the properties of the mouse antihuman CD3 OKT3 antibody. Both antibodies do not readily activate complement in the treated host and are powerfully mitogenic in vitro. Both are immunosuppressive and cause cytokine release in vivo. Thus the 145-2.C11 mAb can be used to probe OKT3-like effects. The original reports concerning 145–2C11 effects used much higher doses and body weight than the clinically used OKT3 doses. This analysis is centered on "low-dose" anti-CD3 effects as means to approach the clinical effects of OKT3.

This study clearly shows that nonlytic doses of anti-CD3 are immunosuppressive. Indeed, splenci lymphoproliferation resulted from anti-CD3 treatment. Moreover, T cells harvested from treated animals proliferated normally to anti-CD3. In a subset of anti-CD3–treated islet cell allografted hosts, "tolerance" results. Nonetheless, in animals that do not reject grafts even long after therapy has ceased, rejection can often be stimulated by an infusion of donor white blood cells. I believe the data indicate that anti-CD3 can effect immunosuppression simply by blocking the T-cell receptor/CD3 complex. Anti-CD3 mAbs do, in fact, cap both TCR and CD3 proteins for the T-cell membrane. I am intrigued by the capacity of donor white blood cells to evoke rejection in "tolerant" hosts. T-cell anergy is not affected anti-CD3 treatment. All antigen-bearing cells are not created equal in terms of effectively stimulating T cells. Antigen density varies among cell types. More important, perhaps, cells vary in their ability to deliver co-stimulatory signals to T cells. Islet cells do not make IL-1, IL-6, IL-7, or express LFA-3 and B7. These are the substances that produce co-stimulatory signals. Hence, anti-CD3 may paralyze alloreactive T cells until the passenger leukocytes perish. Subsequently, immunosuppression may not be required.— T. Strom, M.D.

Differential Role of CD4⁺ Cells in the Sensitization and Effector Phases of Accelerated Graft Rejection

Sablinski T, Sayegh MH, Hancock WW, Kut JP, Kwok CA, Milford EL, Tilney NL, Kupiec-Weglinski JW (Harvard Med School; Brigham and Women's Hosp, Boston)
Transplantation 51:226–231, 1991   13–5

Background.— Many studies have attempted to understand the mechanism of the accelerated graft rejection (ACCR). The recent use of CD4 monoclonal antibodies (MAb) to prolong survival of organ allografts in naive rodents showed the effectiveness of this type of therapy. Some CD4 MAbs markedly prolonged or induced acceptance of skin, pancreatic islet, cardiac, and renal transplants in these animals. A new CD4 MAb, BWH-4, was used in an ACCR model of heart transplant rejection in presensitized rats.

Methods.— Inbred male Sprague-Dawley adult rats were sensitized with skin from Brown Norway rats. Hearts were transplanted to the infrarenal great vessels of the host animal using standard microvascular

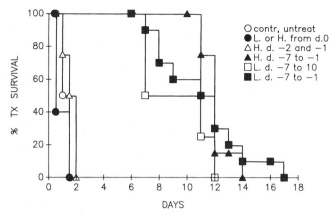

Fig 13–1.—Effects of CD4-targeted therapy on survival of cardiac transplants in LEW rats sensitized with BN skin transplants 7 days earlier. BWH-4 mAb was given intravenously at a dose of 100 μg/day (Ld) or 700 μg/day (Hd) during sensitization phase (before cardiac transplant) and/or effector phase (after cardiac transplant) of ACCR. Four to 10 rats in each group. (Courtesy of Sablinski T, Sayegh MH, Hancock WW, et al.: *Transplantation* 51:226–231, 1991.)

techniques. The antirat BWH-4 MAb is an immunoglobulin (IgG2a) that precipitates a 53kd polypeptide on rat T cells. Lymphocyte-mediated cytotoxicity (LMC) was specifically assayed.

Findings.—In this model of ACCR, associated with cardiac transplant in rats, treatment with the CD4 MAb (IgG2a) BWH-4 stopped fulminant rejection response (< 36 hours) during the sensitization phase of the rejection reaction but not during the effector phase (after the actual heart transplant). This effect prolonged transplant survival for about 11 days (Fig 13–1). These results correlated with the lower amount of CD4$^+$ cells in the circulation, although it did not appear to depend on the total absence of CD4$^+$ cells. The beneficial effects of BWH-4 treatment were also associated with BWH-4 MAb-mediated elimination and depression of antidonor humoral responses and cellular interactions, which were measured by LMC and mixed lymphocyte reaction. Immunoperoxidase studies of the heart transplant in rats who had been preconditioned with BWH-4 demonstrated a reduction in T and B cell activities as assessed by the deposition of humoral mediators, infiltrating cells, interleukin-2 and interferon-gamma elaboration, and cell activation.

Conclusion.—This new method avoids sensitization and ACCR by treating animal heart recipients with CD4 MAb at the time of initial antigenic challenge. These beneficial effects were achieved with relatively low doses of the BWH-4 MAb.

▶ The sensitized host represents a major and increasing problem in the field of kidney transplantation; less so for other solid organs. This study focuses on the role of CD4$^+$ cells in accelerated graft loss. This study shows a beneficial effect of early administration of monoclonal antibody to CD4$^+$ cells. The approach to the sensitized host will by necessity involve multiple treatments. Antibody to CD4$^+$ cells may, for example, be used in conjunction with antibody to CD8$^+$ cells and one of liver antimetabolites.—N.L. Ascher, M.D., Ph.D.

Corticosteroid Inhibition of the OKT3-Induced Cytokine-Related
Syndrome—Dosage and Kinetics Prerequisites
Chatenoud L, Legendre C, Ferran C, Bach J-F, Kreis H (Hôpital Necker, Paris)
Transplantation 51:334–338, 1991   13–6

Background.—The anti-CD3–induced physical reaction seen in patients receiving OKT3 as part of their immunosuppressive regimen is
caused by a massive, transient release of some cytokines. Corticosteroids
must be administered at high dosages to be more effective in reducing the
severity of the OKT3-induced syndrome. The best schedule of high-dose
corticosteroids with the first monoclonal antibody injection in patients
receiving prophylacyic OKT3 treatment was defined in a prospective randomized study.

Methods.—Three groups of patients were studied. The first group consisted of 27 consecutive recipients of cadaver renal allografts treated with
OKT3 as part of their immunosuppressive regimen to prevent rejection
episodes. Corticosteroids, .25 mg/kg/day, and azathioprine, 3 mg/kg/day,
were given along with OKT3, 5 mg/day, for 14 consecutive days. A 1-g
methylprednisolone bolus was also given at the time of the first OKT3
injection but not on a precise schedule: high-dose corticosteroids were
given either at the same time or preceding the first OKT3 injection by 30
minutes to 4 hours. Group 2 included 6 additional patients receiving in-
trafamilial haploidentical renal allografts. The daily dose of corticosteroids was not given in those patients' OKT3 regimen. Three received the
same type of pretreatment as patients in group 1. The third group consisted of 12 consecutive recipients of a cadaver renal allograft enrolled in
a pilot randomized trial who were given high-dose corticosteroids before
or at the time of the first OKT3 injection.

Findings.—When corticosteroids were given in a sufficient amount and
1 hour before the first OKT3 injection, they significantly reduced the release of tumor necrosis factor and interferon gamma. Pretreatment with
corticosteroids may have totally abolished the IL-2 release that OKT3 induces.

Conclusions.—The results suggest that high-dose corticosteroids
should be given along with the first OKT3 injection, preferably 1 hour
before the injection. This schedule effectively reduces the cytokine production responsible for the acute deleterious OKT3-induced clinical syndrome.

▶ In the test tube, OKT3 and other anti-CD3 or anti-TCR mAbs are powerful
mitogens. In vivo, the first and often second dose of OKT3 stimulates the host
to produce a myriad of cytokines, thereby causing a syndrome of fever, myalgia,
and a potentially fatal capillary leak syndrome. The release of tumor necrosis
factor has been implicated as being of special importance in this syndrome.
This analysis indicates that pretreatment of patients about to receive OKT3
with corticosteroids will result in a diminished outpouring of tumor necrosis
factor and interferon gamma (see Fig 2 in the original article). Although
corticosteroid pretreatment was more effective than use of corticosteroids

with OKT3 administration both groups were spared life-threatening OKT3 side effects.— T. Strom, M.D.

Inhibition of Anti-OKT3 Antibody Generation by Cyclosporine—Results of a Prospective Randomized Trial

Hricik DE, Mayes JT, Schulak JA (Univ Hosp of Cleveland, Case Western Reserve Univ)

Transplantation 50:237–240, 1990   13–7

Background.—The best strategy for maintenance immunosuppressive therapy during OKT3 treatment for acute renal allograft rejection has not yet ꞓn established. The effects of cyclosporine (CsA) treatment on the generation of antibodies to OKT3 were studied.

Methods.—Fifty-one renal transplant recipients previously given maintenance therapy of CsA, azathioprine, and prednisone were randomly assigned to 1 of 2 conditions. The 27 patients in group 1 received 50% of their maintenance dose of CsA, and the 24 in group 2 discontinued CsA during the 7 days of OKT3 treatment for acute renal allograft rejection.

Results.—In the month after OKT3 treatment, anti-OKT3 antibodies were found in 11% of group 1 patients and in 42% of group 2 patients. None of the patients in gruop 1 had antibody titers greater than 1:100. By contrast, 4 patients in group 2 had titers of 1:1,000 or more. Ninety-six percent of patients in group 1 had rejection reversal, compared with only 75% in group 2.

Conclusions.—Continued administration of reduced doses of CsA during OKT3 treatment improves the short-term response to this monoclonal antibody. Concurrent CsA and OKT-3 therapy appears to inhibit the generation of anti-OKT3 antibodies and to improve patient responses to this monoclonal antibody (table).

▶ Although the mouse antihuman CD3 mAb OKT3 is a potent immunosuppressive agent, many OKT3-treated patients make anti-OKT3 antibodies. Moreover, a significant proportion of anti-OKT3 antibodies are neutralizing, thereby rendering these patients refractory to OKT3-mediated immunosuppression. By con-

	Incidence and Titer of Anti-OKT3 Antibodies After Treatment With OKT3						
Group	Immediately after OKT3			1 Month after OKT3			Total
	1:100	1:1000	1:10000	1:100	1:1000	1:10000	
1 (n=27)	1	0	0	2	0	0	3/27*
2 (n=24)	6	0	0	2	3	1	10/24†

*Statistically different from group 2 (*P* < .03) by chi-square.
†Two patients in group 2 had positive titers on both occasions.
(Courtesy of Hricik DE, Mayes JT, Schulak JA: *Transplantation* 50:237–240, 1990.)

vention, cyclosporine is not administered during a course of OKT3 because of the potential for over-immunosuppression. This study clearly demonstrates that low-dose CsA inhibits the host immune response against OKT3 (table).—T. Strom, M.D.

Anti-Tac-H, a Humanized Antibody to the Interleukin 2 Receptor, Prolongs Primate Cardiac Allograft Survival
Brown PS Jr, Parenteau GL, Dirbas FM, Garsia RJ, Goldman CK, Bukowski MA, Junghans RP, Queen C, Hakimi J, Benjamin WR, Clark RE, Waldmann TA (Natl Cancer Inst, NIH, Bethesda, Md; Protein Design Labs. Inc, Mountain View, Calif; Hoffmann-La Roche Inc, Nutley, NJ)
Proc Natl Acad Sci USA 88:2663–2667, 1991   13–8

Introduction.—The development of effective, nontoxic immunosuppressive agents continues to be a goal of human allograft research, with the ideal drug being one that eliminates only those T cells that promote rejection. Because high-affinity interleukin 2 receptors (IL-2Rs) appear as the T-cell expressed antigens against foreign bodies, an attempt was made to counter this IL-2R expression using an anti-Tac-M murine monoclonal antibody (mAb) specific for the IL-2R-α chain to stop organ allograft rejection. Unmodified murine anti-Tac and humanized anti-Tac mAb were tested in cynomolgus monkeys.

Methods.—The anti-Tac mAb was produced and characterized. The humanized anti-Tac mAb resulted from a combination of the complement-determining regions (CDRs) of the anti-Tac antibody with the human IgG1 κ framework and constant regions. The 3 experimental groups included 5 animals each: group I had a heterotopic, cardiac allograft but did not receive immunosuppression; group II received anti-Tac-M per kilogram of body weight intravenously on the day of the allograft and every other day until rejection; group III underwent the same protocol as group II, except that the animals received anti-Tac-H rather than anti-Tac-M.

Results.—Pharmacokinetic studies with ^{131}I-anti-Tac-M and ^{125}I-anti-Tac-H showed that the radioactivity remained intravascular, then slowly declined from the plasma exponentially. The 5 monkeys that received no immunosuppressive agents rejected their grafts on or about day 9 after transplantation. The 5 animals that received the unmodified anti-Tac-M had significantly prolonged survival compared with controls. The 5 animals that received anti-Tac-H demonstrated significantly prolonged graft survival compared with both controls and the anti-Tac-M animals in group II. Antibodies to the mAb developed in all 5 animals in group II. In group III antibodies to the mAb did not develop during the 19- to 22-day anti-Tac initiation and graft rejection.

Conclusion.—Anti-Tac-M antibody can increase the mean survival of the cardiac allograft from 9.2 to 14 days. The administration of the anti-Tac-H antibody further increases allograft survival to 20 days; although it cannot do this alone, it may complement the action of other immuno-suppressive agents.

▶ The humanization of murine monoclonal antibody to activation antigens has the theoretical advantage of decreasing neutralization of activity by host development of antimurine antibody. In this monkey cardiac allograft model, humanized antibody had more immunosuppressive effect than mouse monoclonal antibody. Nonetheless, neither had enough effect to be used alone as immunosuppression. These data underscore the need for development of nontoxic immunosuppression and the likely use of multiple agents to achieve adequate immunosuppression.—N.L. Ascher, M.D., Ph.D.

A Randomized Prospective Trial of Anti-TAC Monoclonal Antibody in Human Renal Transplantation
Kirkman RL, Shapiro ME, Carpenter CB, McKay DB, Milford EL, Ramos EL, Tilney NL, Waldmann TA, Zimmerman CE, Strom TB (Brigham and Women's and Beth Israel Hosps, Harvard Med School, Boston; Natl Cancer Inst, Natl Inst of Health, Bethesda, Md)
Transplantation 51:107–113, 1991   13–9

Background.—Researchers continue to search for more effective and less broadly toxic immunosuppressive agents for transplantation. In a previous study of anti-Tac for prevention of rejection in clinical renal transplantation, anti-Tac reduced the frequency of rejection episodes during the treatment period and delayed the time to first rejection episode. Anti-Tac combined with low-dose cyclosporine (CsA), azathioprine, and prednisone was compared with standard-dose cyclosporine-based triple immunotherapy.

Methods.—Recipients of primary cadaver allografts were randomly assigned to receive anti-Tac, 20 mg daily for 10 days beginning day 1 after transplantation, plus low-dose CsA, azathioprine, and prednisone, or conventional triple therapy with a higher dose of CsA. Each group consisted of 40 patients, who were followed for 6 to 26 months.

Results.—Patients in the anti-Tac group had a significant reduction in early rejection episodes. During the 10 days of treatment, 5 anti-Tac–treated patients suffered rejection episodes, compared with 21 control patients. Anti-Tac treatment also significantly delayed time to first rejection; the mean was 12.5 days in the anti-Tac group and 7.6 days in the control group. However, there were no differences in actual or actuarial graft or patient survival between groups. Pneumonia developed in 5 anti-Tac–treated and 4 control patients. In patients with functioning grafts, mean serum creatinine at 3 months was 1.8 and 2 in the anti-Tac and control groups, respectively. The difference between those values continued to be nonsignificant at 12 months. The peak expression of IL-2 receptors on circulating T cells was significantly lower in the anti-Tac group. Seven of 10 tested patients had antimouse immunoglobulin antibodies. Five patients in this and previous anti-Tac studies received OKT3 for acute rejection despite pretreatment antimouse antibodies, with rejection resolution in all cases.

Conclusions.—The prophylactic administration of anti-Tac, a murine monoclonal antibody directed against the human IL-2 receptor, significantly reduces the number of early rejection episodes compared with the standard triple therapy regimen. The overall number of rejection episodes and the number of patients having rejection episodes were also reduced in this series by anti-Tac treatment, although the result was not statistically significant.

▶ The possibility that antigen-activated lymphocytes can be selectively targeted by cytocidal agents directed at the IL-2 receptor has been an interest (obsession?) for years. This study demonstrated that a mouse antibody directed against the alpha chain of the human interleukin-2 receptor can reduce the incidence of early rejection episodes. The effect was not as pronounced as in the similar study of Soulillou et al. (1). In the French study higher doses of corticosteroids were given as adjunctive than in our study. Other first generation murine anti-IL-2 receptor mAbs have had a beneficial effect in liver and bone marrow transplantation, yet the effects fall short of the profound impact that mouse antirat or rat antimouse antibodies deliver in preclinical transplant models. Our own preclinical work has demonstrated that full immunosuppressive effects require use of a "lytic" anti-IL-2R mAb. As in the case of first generation anti-CD4 mAbs, the murine anti-IL-2R antibodies used do not activate human complement or ADCC mechanisms. A fully humanized antibody, now ready for testing, may provide a more potent therapeutic tool. A genetically engineered IL-2 diphtheria toxin-related protein that produces tolerance in murine transplant systems has also entered clinical trials. Initially, this agent was used as a treatment for certain hematopoietic malignancies. However, the drug has shown considerable promise as an immunosuppressive in treatment of methotrexate resistant rheumatoid arthritis and new onset type I diabetes mellitus. Thus, several cytocidal IL-2 receptor-directed therapeutics will soon be available for testing in clinical transplantation.—T. Strom, M.D.

Reference

1. Soulillou JP, et al: *N Engl J Med* 322:1175, 1990.

Use of Yttrium-90-Labeled Anti-Tac Antibody in Primate Xenograft Transplantation
Cooper MM, Robbins RC, Goldman CK, Mirzadeh S, Brechbiel MW, Stone CD, Gansow OA, Clark RE, Waldmann TA (Natl Heart, Lung, and Blood Inst; Natl Cancer Inst, Bethesda, Md)
Transplantation 50:760–765, 1990   13–10

Background.—T cells express interleukin-2 receptor (IL-2R) in the presence of foreign histocompatibility antigens but not normal resting cells. Selective immunosuppression might, therefore, be achieved if the in-

Cardiac Xenograft Survival

Immunosuppression

	None (n=3)	anti-Tac (n=5)	^{90}Y-anti-Tac (n=5)	^{90}Y-UPC-10 (n=4)
Graft survival (days)	6,6,8	2,5,7,8,9	26,32,40,41,53	9,18,23,35
Mean survival (days)	6.7±0.7	6.2±1	38.4±5[a]	21.3±5[b]

*P < .005 vs. no immunosuppression; P < .0005 vs. anti-Tac; P < .025 vs. ^{90}Y-UPC-10.

†P < .05 vs. no immunosuppression; P < .01 vs. anti-Tac.

(Courtesy of Cooper MM, Robbins RC, Goldman CK, et al: *Transplantation* 50:760–765, 1990.)

teraction of IL-2 and IL-2R could be blocked. The use of the murine IgG$_{2a}$ monoclonal antibody, which is specific to IL-2R, with or without yttrium-90, to inhibit rejection in a primate xenograft model was studied.

Methods.—Cardiac xenografts were transplanted from cynomolgus monkey donors to the cervical or abdominal region of rhesus monkey recipients. Group 1 was comprised of 3 animals that received no immunosuppression; group 2 included 5 animals that received unmodified anti-Tac, 2 mg/kg; and group 3 was comprised of 5 animals that received ^{90}Y-anti-Tac, 16 mCi. Four animals, comprising group 4, received the same dose of ^{90}Y bound to UPC-10, another murine monoclonal antibody that does not recognize activated immunoresponsive cells specifically. Immunosuppressive regimens were given in divided doses in the first 2 weeks after transplant.

Results.—Mean rejection time in group 1 was 6.7 days with an increase in soluble IL-2R levels at the time; this indicated generation of Tac-releasing and Tac-expressing cells. Mean survival was 6.2 days in group 2, and that in group 3 averaged 38.4 days. Mean survival was 21.3 days in group 4, but this was significantly less than in group 3, in which half of the radioactive dosage was given in specific fashion by anti-Tac (table). In group 3, the animals had reversible bone marrow supresion without associated toxicity to the kidney or liver, and almost all had antibodies to murine monoclonal.

Conclusion.—[90]Y-anti-Tac therapy directed at IL-2R might have uses in organ transplantation and treatment of neoplastic diseases that express Tac. The inhibitory effect of T suppressor lymphocytes, which are active during acute rejection, appears to be exceeded by the helper/cytotoxic response driven by IL-2. Prolongation of graft survival depends on deleting or killing the activated T cell clones generated, rather than just blocking IL-2R.

14 Cytokines in Allograft Rejection

▶ ↓ Along with increased understanding of the mechanisms of allograft rejection, there is increasing recognition of the role of cytokines in the allograft response. Identification of cytokines is important in diagnosis and particularly in treatment of rejection.—Nancy L. Ascher, M.D., Ph.D.

The Role of Tumor Necrosis Factor in Allograft Rejection: III. Evidence That Anti-TNF Antibody Therapy Prolongs Allograft Survival in Rats With Acute Rejection
Imagawa DK, Millis JM, Seu P, Olthoff KM, Hart J, Wasef E, Dempsey RA, Stephens S, Busuttil RW (Univ of California, Los Angeles School of Medicine; Endogen Corp, Boston; Celltech Ltd, Berkshire, England)
Transplantation 51:57–62, 1991   14–1

Background.—The levels of tumor necrosis factor-alpha (TNF-α) are increased in liver transplant recipients with acute rejection. Studies in a rat model of heterotopic heart transplantation have shown that pretreatment with anti-TNF-α or anti-TNF-β antibodies prolonged graft survival.

Study Design.—Anti-TNF treatment was evaluated in Lewis recipients of cardiac transplants from Buffalo donor rats. Treatment with immunoglobulin G, cyclosporine A, or anti-TNF-α alone or in combination with anti-lymphotoxin (anti-LT) began on postoperative day 4 and was continued for 10 days or until terminal rejection occurred.

Results.—Treatment with both polyclonal anti-TNF-α and polyclonal anti-TNF-β prolonged graft survival nearly as much as cyclosporine. Monoclonal anti-TNF-α was even more effective. Treatment with monoclonal anti-TNF-α combined with cyclosporine extended graft survival to greater than 30 days. In contrast, recombinant TNF-α markedly accelerated graft failure. Histological studies showed that TNF-α increased inflammation, whereas anti-TNF decreased mononuclear-cell infiltration.

Conclusions.—In this model of cardiac heterografting, treatment with a combination of monoclonal anti-TNF-α and low-dose oral cyclosporine forestalled rejection most effectively. This approach could limit the side effects associated with cyclosporine in the clinical setting, and it might also provide more selective immunosuppression.

▶ Cytokines are felt to play a central role in allograft rejection. This group has also shown increased TNF levels in patients with acute allograft rejection, although elevated levels were also seen in patients with viral infections. In these studies, the investigators determine that antibody to TNF is immunosuppressive in a rat cardiac allograft model. These data indicate that antibody to tumor necrosis factor may have ready clinical application. The effect of anti-TNF was additive to the effect of anti-lymphotoxin antibody.—N.L. Ascher, M.D., Ph.D.

Tumor Necrosis Factor, Macrophage Colony-Stimulating Factor, and Interleukin 1 Production Within Sponge Matrix Allografts
Ford HR, Hoffman RA, Wing EJ, Magee DM, McIntyre LA, Simmons RL (Univ of Pittsburgh, Pa)
Transplantation 50:460–466, 1990   14–2

Background.—The rejecting allograft is infiltrated with many different types of cells, such as B and T lymphocytes, monocytes and macrophages, granulocytes, and other inflammatory cells. Research supports the concept that alloimmunity develops initially at the site of the allograft challenge and not in systemic lymphoid depots. Cytokines may play a role in cytotoxic T lymphocyte (CTL) development. The levels of certain cytokines [colony-stimulating factor (CSF), tumor necrosis factor (TNF), and interleukin 1 (IL-1)] in the maturing sponge matrix allograft at various times after grafting were studied.

Methods.—Female BALB/c(H-2^d) mice received implants of polyurethane sponges containing either allogeneic C57BL/6(H-2^d) or syngeneic splenocytes, or splenocyte-free media. At 3, 5, 8, and 13 days after grafting, the sponges were retrieved, and the cells within the grafts were assessed for antidonor cytotoxic activity. The CSF, TNF, and IL-1 levels were measured in the graft exudate fluid.

Findings.—Of the 10^7 allogeneic or syngeneic splenocytes injected into each sponge on day 0, fewer than 10^6 cells were recovered in the grafts after 24 hours, and only 1.4–1.7 million cells were found in the grafts on day 3 postgraft. Cell numbers retrieved increased between days 5 and 8 postgraft, peaking by day 13 in all 3 groups. The cell infiltrates contained mostly polymorphonuclear leukocytes on days 3 and 5 postgraft, and mononuclear cells on day 13 postgraft. Allogeneic grafts harbored significantly greater levels of CSF, TNF, and IL-1 than did the syngeneic or splenocyte-free grafts. Macrophage colony-stimulating factor (M-CSF) was the primary CSF produced in the grafts. The highest TNF levels preceded the highest M-CSF and IL-1 levels. Maximum allospecific CTL activity occurred on day 13, at which time the various cytokine levels were decreasing.

Comment.—Evidence suggests that M-CSF, TNF, and IL-1 may regulate the immunologic events that occur at the site of allograft challenge, but the nature of this regulatory role requires further study.

▶ This study address the regulatory role of cytokines in allograft ejection. Unmodified sponge matrix allografts display significant levels of M-CSF, TNF, and IL-1 relative to syngeneic grafts. Limited by the nonvascular nature of the model, the study nonetheless underscores the potentially important role for cytokine-directed cell activity at the graft site. Modification of cytokine levels has the potential to modify the outcome of the allograft response.—N.L. Ascher, M.D., Ph.D.

Regulation of Alloreactivity In Vivo by IL-4 and the Soluble IL-4 Receptor

Fanslow WC, Clifford KN, Park LS, Rubin AS, Voice RF, Beckmann MP, Widmer MB (Immunex Corp, Seattle, Wash)

J Immunol 147:535–540, 1991   14–3

Background.—Although cytokines are involved in generating alloreactive effector cells in vitro, little is known about their role in vivo. Experiments were done to assess the effects of a soluble ligand-binding form of murine IL-4R (sIL-4R) on survival of heterotopic cardiac allografts and on the lymphoproliferative response to challenge with allogeneic cells.

Methods.—The cDNA encoding both membrane-bound and soluble forms of murine IL-4R were cloned and expressed. Experiments were carried out in female BALB/c and C57BL/6 mice. Hearts from newborn C57BL/6 mice were engrafted in the ear pinnae of BALB/c mice, which were then treated with sIL-4R or mouse serum albumin.

Results.—In BALB/c mice treated with IL-4, the anti-C57BL/6 lymphoproliferative response was slightly augmented compared with that in control mice treated with mouse serum albumin. In mice treated with sIL-4R, the response was suppressed in a dose-dependent way; at a dose of 50 µg/kg/day, the response was nearly completely inhibited. Simultaneous administration of IL-4 reversed the inhibitory effect of sIL-4R. Given at concentrations of 100 to 1,000 times higher than the required amount of sIL-4R, neutralizing antibodies against IL-4 and IL-4R were effective inhibitors. In the heart allograft experiment, grafts in mice treated with sIL-4R survived 4 days longer on the average.

Conclusions.—In vivo alloresponsiveness is inhibited by neutralization of IL-4. The pleiotropic cytokine has a definite regulatory role in allograft rejection, and IL-4 antagonists, alone or combined with other immunosuppressive agents, may have therapeutic value.

▶ Increasing attention has been directed toward the role of cytokines in allograft rejection. This study confirms the role of IL-4 in murine cardiac and skin allograft. The use of a soluble binding form of IL-4 receptor indicates a potential means of preventing rejection.—N.L. Ascher, M.D., Ph.D.

Expression of the Protease Gene HF as a Marker in Rejecting Allogeneic Murine Heart Transplants

Mueller C, Shelby J, Weissman IL, Périnat-Frey T, Eichwald EJ (Univ of Bern, Switzerland; Univ of Utah; Stanford Univ)

Transplantation 51:514–517, 1991.   14–4

Background.—The cells that infiltrate allografts appear to be attracted nonspecifically to the graft; therefore, cell type cannot be used to determine the fate of the graft. Identification of functional effectors of allograft rejection would be extremely useful. One serine protease, HF or granzyme A, appears to be involved in cytolysis and may be a useful marker. The expression of the HF gene was compared in cells infiltrating both allogeneic and syngeneic heart transplants in mice.

Results.—In syngeneic heart transplants, cells expressing the HF gene were detected rarely throughout the entire 10-day posttransplant observation period. However, in allogeneic transplants that eventually were rejected, high numbers of HF-positive cells could be detected as early as the second day after transplantation.

Conclusion.—Expression of HF in cells infiltrating allografts may provide a reliable indication of graft outcome. As an antibody to human HF has been produced recently, this may have clinical significance.

▶ Expression of the gene for serum protease, HF, in cells infiltrating cardiac allografts, predicts for rejection. This may prove an early marker for rejection, although its presence in the absence of tissue may not be accepted until further confirmation is obtained. More importantly, the identification of HF may provide the basis for immunosuppression through antibody to granzyme A.—N.L. Ascher, M.D., Ph.D.

15 Xenotransplantation

▶ ↓ Interest has been rekindled in the field of xenotransplantation as donor organs become more scarce and more patient immunosuppressive drugs are discovered. These articles attempt to delineate mechanisms of xenotransplant rejection and potential therapies.—Nancy L. Ascher, M.D., Ph.D.

Induction of Long-Term Survival of Hamster Heart Xenografts in Rats
van den Bogaerde J, Aspinall R, Wang M-W, Cary N, Lim S, Wright L, White D
(Cambridge University; Quadrant Research Foundation, Cambridge, England)
Transplantation 52:15–20, 1991   15–1

Introduction.—Generally, graft survival is more difficult to achieve across a concordant xenogeneic than an allogeneic barrier. In rodent models, allograft survival was extended by in vivo treatment of recipients with monoclonal antibodies to the CD4 molecule. The effect of specific T-cell immunosuppression on survival of vascularized hamster heart xenografts in rats was investigated.

Methods.—Syrian hamster hearts were grafted into the necks of rats, joining the aorta to the carotid artery and the pulmonary artery to the jugular vein. Monoclonal antibodies were selected which recognize the overlapping epitopes of the rat CD4 molecule, that bind to the rat CD8 molecule, and which recognize an epitope on all rat T-cell receptors. Animals were also treated with cobra-venom factor, which has been shown to deplete complement in vivo combined with CsA. The CH50 assay, which measures antihamster lytic antibody levels, and immunohistochemistry studies were performed.

Results.—Depletion of CD4-positive T cells in recipients did not extend survival of the xenograft, nor did survival improve by suppression of T-cell immunity using the other monoclonal antibodies or cyclosporine. Xenograft survival was prolonged only by depletion of complement with cobra-venom factor. After transplantation, the rats showed high-antibody titers to hamster cells. Xenograft rejection appeared to be mediated mainly by antibody-complement mechanisms. The production of antihamster antibodies without T-cell help suggested that suppression or depletion of T cells could not inhibit antibody-mediated destruction of the graft.

Conclusion.—Rejection of concordant organ grafts may depend on antibody complement-mediated mechanisms. It will be difficult to inhibit antibody production to concordant xenogeneic transplants in human beings merely by suppressing T-cell immunity. Inclusion of complement-depleting agents such as cobra-venom factor should be considered in therapy for concordant xenografting.

▶ This study represents an increasing interest and knowledge regarding xenotransplantation. Although transplantation between concordant species does not result in hyperacute rejection, successful outcome can only be achieved using agents to deplete complement in combination with cyclosporine. Monoclonal antibodies to deplete CD4 and/or CD8 cells did not have an impact on xenotransplant survival. The antibody response in concordant combinations is important despite the absence of naturally occurring xenoantibodies. For this antibody, titers rise rapidly after transplantation. Insufficient organs move the transplantation community toward the use of xenotransplants. These data indicated that the use of concordant series to take advantage of the lack of naturally occurring xenoantibodies will not obviate the need for anti-antibody treatment.—N.L. Ascher, M.D., Ph.D.

Prevention of Xenograft Rejection by Masking Donor HLA Class I Antigens
Faustman D, Coe C (Massachusetts Gen Hosp, Boston)
Science 252:1700–1702, 1991   15–2

Introduction.—Activation of cytotoxic T cells (CTLs) underlies the xenogeneic response leading to rejection of transplants, and presumably to

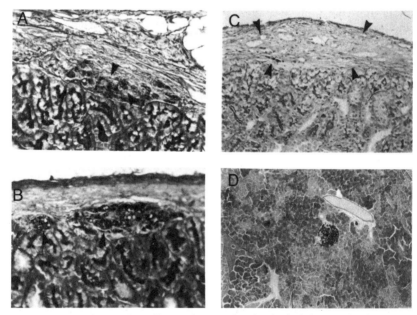

Fig 15–1.—Histologic analysis of human islets transplanted under the kidney capsule of BALB/c recipients. A, human islet xenograft 30 days after implantation of islets that had been treated with W6/32 F(ab')$_2$ fragments. The aldehyde-fuchsin stain (×212) shows well-granulated islets under the kidney capsule. B, human islet xenograft 200 days after implantation of islets that had been treated with W6/32 F(ab')$_2$ fragments. Well-granulated islets are present under the kidney capsule. C, a control BALB/c mouse was transplanted with untreated fresh human islets and then killed at day 30. No donor islets can be detected, but subcapsular fibrosis in the area where the islets were transplanted is apparent. D, aldehyde-fuchsin stain of a mouse islet in the mouse pancreas, demonstrating the characteristic purple granulation of healthy β cells. (Courtesy of Faustman D, Coe C: *Science* 252:1700–1702, 1991.)

autoimmune rejection of tissues. Many methods of interfering with T cell–target cell adhesion have produced recipient immune responses that interfere with treatment. An alternative approach is to treat the target cell to avoid T-cell adhesion and activation, precluding the need to treat the host.

Methods.—This approach was used to conceal HLA class I antigens on pancreatic islets before their transplantation. Human islets lack large amounts of 2 adhesion epitopes, and for this reason there is less of a need to conceal them from CTLs. Thus, the HLA class I antigens become the chief candidates for masking. Mice were given transplants of human islets treated with antibody to HLA class I, polyclonal antibodies to islet cells, or antibody to CD29.

Results.—Treatment of donor xenogeneic islets with antibody to HLA class I led to total survival of the islets (Fig 15–1). Large islet clusters were well granulated. Untreated islets were rejected within 1 week. It appeared necessary to remove the Fc domain from the antibody to circumvent complement lysis. Mice given islets coated with HLA class I antibody had increased C peptide levels. Immunofluorescence studies confirmed that prolonged islet survival resulted from antigen masking by F(ab')$_2$ fragments of the antibody.

Conclusion.—Concealing foreign HLA class I determinants permits prolonged survival of islet xenografts without the need to treat the recipient. An intact immune system is preserved.

▶ These data confirm the importance of MHC class I antigen in eliciting xenograft rejection. Faustman has previously studied the role of MHC class II in islet allograft rejection. It is noteworthy that xenoantibody plays no apparent role in the response to xenogeneic islets. Islets have been found to be deficient in adhesion molecules. It may be under that setting that class I antigen assumes a greater role.—N.L. Ascher, M.D., Ph.D.

An ELISA Assay for Xenoreactive Natural Antibodies
Platt JL, Turman MA, Noreen HJ, Fischel RJ, Bolman RM III, Bach FH (Univ of Minnesota, Minneapolis)
Transplantation 49:1000–1001, 1990   15–3

Introduction.—Antibodies that react against xenogeneic tissue may serve as important factors in initiation of interspecies hyperacute rejection. The presence and quantity of natural antibodies are usually measured by hemagglutination or lymphocytotoxicity methods. Porcine endothelial cells are recognized by human natural antibodies. An immunoassay using cultured porcine aortic endothelial cells as the target for human and nonhuman primate natural antibodies was evaluated.

Methods.—Aortic endothelial cells from pigs were cultured and used within 7 days of plating. Pooled sera from normal persons and from rhesus monkeys were assayed. The porcine aortic endothelial cells in plate wells were washed and diluted serially with PSA buffer. The secondary antibody in the assay consisted of goat antihuman IgM conjugated to alkaline phosphatase or goat antihuman (Ig) similarly conjugated.

Results.—Using the anti-IgM reagent, an essentially linear titration with an absorbance at a dilution of 1:1024 was demonstrated. Results of 6 experiments using pooled human sera and 7 experiments with individual human sera demonstrated positive reactions even at a dilution of 1:256. The reactivity of the porcine serum, however, was not significantly higher than background. In the experiment using the natural circulation of a rhesus monkey by placing porcine kidneys onto an arteriovenous shunt, the natural antibodies in the circulation decreased significantly after only 10 minutes. After 30 minutes, the natural antibodies virtually disappeared from the circulation. Later, with or without any following transplants, the natural antibodies returned as demonstrated by the enzyme-linked immunosorbent assay.

Conclusion.—These findings support the use of this assay as a sensitive method for natural antibodies that are considered participants in the organ transplant rejection.

▶ A reliable assay for xenoreactive natural antibodies may be important in the development of xenotransplantation. This ELISA assay will allow for ready monitoring of the efficacy of systems used to remove these antibodies. The cellular response to the xenograft will also require specialized survey; this area awaits development.—N.L. Ascher, M.D., Ph.D.

Production of Marked Prolongation of Islet Xenograft Survival (Rat to Mouse) by Local Release of Mouse and Rat Antilymphocyte Sera at Transplant Site
Aebischer P, Lacy PE, Gerasimidi-Vazeou A, Hauptfeld V (Brown Univ, Providence, RI; Washington Univ, St Louis)
Diabetes 40:482–485, 1991   15–4

Introduction.—Rejection of rat islet xenografts can be prevented by low-temperature culture of donor rat islets, by alteration of antigen-presenting cells, and by the injection of mouse (M) and rat (R) antilymphocyte sera (ALS). The RALS were found to damage and destroy islet cells, however. Polymer rods were used to incorporate the lypholized MALS or RALS particles, which were implanted in the kidney capsule next to the islet grafts. This system allowed for the slow release of ALS.

Methods.—Male Wistar-Furth rats provided the islets. Diabetes was induced in male C57BL/B6 mice through streptozocin injection. The donor islets were cultured and then transplanted in the diabetic mice. The animals' diabetic states were evaluated by monitoring nonfasting plasma glucose levels. The MALS or RALS, in the form of a fine powder, was impregnated into the polymer rods, which were then implanted under the kidney capsule before islet transplantation.

Results.—Control polymer rods without ALS had no effect on islet graft survival. Neither the MALS- nor the RALS-impregnated polymer rods prolonged graft survival. When the MALS and the RALS rods were used at the transplant site, allograft survival was significantly prolonged compared with that in controls. When the rods were implanted containing a slightly higher (30%) concentration of either MALS or RALS, a further significant prolongation of graft survival occurred. One animal in this last experiment remained normoglycemic at 100 days. Histologic studies determined that the tissue reaction to the rods remained minimal. The mean survival time of grafts was significantly greater in animals in which the MALS or RALS rods were implanted in the same kidney next to the islet groups, rather than under the opposite kidney.

Conclusion.—Marked prolongation of rat islet xenograft survival can occur during the local release of MALS or RALS at the transplantation site. The polymer rods can be coated with various layers of pure polymer, thereby further slowing the release of RALS or MALS to provide indefinite xenograft survival.

▶ This study is another demonstration of the potential usefulness of local immunosuppression and the possibility of separating local from systemic immunity. The application to human transplantation will depend on the development of a reliable method of drug delivery.—N.L. Ascher, M.D., Ph.D.

16 Role of MHC Antigen Expression and Mechanisms of Rejection

▶ ↓ It has been widely assumed that cytokine-induced expression of class II major histocompatibility complex (MHC) molecules would always incite increased immunologic activity against the organ. Hence, it is of considerable interest to note in the report of Shoskes et al. (Abstract 16–1) that acute tubular necrosis results in increased MHC antigen expression on the ischemic kidney. Before we conclude that increased MHC expression is always harmful, it is important to recognize that antigen recognition is only the first, albeit prerequisite, step in T-cell activation. Other co-stimulatory signals provided by antigen-presenting cells (APC) are also needed to stimulate T cells into the full activation state that is associated with stable transcription of the IL-2 gene. Indeed, if immunologically virgin T cells are stimulated with antigen in the absence of co-stimulatory mitogenic signals, they become paralyzed. Thus, it is with extreme interest that I read the two articles by Halttunen (Abstracts 16–2 and 16–3). He points out that purified renal cellular components fail to incite allograft immunity in vitro. This work, which may seem counterintuitive, in fact makes a great deal of sense. This work imparts a message similar to that delivered in a series of articles dealing with tissue-specific "foreign" MHC class II expression on nonlymphoid tissues. When these MHC class II-expressing parenchymal tissues do not have APC capacity, the transgenic mouse is rendered anergic to the MHC component expressed solely on parenchymal cells. In this regard, it is also interesting to note that Larsen et al. (Abstract 16–4) have found that dendritic cells, an extremely potent APC, failed to migrate from the blood into tissue allografts. This work would infer that the hematopoietic elements that are contained in the allograft may be totally responsible for immunogenicity. Dendritic cells cannot be recruited from the circulating blood.— Terry Strom, M.D.

Increased Major Histocompatibility Complex Antigen Expression in Unilateral Ischemic Acute Tubular Necrosis in the Mouse
Shoskes DA, Parfrey NA, Halloran PF (University of Alberta, Edmonton, Canada)
Transplantation 49:201–207, 1990   16–1

Background.—Although acute tubular necrosis (ATN) predisposes to a higher rate of graft loss in kidney transplant recipients, the mechanism is unknown. This observation may be related to increased immunogenicity of the graft. A mouse model of ischemic ATN was used to study expression of major histocompatibility complex (MHC) antigens in kidneys damaged by ischemia.

Methods.—Acute tubular necrosis was induced in the left kidney of male CBA mice by clamping the vascular pedicle for 15, 45, or 60 minutes. After 1 day to 35 days, class I and II MHC expression was quantified by the extent of binding of the monoclonals in radioimmunoassay. Indirect immunoperoxidase staining was done to localize MHC induction, and Northern blot analysis using ^{32}P-labeled probes was done to quantify specific steady state messenger RNA for β-2 microglobulin and class II MHC. The injured left kidney and control right kidney were compared to evaluate the changes in MHC expression.

Results.—Histological signs of ATN were present at 1 day, but changes in MHC expression were not. However, by day 3, class I MHC expression was increased threefold to sixfold in the injured kidney, compared with the uninjured kidney. The increase in class I expression was localized to the tubular epithelial cells. Class II expression was increased by 1.5 times to 3 times in the ischemic kidney beginning on day 7 and continuing to day 35. This increase was seen not only in the interstitial cells, but also in the primary cells; it was associated with the expression of Thy 1.2-positive cells in the interstitial area. Increased steady state mRNA was noted before antigen expression increased.

Conclusions.—Studies in mice suggest that unilateral ischemic ATN increases MHC expression in tubular cells and causes accumulation of an inflammatory infiltrate. Both of these changes may play a role in the increased incidence of rejection and graft loss in kidneys with ischemic injury. These changes might be part of a greater process in which the host responds to tissue injury by inflammatory cell accumulation and cytokine release, probably through non-T cells.

▶ Excessive graft loss has been noted by many centers in patients with postoperative ATN. This loss has been attributed to rejection mediated injury. This study documents increased tubular MHC expression in the injured kidney in a unilateral ATN model. A quick "read" of this scenario supports the notion that this increase in antigenicity causes the kidney to become rejection prone. I favor an alternative nonimmunologic interpretation. Kidneys damaged by ATN are less able to withstand rejection than a normal kidney afflicted with an equal dose of rejection. Increased expression of tubular MHC may not automatically render the tissue more immunogenic because the increase in antigenicity is not necessarily accompanied by parallel changes (i.e., expression of LFA-3, IL-6, etc.) that allow the kidney to deliver comotogenic signals.—T. Strom, M.D.

Failure of Rat Kidney Nephron Components to Induce Allogeneic Lymphocytes to Proliferate in Mixed Lymphocyte Kidney Cell Culture
Halttunen J (Helsinki University Central Hospital, Finland)
Transplantation 50:481–487, 1990   16–2

Background.—In previous studies of mixed lymphocyte kidney cell culture (MLKC), in both animals and humans, dissociated cells evoked a lymphoproliferative response when mixed with allogeneic lymphocytes, though weaker than allogeneic lymphocytes. Human kidney cells were poor allostimulators even after treatment with γ-interferon (gIFN). The ability of isolated rat kidney cells to induce proliferation of allogeneic spleen lymphocytes in MLKC was investigated.

Methods.—After Wistar Furth rat glomerular mesangial, glomerular epithelial, and tubular epithelial cells were isolated in nearly pure form in culture, MLKC assays were done. The responses were compared with those induced by allogeneic endothelial cells or spleen lymphocytes in the same strain combination. Some of the stimulator cells were treated with gIFN, which increases the MHC class II and class I expression of the stimulator cells.

Results.—The isolated nephron components were incapable of inducing lymphoproliferation in the MLKC. On the other hand, in mixed lymphocyte endothelial cell cultures (MLEC), rat heart endothelial cells and allogeneic spleen cells strongly induced lymphoproliferation. Although gIFN treatment caused an obvious antiproliferative effect, endothelial cells treated with gIFN had an effect comparable to that of native cells in MLEC.

Conclusions.—Kidney parenchymal cells appear incapable of functioning on their own as antigen-presenting cells; however, they are known to be immunogenic in vivo. Although they express class II antigens, these cells appear to serve only as targets for cytotoxic T cells.

▶ All cells were not created equal in their ability to elicit an immune response. This fascinating study demonstrates that a mixture of cultured allogeneic glomerular epithelial, glomerular mesangial, and tubular epithelial cells are weak immunogens. Following incubation with gamma-interferon, expression of class II MHC molecules is enhanced, but these cells still fail to stimulate allogeneic T cells. Why? Antigen is necessary but not sufficient to stimulate T-cell proliferation. A second co-stimulatory signal derived from certain cytokines or T-cell protein to stimulating cell protein interactions are required to stimulate T-cell proliferation. Provision of antigen alone actually anergizes or paralyzes the responding T cells. One conclusion to be derived from this analysis is that cultured kidney parenchymal cells do not deliver a co-stimulatory signal. My guess is that they actually paralyze the responding T cell in a state of anergy. What causes rejection? The cellular components that were lacking from intact allografts are endothelial cells and passenger leukocytes. Both of these cell types are able to deliver co-stimulatory signals. Nonetheless, this work calls attention again to the importance that passenger leukocytes are likely to play in stimulating rejection. In the works are plans to destroy passenger leukocytes at the time of transplantation to diminish graft antigenicity. At least one pilot trial using anti-CD45 mAbs showed considerable promise.—T. Strom, M.D.

Immunogenicity of Rat Renal Allograft Nephron Components In Vivo: Lack of Correlation Between MHC Expression and Immunogenic Potential
Halttunen J (University of Helsinki, Finland)
Transplantation 50:150–155, 1990   16–3

Background.—Immunogenicity is the property of a substance or cell to induce an immune response, or, in transplantation, to induce rejection. The in vivo immunogenicity of cultured rat nephron components and of cultured rat heart endothelial cells was compared using the primed rejection assay.

Methods.—Rat tubular cells, glomerular mesangial cells, and glomerular epithelial cells were compared with rat heart endothelial cells. Gamma interferon (gIFN) was used to regulate the class I and II major histocompatibility complex antigen expression of the cells.

Results.—The heart endothelial cells were the only cell type able to induce a maximal rejection response in the native state, achieved with a cell number of 10^6 when the survival of a subsequent heart allograft from a relevant donor was decreased from 5 to 3 days. All the kidney nephron components were immunogenic in the primed rejection assay but not nearly as much as the endothelial cells. With a cell number of 10^6 cells, graft survival was reduced from 5 to 4 days, with no immunogenic effect in smaller cell numbers. The gIFN-treated endothelial cells were more potent than endothelial cells that were not treated. They decreased graft survival to 4 days with a cell number of 10^3. They also cause a maximal decrease in survival to 3 days, with a cell number of 10^5. The nephron components did not increase their immunogenicity after 3 days of gIFN treatment, irrespective of a high elevation in their class I and II expression rates.

Conclusions.—In contrast to endothelial cells, none of the nephron components studied appears capable of acting as an antigen-presenting cell on its own. In vitro experiments using mixed kidney cell lymphocyte culture conditions are needed to clarify this issue. The ability of the nephron components to produce interleukin-1 must also be assessed.

Failure of Mature Dendritic Cells to the Host to Migrate From the Blood Into Cardiac or Skin Allografts
Larsen CP, Barker H, Morris PJ, Austyn JM (University of Oxford, John Radcliffe Hospital, Oxford, England)
Transplantation 50:294–301, 1990   16–4

Background.—The exact location of sensitization after transplantation is unknown. It has been assumed that sensitization to skin grafts occurs centrally in the draining lymph nodes. However, sensitization to fully vascularized organs is believed to occur peripherally within the graft itself. In previous work the authors showed that mature dendritic cells (DC) migrate from the blood into the spleens of normal mice in a T cell–

dependent fashion, which suggests that circulating host dendritic leukocytes may be recruited from the blood into allografts where T cells accumulated. This would suggest peripheral sensitization after transplantation.

Methods and Results.—Whether [111]indium-labeled mature DC of host strain could migrate from the blood into cardiac or skin grafts was studied. Migration into either allografts or isografts of these tissues could not be detected. Instead, the cells migrated to the spleen as in unmanipulated animals. This occurred even though accumulation of resting T cells was readily shown in cardiac or skin allografts. In addition, T cells sensitized against donor or third-party alloantigens had equal access to cardiac allografts, which suggests that their migration into transplants is independent of their antigen specificity.

Conclusions.—Mature host strain DC do not have access to cardiac or skin grafts when the animal is becoming sensitized to graft antigens, even though T cells have entry to these sites. Allograft rejection may be mainly initiated centrally in host lymphoid tissues.

Tolerogenic Ability of Thymocytes in Organ-Cultured Thymus Lobes

Matsuhashi N, Kawase Y, Suzuki G (National Institute of Radiological Sciences, Anagawa, Japan)
J Immunol 146:444–448, 1991   16–5

Background.—There is increasing evidence that interactions between T cell receptors on developing thymocytes and major histocompatibility complex (MHC) molecules on stromal thymic cells are critical in both positive and negative selections of thymocytes.

Objective.—To assess the tolerogenic ability of thymic thymocytes, Thy-1 bright developing thymocytes were colonized into allogenic thymus glands in vitro. It was then determined whether precursor cytotoxic T lymphocytes in the thymic lobes were tolerant to class I MHC molecules of the donor haplotype.

Findings.—Thymocytes recovered from repopulated thymic lobes were tolerant to class I, but not to class II MHC of the donor haplotype, suggesting that class I molecules expressed on the thymocytes acted as tolerogen. In those thymic lobes made parabiotic from day 5, the cytotoxic T lymphocytes were tolerant to class I, but not to class II MHC.

Conclusions.—The interactions among developing thymocytes are apparently sufficient to induce class I tolerance of cytotoxic T lymphocytes.

▶ The mechanisms by which interaction between T-cell receptor and MHC molecules positively and negatively select within the thymus are addressed by this group. Although macrophages and dendritic cells have been thought to be the essential cells in negative selection, Thy-1 bright cells expressing class I molecules can act as tolerogens.—N.L. Ascher, M.D., Ph.D.

Failure of Cell Surface Expression of a Class I Major Histocompatibility Antigen Caused by Somatic Point Mutation

Zeff RA, Nakagawa M, Mashimo H, Gopas J, Nathenson SG (Univ of Connecticut, Farmington; Albert Einstein College of Medicine, Bronx, NY)

Transplantation 49:803–808, 1990

16–6

Introduction.—Cell survival may be expected to improve if the cells involved could down-regulate the expression of their major histocompatibility complex class I antigen on the allografts before the actual transplantation procedure. Characterization of the molecular basis for the attenuated MHC class I gene expression could provide an understanding of how tumor cells are not detected by the immune system. The authors have characterized the H-2K^b surface null somatic cell variants derived from an H-2 heterozygous tumor cell line (H2^b × H-2^d) to determine the genetic mechanisms responsible for the attenuation of the MHC class I antigen expression.

Methods.—Cytotoxic T cells that act against H-2K^b were produced by immunization of BALB.G mice. The live cells were harvested after 5 days and then grown in culture. A genomic DNA library was prepared and the mutant H-2K^b gene was cloned, and its DNA was sequenced using genomic DNA hybridization analysis and transfection and cytofluorometric methodologies.

Results.—The parental cell lines were efficiently lysed by the primary CTL at many killer target ratios; however, this type of cell killing was not seen for the variant cell line. The mutant H-2K^b gene was successfully transfected into the L cells. Analysis of these H-2K^b mRNA-positive clones demonstrated no detectable expression of the H-2K^b antigen on the surface of the cells. The H-2K^b antigen was detected on the cell surface of L cells transfected with the wild-type H-2K^b gene. The complete coding sequence (exons 1–8) of the mutant H-2K^b gene showed only a single nucleotide change (G→A transition) that caused a TGC conversion to TAC at codon 164, which produced an RsaI restriction enzyme site (GTGC→GTAC).

Conclusion.—The anti-H-2K monoclonal antibody 5F1.2.14 did not react with this mutant H-2K^b molecule, probably because of the profound nature of this mutation. In addition, a genetic event as small as a single somatic point mutation can eliminate the expression of an MHC class I antigen. Protein folding is important in the cell surface expression of the MHC class I molecules.

▶ Although most approaches to immunosuppression involve modification of the host, another avenue involves modification of donor immunogenicity. This study demonstrates decreased immunogenicity of mutant cells that fail to express MHC class I antigen. The challenge will be to achieve decreased MHC antigen expression without compromising the function of cells and organs.—N.L. Ascher, M.D., Ph.D.

Reassociation With β₂-Microglobulin is Necessary for Kᵇ Class I Major Histocompatibility Complex Binding of Exogenous Peptides

Rock KL, Rothstein LE, Gamble SR, Benacerraf B (Dana-Farber Cancer Inst, Boston; Harvard Med School, Boston)

Proc Natl Acad Sci USA 87:7517–7521, 1990   16–7

Background.—Cytotoxic T lymphocytes recognize endogenous antigenic peptides in association with major histocompatibility complex (MHC)-encoded molecules. Peptides in the extracellular fluid are associated with class I and class II MHC molecules. Although there is considerable similarity in the peptide motifs that bind to these 2 sets of molecules, there are marked operational differences in the way peptides bind to class I and class II MHC molecules.

Observations.—Cell culture studies showed that mature Kᵇ class I MHC molecules bind peptides when their light chains are dissociated and reassociated. Unlike class II MHC molecules, intact Kᵇ heterodimers were not very receptive to binding peptides. Exogenous β₂-microglobulin strongly influenced the association of peptides with Kᵇ molecules.

Conclusions.—The differences in how peptides bind to class I and class II MHC molecules may help maintain segregation of class I and class II MHC-restricted peptides. Class I MHC molecules appear to be relatively nonreceptive to exogenous peptides in vivo because the level of free β₂-microglobulin is low.

► These data indicate that MHC class I molecules are relatively resistant to exogenous peptide binding and may be closely linked to free β₂ microglobulin in the media. With higher levels of free β₂ microglobulin, binding is enhanced. An alternative pathway involving incorporation of peptide into the cell with de novo synthesis of MHC class I and binding may also operating. These data are important in understanding the differences in response related to class I versus class II molecules.—N.L. Ascher, M.D., Ph.D.

Mutations Affecting Antigen Processing Impair Class II-Restricted Allorecognition

Cotner T, Mellins E, Johnson AH, Pious D (Univ of Washington, Seattle; Georgetown Univ)

J Immunol 146:414–417, 1991   16–8

Background.—The major histocompatibility complex (MHC) class I and class II proteins function as carrier molecules for antigens (Ag) that interact with T cells in the form peptide-MHC complexes. Several B cell mutants were characterized that could not present intact protein Ag to MHC class II-restricted T cells even though these B cell mutants presented antigenic peptides normally. The ability of alloreactive T cells to recognize the MHC class II molecules on the Ag processing and presentation defective mutants was examined.

Methods.—The Ag-processing mutants 9.5.3 and 9.10.3 were selected from B lymphoblastoid cell lines for the loss of a polymorphic determinant defined by monoclonal antibody 16.23. B-cell surface markers were quantitatively assessed on a fluorescence-activated cell sorter. Four DR3-specific T cell clones were derived and characterized and their proliferation measured.

Results.—Three alloreactive anti-DR3-specific clones were produced by either repeated stimulation in vitro using an HLA-DR3 β lymphoblastoid cell line or by a mixed lymphocyte reaction. T cells were cloned by limiting dilution. Four of these clones were specific for DR3β chains. Both of the Ag presentation mutants tested (9.5.3 and 9.10.3) could not stimulate the 3 T-cell clones specific for DR3β1, while the fourth clone (C6) was stimulated by both presentation-defective antigen processing cells. The inability of the presentation-defective antigen processing cells to stimulate the 3 DR3β 1 allospecific clones appeared to be an absolute characteristic. The failure of the mutants to stimulate the DR3β 1 allospecific clones was not related to the loss of expression of accessory molecules ICAM-1 or LFA-3 because the levels of these 2 molecules remained equivalent in progenitor and mutant cells.

Discussion.—A link has been established between the ability of stimulator cells to produce class II-peptide complexes and their ability to be recognized by some class II-restricted alloreactive T cells. The inability of the β-cell mutants to stimulate 3 of 4 alloreactive T-cell clones suggests that polymorphic residues in the class II protein molecules alone cannot initiate all alloreactive T cells. It is possible that a peptide could participate directly in allorecognition or indirectly through the effect of peptide binding on the class II molecular conformation.

Heterogeneity of CD4[+] T Cells Involved in Anti-Allo-Class I H-2 Immune Responses: Functional Discrimination Between the Major Proliferating Cells and Helper Cells Assisting Cytotoxic T Cell Responses

Kitagawa S, Sato S, Azuma T, Shimizu J, Hamaoka T, Fujiwara H (Osaka University Medical School, Japan)
J Immunol 146:2513–2521, 1991   16–9

Background.—Immune responses to alloantigens begin with the recognition of alloantigens by Th cells. Three distinct Th paths exist for activating anti-allo cytotoxic T-lymphocyte (CTL) precursors, and at least 2 subsets of Th function to start immune responses to class I H-2 alloantigens.

Objective.—A single intravenous presensitization with class I H-2 disparate allogeneic cells was examined for its effects on the ability of CD8[+] and CD4[+] Th to proliferate and produce interleukin-2 (IL-2), to aid CTL responses, and to initiate graft rejection in various class I H-2 disparate combinations. Several strains of mice were used in the studies.

Observations.—Administration of class I-disparate allogeneic spleen cells nearly abrogated the anti-class I proliferative ability of both CD4[+] and CD8[+] cells. There also was a marked reduction in ability to produce

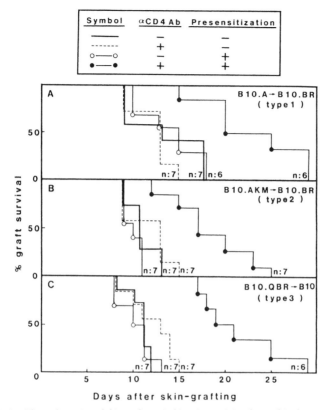

Fig 16–1.—The prolongation of skin graft survival in mice receiving the combined treatment in various types of class I H-2-disparate combinations. Mice received skin grafts 2 weeks after initiation of treatment. Three distinct types of combinations were used: **A**, type 1 (B10.BR anti-B10.A); **B**, type 2 (B10.BR anti-B10.AKM); and **C**, type 3 (B10 anti-B10.QBR). (Courtesy of Kitagawa S, Sato S, Azuma T, et al: *J Immunol* 146:2513–2521, 1991.)

IL-2 after stimulation with relevant class I alloantigens. Nevertheless these animals were able to mount graft rejection responses comparable to those induced by nonpresensitized mice. Graft survival was prolonged when anti-CD4 antibody was given to presensitized mice (Fig 16–1).

Discussion.—These findings demonstrate functional heterogeneity in CD4$^+$ T cells responding to allo-class I H-2 antigen. Some cells proliferate strongly and produce lymphokine. Others lack proliferative capacity but can support graft rejection and CTL responses. Studies in progress are intended to show whether the exact allo-class I target antigens recognized by functionally distinct CD4$^+$ T cells are the same or different.

▶ These authors provide further evidence of distinct helper subsets. The differentiation of CD4$^+$ cells into a Th1 and Th2 subset is taken a step further with the identification of cells of varying capacity to proliferate and to produce lymphokines in response to class I antigen stimulation.—N.L. Ascher, M.D., Ph.D.

Cellular Basis of Skin Allograft Rejection Across a Class I Major Histocompatibility Barrier in Mice Depleted of CD8$^+$ T Cells In Vivo

Rosenberg AS, Munitz TI, Maniero TG, Singer A (Ctr for Biologics Evaluation and Research, Food and Drug Administration; Natl Insts of Health, Bethesda, Md)

J Exp Med 173:1463–1471   16–10

Introduction.—Skin allograft rejection often results from the large tissue injury caused by immunocompetent cytolytic T cells responding to the allogeneic histocompatibility of the antigens produced from the graft itself. The rejection of major histocompatibility complex (MHC) class I disparate skin grafts in mice results from the action of CD8$^+$ cells lacking CD4$^+$ T cells. An attempt was made to identify the cellular mechanisms whereby mice without CD8$^+$T cells reject the MHC class I disparate skin grafts.

Methods.—Experimental CD8$^-$ mice underwent depletion of CD8$^+$ cells through adult thymectomy (ATX) followed by the in vivo treatment with anti-CD8 monoclonal antibody (mAb). The anti-CD8 mAb was produced in the hybridoma cell line 2.43, a rat IgG$_{2b}$ antibody. Mice received the skin grafts within 3 weeks of antibody depletion.

Results.—The spleen cell populations from mice that rejected the B10.YBR skin grafts did not demonstrate any CD8$^+$T cells. The CD8$^-$ B6.K1 and B6.T1a^a mice rejected the bm1 skin grafts, but the CD8$^-$ B6 animals did not reject these grafts. All 3 strains of mice rejected the B10.YBR skin grafts. The bm1-specific effector cells from the untreated B6.K1 mice are CD8$^+$, based on their elimination by anti-CD8 and C' treatment. The cytolytic T lymphocyte (CTL)-mediating anti-bm1 activity of the CD8$^-$ B6.K1 mice appeared as CD8$^+$ also. In contrast to normal mice, the bm1-specific CTL in the CD8$^-$ mice remained after the addition of the anti-CD8 mAb to the effector cell culture. The CD8$^-$ mice produced CD8$^+$ effector cells specific for the B10.YBR and the bm1 target cells, but the bm1 and the B10.YBR specific CTL effectors were not blocked by the anti-CD8 mAb. The alloantigens co-expressed on the MCH class I disparate grafts related to graft rejection in the CD8-depleted animals could be MCH-linked or not. The alloantigens operated as activators to third-party specific CD4$^+$ helper (Th) cells to generate CD8$^+$ anti-CD8 resistant CTL effector cells.

Conclusion.—Mice without CD8$^+$ cells have a group of unique precursor cells that can produce anti-CD8 resistant CD8$^+$ effector cells. These effector cells can mediate the anti-MHC class I responses both in vivo and in vitro, although they need third-party Th cells to accomplish this.

▶ This study attests to the myriad of pathways by which allograft rejection can occur. Modification of the host to inhibit a given pathway may elucidate the presence of a separate pathway. It is noteworthy that methods used to deplete a host of CD8$^+$ cells (thymectomy and monoclonal antibody) leave a subset of functionally active CD8$^+$ cells. The relative importance of this cell group in the context of the intact host remains unclear.—N.L. Ascher, M.D., Ph.D.

Dissociation of Tissue Destruction Induced by Cytolytic T Cells in Vivo and Cytotoxicity as Measured In Vitro

Steinmuller D, Snider ME, Noble RL, Waldschmidt TJ (Univ of Iowa, Iowa City)
Transplantation 50:663–668, 1990   16–11

Introduction.—The transfer reaction (TrR) and the bystander reaction (ByR) have been used to assay the local cutaneous graft-vs.-host reaction. Both TrR and ByR are induced by CD8$^+$ T cells. These 2 reactions were used to assay the in vivo activity of cytolytic T cells in several antigen systems and mouse strain combinations.

Methods.—Inbred mouse strains were used for both reactions. The cytotoxic T-lymphocyte (CTL) specific for both MHC and non-MHC antigens were generated. In the immune lymphocyte TrRs, the CTLs were injected intradermally into allogenic hosts to which they had been sensitized. In the ByRs, the CTLs were combined with target cells and the mixture injected into hosts syngeneic to the CTL.

Results.—The in vitro assays of the CTLs did not predict of the ability of the CTLs to induce ulcerative TrRs and ByRs. All the TrRs induced by the CTLs increased to grade 5+, but the SL values for the 17 CTL effector groups ranged from 0% to 71%. The incidence and severity of ByRs varied from strain to strain, indicating that the ByR induced by CTL is under genetic control. These variations were not reflected in CML activity in vitro (table). All experiments were performed with unpurified bulk culture CTL populations, which can lead to such variability in results. Poor correlations between in vitro and in vivo activity were observed in tests with cloned CTL. Clone 58, a non-MHC-specific CD8$^+$ clone from

	Antigen differences			
Bystander reaction: incidence and severity*	H-2 and non-H-2		Non-H-2 only	
	No. assays	% Specific lysis at 25:1	No. assays	% Specific lysis at 25:1
High	22	64.9±16.2 †	102	49.7±22.3
		33.0—(64.1)—92.6 ‡		0—(51.5)—100
Moderate	11	62.2±18.9	28	54.1±20.9
		27.8—(66.2)—89.0		13.5—(49.9)—91.6
Low to null	20	80.1±15.9 §	8	58.3±21.6
		31.3—(84.5)—100		14.8—(58.3)—85.6

Levels of Cytotoxicity Mediated in Vitro by Cytolytic T Cells That Induced Bystander Reactions of Different Incidence and Severity in Vivo

*Persistent swelling at least 5 mm in diameter (i.e., grade 3+ or higher) for more than 3 days and ulceration (grade 5+) at the injection site in 60% to 100% (high) 20% to 50% (moderate), 10% to 15% (low), or 0% (null) of the hosts.

†Mean ± SD.

‡Minimum—(median)—maximum.

§Significantly different from the values for the high ($P = .004$) and moderate ($P = .054$) groups.

(Courtesy of Steinmuller D, Snider ME, Noble RL, et al: *Transplantation* 50:663–668, 1990.)

cells extracted from a sponge matrix allograft, ceased to show CML activity, but continued to induce necrotizing TrRs and ByRs.

Conclusion.—The CML reaction has served as the in vitro indicator for allograft rejection. However, these results challenge the reliability of CML in predicting the ability of mouse CTL to cause the tissue destruction observed with allograft rejection.

▶ This group used 2 assays, the transfer reaction and the bystander reaction, to delineate the specific and nonspecific effect of cytolytic T cells in graft vs. host disease. They found that in vitro cytolytic activity correlated poorly with tissue damage. These findings raise questions regarding the predictive value of in vitro cytolytic assays. Nonspecific tissue damage by cytolytic cells may be of vital importance in allograft damage.—N.L. Ascher, M.D., Ph.D.

17 Donor Selection and Matching

Frequency Analysis of HLA-Specific Cytotoxic T Lymphocyte Precursors in Humans
Breur-Vriesendorp BS, Vingerhoed J, van Twuyver E, de Waal LP, Ivanyi P (University of Amsterdam, The Netherlands)
Transplantation 51:1096–1103, 1991   17–1

Background.—It is important to quantify HLA-specific cytotoxic T lymphocyte precursors (CTLp). Extensive studies of the frequency distribution of HLA-specific CTLp in healthy blood donors, however, have been quite limited.

Methods.—The frequency of HLA class I-specific CTLp was examined in 33 individual responders by using 115 responder-stimulator combinations. In each combination there was a single HLA-A or HLA-B antigen mismatch.

Findings.—A wide range of CTLp frequencies was found for most A and B locus antigens. The A locus antigens differed more in immunogenicity. The HLA-specific CTLp frequencies of cross-reactive and subtype antigens were not significantly lower than the CTLp frequencies against non–cross-reactive antigens. A high frequency of CTLp was consistently found in combinations with multiple HLA antigen differences.

Conclusions.—Variations in the frequency of HLA-specific CTLp suggest that such estimates may help in selecting appropriate donor-recipient pairs in clinical transplantation. Enlarging panels of potential marrow donors make HLA antigen matching more likely and also permit the selection of donors with low or very low CTLp frequency in pairs with known or suspected HLA-A, -B incompatibility.

▶ Matching for HLA structural variations alone may not adequately predict alloimmune responses in transplant patients if there are significant differences in the way individuals respond to a given antigen mismatch. This study describes cytotoxic T lymphocyte precursor (CTLp) frequencies measured in normal blood donors in response to selected stimulator cells mismatched for single HLA-A and -B antigens. The results demonstrate a wide range in the frequency of CTLp. Certain antigens appeared to function as stronger target antigens than others. The strength of the CTLp response, however, was not significantly less when mismatching for antigens of the same serologically defined cross-reactive groups (CREG), suggesting that the structural polymorphisms recognized by B cells are not necessarily the same as those recognized by T cells. These results suggest that preferential matching for CREG, the so called "minor mismatches," may not predict the strength of T cell responses in vivo. The CTLp frequency assay may be of value in donor selection, as suggested by Kaminski et al. (1); however, a substantial amount of the CTLp measured may represent responses to unrecognized class I and class II antigen disparities (see Abstracts 17–2 and 17–3). The in vitro data presented by Breur-Vriesendorp et al. should give impetus for further studies designed to determine whether the use of this functional test in patients and potential donors thoroughly typed for HLA alleles and molecular variants can predict for GVHD and thereby improve the outcome of clinical transplantation.—J.A. Hansen, M.D.

Reference

1. Kaminski E, et al: *Transplantation* 48:608, 1989.

Bone Marrow–Allograft Rejection by T Lymphocytes Recognizing a Single Amino Acid Difference in HLA-B44

Fleischhauer K, Kernan NA, O'Reilly RJ, Dupont B, Yang SY (Mem Sloan-Kettering Cancer Ctr, New York)
N Engl J Med 323:1818–1822, 1990   17–2

Background.—Bone marrow from unrelated donors is increasingly used in transplantations for various disorders. Although this has led to the establishment of national and international HLA-typed volunteer donor registries, graft rejection appears more likely when unrelated donors are used. Marrow-graft rejection occurred in a patient with leukemia after transplantation of unrelated T-lymphocyte-depleted bone marrow.

Case Report.—Man, 29, with chronic myelogenous leukemia, received a bone marrow transplant from an unrelated, HLA-identical and compatible female donor. The patient's HLA genotype was HLA-A3, B7, DR2/HLA-A2, B44, DR7; only the HLA phenotype of the donor was known. The patient underwent cytoreduction before transplantation. Thirteen days later, the patient's white blood cells increased from none to .9/m^3 with a 98% lymphocyte count. The lymphocytosis cleared on day 15, but pancytopenia and marrow aplasia persisted. The patient died of multiple organ failure 68 days after transplantation.

Findings.—Cells from both the patient and donor were characterized and assayed using various biochemical, direct cytotoxicity, and oligonucleotide typing techniques. A specific B-lymphoblastoid cell line transfected with HLA-B44.1 was generated and identified. Isoelectric focusing (IEF) analysis of HLA-B44 showed that the donor carried the basic IEF B44.1 subtype, but the patient expressed the more acidic HLA-B44.2 subtype. Peripheral blood mononuclear cells from the patient demonstrated specific cytotoxic action against target cells expressing the B44.1 IEF subtype but not against the B44.2 IEF subtype. Cells transfected with the DNA-library-derived HLA-B (from the SKPB1 clone) expressed the IEF band corresponding to the HLA-B44.1 antigen, which differed from the HLA-B44.2 antigen by a single amino acid encoded by codon 156 of the α_2 domain.

Implications.—The patient's peripheral blood mononuclear cells lysed only the cells that expressed HLA-B44.1, even those transfected with CIR B-lymphoblastoid cell lines. Thus a structural HLA class I incompatibility, even if limited to a single amino acid change, can lead to a major histocompatibility barrier when using an unrelated donor for bone marrow transplantation. It is recommended that HLA typing for common HLA-B antigens be performed to optimize HLA matching with unrelated marrow donors.

▶ This case report described the appearance in a patient following marrow allograft rejection of cytotoxic T lymphocytes (CTL) that reacted specifically with an HLA-B44 variant present in the unrelated donor but not in the patient. Both patient and donor typed as B44 by standard serology, but these antigens were not the same when compared by IEF analysis. Primary sequencing reveals that these two IEF-defined variants, B44.1 and B44.2, differ by only a single amino acid. It is clear from in vitro studies that this minimal structural change can be recognized by T cells, and assuming that B44.1 was the specific target for rejection in this patient (who received a T cell-depleted marrow graft) it is apparent that at least in some patients the requirements for HLA matching may be very stringent.—J.A. Hansen, M.D.

Cytotoxic T Lymphocyte Precursor (CTL-p) Frequency Analysis in Unrelated Donor Bone Marrow Transplantation: Two Case Studies

Kaminski ER, Hows JM, Bridge J, Davey NJ, Brookes PA, Green JE, Goldman JM, Batchelor JR (Royal Postgraduate Medical School, London)
Bone Marrow Transplant 8:47–50, 1991   17–3

Background.—Compared to HLA-identical sibling bone marrow transplantation (BMT), HLA "matched" unrelated BMT carries an increased risk and severity of acute graft-vs.-host disease. In a previous study, a correlation was found between cytotoxic T lymphocyte precursor (CTL-p) frequency and HLA disparity between responder and stimulator, as well as between CTL-p frequency and incidence of acute graft-vs.-host disease after HLA A, B, DR matched unrelated donor BMT. The specificity of the CTL response in 2 patients with HLA mismatched donors was examined.

Methods.—The subjects were 2 patients scheduled to receive BMT from a HLA "matched" unrelated donor. Donors were selected by serotyping for HLA A, B, and DR antigens and a mixed lymphocyte response of less than 35% RRI in each direction. A limiting dilution analysis was then used to quantitate the CTL-p frequencies.

Results.—Single HLA antigenic mismatches were detected by allogenotyping or isoelectric focusing, but not by HLA serology. The CTL-ps were directed specifically against the mismatched antigens. In one case the CTL-p assay detected a class I HLA-A locus variant and in the second case the assay detected a class II HLA-OR variant.

Conclusions.—High CTL-p frequencies in HLA "matched" unrelated pairs appear to point out antigenic variants that are undetected by serologic study but detected by molecular typing. The assay is thus valuable in predicting acute graft-vs.-host disease in patients undergoing BMT. This assay system could be used to assist in donor selection for patients undergoing BMT from an unrelated HLA matched or related HLA mismatched donor.

▶ This study adds to previous reports from this group (1, 2) demonstrating that the frequency analysis of cytotoxic T lymphocyte precursors is a functional assay that may contribute significantly to donor selection when the available standard typing techniques such as serology are unable to detect certain structural variants of the HLA class I and class II molecules. It remains to be seen, however, whether frequency assays can further improve donor selection or molecular typing methods can reliably predict matching for individual alleles (i.e., perfect matching at the structural level).—J.A. Hansen, M.D.

References

1. Kaminski E, et al: *Bone Marrow Transplant* 3:149, 1988.
2. Kaminski E, et al: *Transplantation* 48:608, 1989.

Influence of HLA-DP Mismatches on Primary MLR Responses in Unrelated HLA-A, B, DR, DQ, Dw Identical Pairs in Allogeneic Bone Marrow Transplantation
Cesbron A, Moreau P, Milpied N, Muller JY, Harousseau JL, Bignon JD (Laboratoire HLA; Hématologie Clinique, Nantes, France)
Bone Marrow Transplant 6:337–340, 1990   17–4

Background.—Matching of class I and II HLA identity between donor and recipient is important to the success of bone marrow transplantation. However, no studies have established the effect of DP mismatches on primary mixed lymphocyte reaction (MLR I) responses. The results of HLA-DP typing and correlation with MLR I responses were examined.

Methods.—The subjects were 10 patients and 22 selected potential donors. The patients and donors were HLA-A, B, DR, DQ, Dw identical, according to serologic, restriction fragment length polymorphism, and oligotyping methods. All subjects underwent HLA-DP typing by a restriction fragment length polymorphism method. The results of this match were then compared to MLR I responses obtained in 22 HLA-A, B, DR, DQ, Dw identical donor-recipient pairs and in 30 HLA-A, B, DR, DQ, Dw identical-donor pairs used as a control series.

Results.—When patients' cells were tested as the responder cell, MLR I responses were always lower than when control cells were involved. Mixed lymphocyte reaction I responses were influenced by DP mismatches and the responses especially of the donors stimulated by the patient (the GVHD direction) were stronger for 2 compared to 1 DP mismatch. Response values, however, were greatly scattered. No proliferative response was seen when there was no DP mismatch.

Conclusions.—Histocompatibility leukocyte antigen-DP mismatches, other than the recognized HLA specificities, do not appear to be detected by conventional technical conditions of MLR I. There is a lack of linkage between DR, and DP loci, that might explain the higher incidence of graft-vs.-host disease observed in unrelated donor non-T cell-depleted marrow transplant recipients.

▶ This study demonstrates that unrelated individuals phenotypically matched for HLA-A, B, DR, DQ, and Dw are likely to be mismatched for DP, and furthermore that mismatching for 0, 1, or 2 DP antigens correlates with the level of T cell response as measured in vitro in the mixed lymphocyte culture (MLC) test. In the absence of DP disparity, the MLC was essentially nonreactive, suggesting that there are no genetic factors other than the HLA antigens for which these unrelated individuals were matched that are capable of eliciting an MLC response. The authors suggest that DP disparity might be a factor responsible for the increased GVHD known to occur in HLA-A, B, DR, DQ, and Dw matched unrelated donor transplants. The available data however do not address this important question.—J.A. Hansen, M.D.

HLA-DP Incompatibilities and Severe Graft-Versus-Host Disease in Unrelated Bone Marrow Transplants

Kato Y, Mitsuishi Y, Cecka M, Hopfield J, Hunt L, Champlin R, Terasaki PI, Gajewski JL (Univ of California at Los Angeles)
Transplantation 52:374–386, 1991   17–5

Introduction.—With the advent of large registries of HLA-typed volunteer donors, bone marrow transplants (BMT) from phenotypically matched but genetically unrelated donors have increased. In these transplants, there is an increased incidence of acute graft-vs.-host disease (aGvHD) and graft failure compared with transplants from HLA-identical siblings. Although typing is performed for several antigens, it is not routinely performed for HLA-DP.

Methods.—Unrelated bone marrow transplants were retrospectively analyzed for HLA-DP compatibility using a polymerase chain reaction/restriction fragment length polymorphism technique. Immunologic outcome and the incidence of aGvHD were compared.

Results.—In 22 transplants, 2 patients who were HLA-DP identical did not have severe aGvHD. The 11 patients who had severe aGvHD were mismatched at HLA-DP in the graft-vs.-host direction. Of 11 patients with mild or no aGvHD, only 6 were mismatched. Of 6 patients with grade 0–I aGvHD, 6 were matched for HLA-DP, of 5 patients with grade II GvHD, 2 were matched.

Conclusion.—There is a significant correlation between HLA-DP matching and a favorable outcome. The HLA-DP antigen mismatches contribute to the incidence of severe aGvHD in recipients of bone marrow transplantation from unrelated donors. If these preliminary results are confirmed, they suggest that identifying immunologic hierarchies that relate to specific regions of the molecules may be more important than counting allelic differences in unrelated donors.

▶ This preliminary study in contrast to the study of Cesbron et al. (Abstract 17–4) suggested an association between DP mismatching and risk of severe acute GVHD. Although the analysis was limited to 22 unrelated donor transplants, this study has the advantage of having typed for 15 different DPB alleles. Some of the increased GVHD observed, however, may have been attributable to mismatching for HLA-A, B, or DR. It may not be possible to adequately evaluate the effect of host DP incompatibility on GVHD until a sufficiently large group of unrelated donor transplants proven to be matched for HLA-A, B, DR, and DQ are available for analysis.—J.A. Hansen, M.D.

Lack of Association Between the Frequencies of HLA-DR or HLA-DP Alleles and the Occurrence of Chronic Graft-Versus-Host Disease
Pawelec G, Müller C, Haen M, Schaudt K, Ehninger G (University of Tübingen, Tübingen Germany)
Transplantation 51:917–918, 1991   17–6

Introduction.—Up to 50% of all patients who survive more than 100 days after undergoing HLA-matched allogeneic bone marrow transplantation (BMT) have chronic graft-vs.-host disease (cGVHD). The causes of cGVHD remain unknown, but differences between donor and recipient at minor histocompatibility loci may be involved. A recent preliminary study reported an increased frequency of HLA-DR4 in patients with cGVHD. The role of HLA specificities in the development of cGVHD was further examined.

Methods.—The study population consisted of 116 patients undergoing HLA-matched BMT for severe aplastic anemia, chronic myelogenous leukemia, or acute lymphoblastic or nonlymphoblastic leukemia. Histocompatibility leukocyte antigen-DR serologic typing was performed for all 116 patients, and HLA-DP typing was performed for 65 patients. Forty-six patients (40%) had cGVHD after BMT.

Results.—There was little or no difference in the frequencies of DR or DP alleles between patients with and without cGVHD. The frequency of HLA-DP4 in BMT patients with cGVHD was slightly increased compared with those without cGVHD, but the difference did not reach statistical significance. The frequencies of HLA-DR specificities among BMT patients did not differ from those among the normal population.

Conclusion.—The occurrence of cGVHD after HLA-matched allogeneic BMT does not appear to be associated with an increased frequency of HLA-DP or HLA-DR alleles.

▶ Although chronic GVHD has features in common with certain autoimmune diseases (1, 2), this study failed to demonstrate any association between chronic GVHD and DR antigen (e.g., DR3 or DR4). In addition, this study demonstrates that the DP allospecificities DP1-DP5 are not risk factors for chronic GVHD.—J.A. Hansen, M.D.

References

1. Sullivan KM, et al: *Blood* 57:267, 1981.
2. Santos GW, et al: *Immunol Rev* 88:169, 1985.

Minor Histocompatibility Antigens
Perreault C, Décary F, Brochu S, Gyger M, Bélanger R, Roy D (Maisonneuve-Rosemont Hospital, Montreal; Canadian Red Cross, Montreal)
Blood 76:1269–1280, 1990   17–7

Introduction.—A distinction between major (MHC) and "minor" histocompatibility antigens (MiHA) based on immunogenicity alone is imprecise; some MiHA are neither weak nor minor in effect, whereas some MHC antigens are weak immunogens. A major role for MiHA in clinical transplantation has been increasingly acknowledged. In addition, these antigens contribute to the definition of immunologic "self" and help shape the T-cell repertoire.

Immunology of MiHA.—The total number of MiHA loci is unknown, but several hundred exist. Responses to MiHA are strictly T cell–mediated, in contrast to MHC antigens, which can be recognized by both B and T lymphocytes. The T cells recognize MiHA only in the context of MHC molecules on both antigen-presenting cells and target cells. Minor histocompatibility antigens probably are small peptides. Their expression appears not to be ubiquitous; some apparently are tissue-specific or differentiation antigens. It has been suggested that viruses may have a role in the generation of MiHA mutants.

Clinical Aspects.—Some MiHA are expressed on the kidney, where they are able to trigger renal graft rejection. Studies of heart and skin transplants in mice have shown that incompatibility at a single MiHA locus can cause rejection. The immunogenicity of some—but not all—MiHA is additive. Graft-host tolerance is observed in many MiHA-incompatible marrow graft recipients. There are suggestions that anti-MiHA cytotoxic T lymphocytes might prove helpful in eradicating leukemic cells.

▶ This is an interesting and timely review summarizing current knowledge about minor histocompatibility antigens. Major topics addressed include the role of minor histocompatibility antigens in self-tolerance, selection of the anti-minor T-cell repertoire and transplantation. The discussion about how T-cell responses to minor histocompatibility antigens might be harnessed for immunotherapy of hematologic malignancies is provocative. The references are comprehensive and provide ready access to a more detailed examination of the subject.—J.A. Hansen, M.D.

Effector Mechanisms in Graft-Versus-Host Disease in Response to Minor Histocompatibility Antigens: I. Absence of Correlation With Cytotoxic Effector Cells

van Els CACM, Bakker A, Zwinderman AH, Zwaan FE, van Rood JJ, Goulmy E
(University Hospital Leiden, The Netherlands)
Transplantation 50:62–66, 1990   17–8

Background.—Unfortunately graft rejection and graft-vs.-host disease (GVHD), both T cell-mediated host-graft interactions, are related in a mutually exclusive manner so that attempts to prevent GVHD probably increase the risk of rejection, and vice versa. Anti-host–specific cytotoxic T cells probably act as effector cells in GVHD induced to minor histocompatibility antigens.

Objective and Methods.—Anti-host–specific Tc cell reactivities were studied sequentially in 16 patients given bone marrow transplants from compatible sibling donors. The 15 leukemic patients received cyclophosphamide and total-body irradiation as conditioning for transplantation. All patients survived for at least 100 days after marrow transplantation. Acute GVHD developed in 10 patients, 5 of whom later developed chronic disease. Methotrexate and cyclosporine were given after grafting, and GVHD was treated with steroid and/or azathioprine.

Findings.—Significant cytotoxicity against host target cells was observed in 39 of 60 host-sensitized T-cell cultures. No cultures exhibited Tc cell activity against the donor. Anti-host Tc cell reactivity usually could not be generated in vitro. In most patients the degree and kinetics of anti-host Tc cell activity varied considerably. In time the Tc cell response to HLA alloantigens was functionally restored in all instances. Anti-host–specific Tc cell activity did not correlate with the occurrence of acute or chronic GVHD.

Implication.—These findings do not support an association of anti-host Tc cells with the development of GVHD, although they do not exclude an effector-cell role for Tc cells.

▶ Anti-host cytotoxic T lymphocytes (CTL) specific for non-MCH minor histocompatibility antigens (mHA) can be demonstrated in both murine and human recipients with acute GVHD after transplantation of MHC matched marrow allografts(1, 2). Patients with chronic GVHD have also demonstrated CTL specific for host mHA (3). In the current study, the Leiden group demonstrated that host-specific mHA can also be detected in patients without GVHD, thus calling into question the role of these CTL in the pathogenesis of GVHD. The frequent occurrence of immune T cells would suggest that the in vivo donor immune response to mHA is very efficient, but the presence of these genetic differences and the generation of specific CTL after transplantation does not necessarily represent a sufficient cause for the clinical syndrome called acute and chronic GVHD.—J.A. Hansen, M.D.

Reference

1. Hamilton BL, et al: *J Immunol* 126:621, 1981.
2. Goulmy E, et al: *Nature* 302:159, 1983.
3. Van Rood JJ, et al: *Exp Hematol* 11:61, 1983.

Bone Marrow Transplantation for Related Donors Other Than HLA-Identical Siblings: Effect of T Cell Depletion
Ash RC, Horowitz MM, Gale RP, van Bekkum DW, Casper JT, Gordon-Smith EC, Henslee PJ, Kolb H-J, Lowenberg B, Masaoka T, McGlave PB, Rimm AA, Ringdén O, van Rood JJ, Sondel PM, Vowels MR, Bortin MM (Med College of Wisconsin, Milwaukee; Univ of California, Los Angeles; Radiobiological Institute, Rijswijk, The Netherlands; St. George's Hospital Medical School, London; Univ of Kentucky, Lexington, et al)
Bone Marrow Transplant 7:443–452, 1991   17–9

Background.—About two thirds of potential bone marrow transplant (BMT) recipients lack an HLA-identical sibling donor. It is reported that patients who undergo alternative donor transplants have an increased risk of severe acute graft-vs.-host disease (GVHD), for which reason many centers use T cell depletion. Data from a transplantation registry were analyzed to identify factors associated with outcome of alternative donor transplants and to determine whether T cell depletion improved the results.

Methods.—During an 8-year period, 470 patients receiving BMT from alternative related donors for leukemia or aplastic anemia were reported to the International Bone Marrow Transplant Registry. Of those, 198 received T cell-depleted marrow, a rate of 42%. The characteristics and outcome of those patients were compared with those of 3,468 patients who had transplants from HLA-identical donors.

Results.—Patients who received alternative donor transplants had an increased incidence of graft failure and acute GVHD and a lower disease-free survival. As donor-recipient HLA disparity increased, so did the likelihood of an adverse outcome. On multivariate analysis of alternative related donor transplants, relative risks (RRs) of treatment failure were calculated. Donor age of 30 years or more carried an RR of 1.7, intermediate leukemia an RR of 1.5, advanced leukemia an RR of 1.6, pretransplant infection an RR of 1.7, and 2- to 3-locus donor-recipient HLA disparity an RR of 1.3. Forty-three patients with alternative donor transplants had none of those adverse prognostic features. Their 2-year probability of leukemia-free survival was 44%, compared with 56% for 868 similar patients receiving HLA-identical sibling transplants. Graft failure was more likely and acute GVHD less likely after T cell depletion; there was no effect on leukemia-free survival.

Conclusions.—Some patients undergoing alternative related donor BMT achieve long-term disease-free survival, but the risks of graft failure, acute GVHD, and other complications are increased. If patients with advanced leukemia are being considered for such treatment, it should be done early in the course of the disease. Outcome is not improved by T cell depletion.

▶ Graft failure and graft-vs.-host disease (GVHD) are increased in patients receiving unmodified (non-T cell–depleted) marrow grafts when donor and recipient are HLA incompatible. Risk of GVHD correlates with degree of recipient incompatibility (1). The risk of graft failure correlates with donor incompatibility; however, a positive lymphocyte crossmatch is the major risk factor for graft failure (2). The probability of graft failure and GVHD are also significantly affected by the type and intensity of the pretransplant and posttransplant immunosuppression therapy. Pretransplant conditioning regimens for patients with malignant disease are designed primarily for their anti-tumor activity and they may have variable immunosuppressive activity. The different approaches to GVHD prophylaxis currently used fall into 1 of 2 categories: the use of immunosuppressive drugs, usually in combination; or T-cell depletion of donor marrow.

The major finding of this analysis involving data from multiple centers by the International Bone Marrow Transplant Registry (IMBTR) is the observation that T-cell depletion of donor marrow significantly decreased GVHD; however, disease-free survival at 2 years was not different for T-cell depleted and non-T cell–depleted transplants. Improved control of GVHD remains a predominant issue in marrow transplantation and is the limiting factor in achieving successful HLA mismatched transplants.—J.H. Hansen, M.D.

References

1. Beatty PG, et al: *N Engl J Med* 313:765, 1985.
2. Anasetti C, et al: *N Engl J Med* 320:197, 1989.

Marrow Transplantation from HLA-Matched Unrelated Donors for Treatment of Hematologic Malignancies
Beatty PG, Hansen JA, Longton GM, Thomas ED, Sanders JE, Martin PJ, Bearman SI, Anasetti C, Petersdorf EW, Mickelson EM, Pepe MS, Appelbaum FR, Buckner CD, Clift RA, Petersen FB, Stewart PS, Storb RF, Sullivan KM, Tesler MC, Witherspoon RP (Fred Hutchinson Cancer Res Ctr, Seattle; Puget Sound Blood Ctr, Seattle; Univ of Washington, Seattle)
Transplantation 51:443–447, 1991   17–10

Background.—An HLA-matched relative donor is available for less than 40% of patients who might benefit from marrow transplantation. Many centers have therefore used marrow grafts from HLA-identical unrelated donors.

Patients.—Of 478 patients for whom an unrelated donor search was conducted over a 4-year period, HLA-A, B, DR phenotypically identical donors were found for 115. Sixty-three patients were HLA-Dw matched and MLC compatible with at least 1 donor. Fifty-two patients underwent

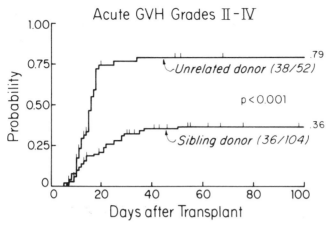

Fig 17–1.—The probability of clinically significant (grades II to IV) GVHD is shown as a function of time after transplantation. Patients were censored at death if they had no significant acute GVHD. (Courtesy of Beatty PG, Hansen JA, Longton GM, et al: *Transplantation* 51:443–447, 1991.)

the transplantation procedure. Results were analyzed by matching each patient to 2 patients with similar disease, disease stage, and age who received marrow from an HLA-genotypically identical sibling donor.

Results.—Grade II to IV acute graft-vs.-host disease (GVHD) occurred in 79% of patients receiving transplants from unrelated donors and in 36% of those receiving transplants from related donors (Fig 17–1). The unrelated group also had a higher risk of grade III to IV GVHD (Fig 17–2). There was no significant difference, however, in the probability of relapse-free survival in the 2 groups at 1 year. One-year survival rates were 41% in the unrelated group and 46% in the related group.

Conclusions.—Use of marrow from HLA-matched unrelated donors should be considered for most patients for whom transplantation is indi-

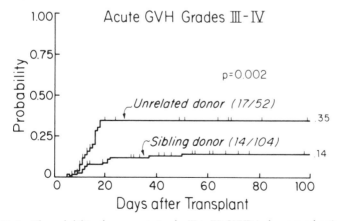

Fig 17–2.—The probability of severe acute (grades III to IV) GVHD is shown as a function of time after transplantation. Patients were censored at death if they had no severe acute GVHD. (Courtesy of Beatty PG, Hansen JA, Longton GM, et al: *Transplantation* 51:443–447, 1991.)

cated but an HLA-matched sibling is unavailable. Patients transplanted with unrelated marrow have a higher incidence of GVHD, but there was no apparent difference in relapse-free survival in the unrelated donor group compared with case-matched controls. The availability of an HLA match, however, remains a major impediment.

▶ This study demonstrates the feasibility and efficacy of HLA-matched unrelated donor marrow transplants for patients with hematologic malignancy. The diagnoses of these unrelated donor transplants included patients with both acute and chronic leukemia and patients at high risk of posttransplant relapse. All received unmodified (non-T cell–depleted) marrow grafts, and combination therapy for graft-vs.-host disease (GVHD) prophylaxis using methotrexate and cyclosporine. Although patients and their unrelated donors were matched for HLA-A, B, DR, and Dw, the probability of acute GVHD was substantially greater than HLA genotypically identical sibling transplants. Survival and relapse-free survival were compared with rates for case-matched controls transplanted from an HLA genotypically identical sibling. There was a trend toward a lower survival and relapse-free survival at 1 year in the unrelated transplant group, but these apparent differences were not statistically significant. Similarly, there was a trend toward a lower relapse rate in unrelated transplants, which was not statistically significant. The need for improved methods for GVHD prevention are clearly demonstrated.—J.A. Hansen, M.D.

18 Hematopoietic Stem Cells, Pretransplant Immunosuppression, and Engraftment

Molecular Basis of Homing of Intravenously Transplanted Stem Cells to the Marrow
Tavassoli M, Hardy CL (Veterans Affairs Med Ctr, Jackson, Miss)
Blood 76:1059–1070, 1990   18–1

Introduction.—Homing is the process whereby hematopoietic stem cells and other progenitor cells are recognized by the marrow stroma after being intravenously administered. It is mediated by membrane interactions between progenitor and stromal cells.

Molecular Mechanisms.—Mechanisms of homing have been studied using synthetic neoglycoprotein probes that lack toxicity both in vivo and in cell culture systems. Studies in irradiated mice suggest that homing is mediated by a lectin-carbohydrate interaction. The carbohydrate involved appears to be a galactosyl or mannosyl moiety. The binding of progenitor cells to stromal cells probably involves an interaction between a membrane lectin on the progenitor cell with the carbohydrate moiety on the stromal cell. Much remains to be learned about how progenitor cells arriving in the marrow are recognized by and interact with the luminal endothelial surface.

Lymphocyte Homing.—Similar mechanisms may regulate lymphocyte traffic. Monoclonal antibody studies have identified a number of homing molecules on the surfaces of murine and human lymphocytes (lymphocyte homing receptors). The lymphocyte receptors have their ligand counterparts—vascular addressins—on the endothelium to which they bind.

▶ This comprehensive review addresses an important aspect of the biology of hematopoietic stem cells (HSC). Interactions between HSC cell surface receptors and organ-specific ligands are integral to the process of homing and achieving sustained engraftment. The latter cannot occur until HSC reach the hematopoietic microenvironment. A better understanding of these mechanisms may open the way to more efficient methods for grafting HSC.—J.A. Hansen, M.D.

Circulation and Mobilization of Hematopoietic Stem Cells in Peripheral Blood

▶ ↓ Previous experimental work has demonstrated that early progenitor cells are mobilized into peripheral blood of mice after the infusion of recombinant human granulocyte colony-stimulating factor (rHuG-CSF) (1, 2). Previous clinical studies have demonstrated that peripheral blood cells collected in the recovery phase after marrow suppressive chemotherapy or radiation function as stem cells in autologous transplantation (3–5). Remarkably, these autologous peripheral blood stem cell grafts show a more rapid recovery of peripheral blood counts than autologous marrow grafts.

The following 2 papers demonstrate the transplantation potential of circulating hematopoietic progenitor cells. Molineux et al. (Abstract 18–2) present critical information demonstrating that peripheral blood mobilized progenitor cells can support hematopoietic engraftment after transplantation and thus function like true stem cells. Lopez et al. (Abstract 18–3) suggest another application of circulating progenitors by showing that even the addition of relatively small numbers of peripheral blood leukocytes collected by pheresis to purged or nonpurged autologous marrow grafts can accelerate the rate of recovery.—John A. Hansen, M.D.

References

1. Duhrsen U, et al: *Blood* 72:2074, 1988.
2. Molineux G, et al: *Blood* 75:563, 1990.
3. Juttner CA, et al: *Br J Haematol* 61:739, 1985.
4. Reiffers J, et al: *Exp Hematol* 14:312, 1986.
5. Kessinger A, et al: *Blood* 74:1260, 1989.

Transplantation Potential of Peripheral Blood Stem Cells Induced by Granulocyte Colony-Stimulating Factor
Molineux G, Pojda Z, Hampson IN, Lord BI, Dexter TM (Holt Radium Institute, Manchester, England)
Blood 76:2153–2158, 1990   18–2

Introduction.—The cytokine granulocyte colony-stimulating factor (G-CSF) plays a role in hematopoietic cell development. Recombinant human G-CSF (rHuG-CSF) promotes the recovery of neutrophils after myeloid suppression caused by cytotoxic events or bone marrow transplantation. The potential of the peripheral blood stem cells, known as spleen colony-forming units (CFU-S), to promote the reconstitution of hematopoiesis was investigated in irradiated transplant animal recipients.

Methods.—Male B6D2F$_1$ mice were treated with G-CSF or carrier alone; female mice served as graft recipients. Transplant recipients were irradiated before experimentation. Animals were killed 8–10 days after irradiation. Their spleens were excised and colony numbers recorded. The rHuG-CSF diluted in phosphate-buffered saline supplemented with

.1% bovine serum albumin was injected subcutaneously into male mice at 12-hour intervals for 4 days to rescue lethally irradiated animals.

Findings.—Mice receiving 10^5 normal bone marrow cells demonstrated a survival of 92% (46 of 50 animals). All 70 mice receiving 50 μL of blood from G-CSF donors survived. However, only 3 of 50 animals lived longer than 1 month if they received no graft. Of the animals receiving 10 μL of G-CSF-induced blood, 69 of 70 survived. Animals receiving 500 μL of blood cells from control mice had poor survival (3 of 70), whereas mice receiving sixfold more normal blood cells had a survival rate of 100%. Analysis of recognizable bone marrow cells demonstrated that erythropoiesis was increased at the expense of granulopoiesis when comparing grafted to nongrafted animals. Using a molecular probe to the Y chromosome, donor cells were found in the spleen, thymus, bone marrow, and blood of animals receiving bone marrow or blood grafts from normal donors and of animals receiving blood grafts from G-CSF donors. Animals that survived because of receipt of marrow cells, high normal blood cells, or G-CSF-induced blood cells had a normal complement of marrow CFU-S, whereas mice receiving blood from control animals had about 30% of host-derived CFU-S.

Conclusions.—These results indicate that a graft of peripheral blood cells from rHuG-CSF-treated mice is as effective as a graft from normal bone marrow cells in reconstituting long-term hematopoiesis in irradiated recipients. Donor cell distribution and their production of CFU-S suggests that blood cells from G-CSF–treated patients may serve as a source of stem cells for autologous and allogeneic bone marrow transplantation.

Acceleration of Hemopoietic Recovery After Autologous Bone Marrow Transplantation by Low Doses of Peripheral Blood Stem Cells
Lopez M, Mortel O, Pouillart P, Zucker JM, Fechtenbaum J, Douay L, Palangie T, Michon J, Salmon D, Gorin NC (INSERM, Fondation Nationale de Transfusion Sanguine; Institut Curie; Unité de Recherche sur les greffes de cellules souches hématopoïétiques, Paris)
Bone Marrow Transplant 7:173–181, 1991   18–3

Background.—Transplantation with autologous peripheral blood cells (PBSC) is an alternative to bone marrow transplantation. The minimum dose of colony-forming unit granulocyte macrophage assumed to be necessary to ensure engraftment ranges from 1 to 3 × 10^5/kg body weight. However, this is not always reached in patients with solid tumors who have been heavily pretreated. The possible use of low doses of PBSC to shorten the duration of aplasia after autologous bone marrow transplantation, with purged or unpurged marrow, was explored.

Methods.—Twenty patients with advanced malignant disease underwent autologous bone marrow transplantation. Marrow was unpurged in 10 cases and purged in vitro with mafosfamide in the other 10. All patients had had ablative chemotherapy. The patients received autologous

PBSC collected during 1- to 3-hour cytapheresis procedures. The kinetics of the hematologic recovery of those patients were compared with those of patients with similar diseases who had grafts at the same center with either unpurged marrow only or marrow purged in vitro with mafosfamide.

Results.—In patients transfused with both autologous bone marrow and PBSC, the median times to reach 10^9/L leukocytes, $.5 \times 10^9$/L polymorphs, and 50×10^9/L platelets were reduced by 10, 10, and 13 days, respectively, compared with those receiving bone marrow only. Patients with grafts of bone marrow and PBSC also had a reduced number of days in the hospital after transplantation and of days of fever greater than 38° C. Their numbers of platelet and red blood cell transfusions were also decreased.

Conclusions.—Infusion of low doses of PBSC with bone marrow may be considered an alternative in some cases and should be tested in a prospective, randomized study. It would be especially useful in patients with diseases such as acute myeloid leukemia, for which the infusion of hematopoietic growth factors may be hazardous because of the risk of stimulating tumor cell proliferation.

Identification of Hematopoiesis Stem Cells in Bone Marrow and Peripheral Blood

Tumor Necrosis Factor-Alpha Strongly Potentiates Interleukin-3 and Granulocyte-Macrophage Colony-Stimulating Factor-Induced Proliferation of Human CD34+ Hematopoietic Progenitor Cells

Caux C, Saeland S, Favre C, Duvert V, Mannoni P, Banchereau J (Schering-Plough (UNICET), Dardilly, France; INSERM U119 and Centre Regional Anticancereux, Marseille, France
Blood 75:2292–2298, 1990   18–4

Introduction.—In previous studies, tumor necrosis factors have been shown to inhibit the proliferative effects of crude or purified colony-stimulating factors (CSFs) on low-density human bone marrow cell fractions. The effect of tumor necrosis factor-alpha (TNF-α) on the growth of CD34+ human hematopoietic progenitor cells (HPC) in response to recombinant CSFs was investigated.

Results.—Results showed that tumor necrosis factors strongly potentiate the proliferative effects of IL-3 and GM-CSF on CD34+ HPC. The potentiation is not a consequence of an IL-3-dependent generation of cells proliferating in response to TNF-α alone. A direct effect of TNF-α on its target cells was demonstrated.

Conclusion.—Tumor necrosis factor-alpha has been described as an inhibitor of hematopoiesis. In this study, TNF-α strongly enhanced the early stages of myelopoiesis.

Engraftment After Infusion of CD34⁺ Marrow Cells in Patients With Breast Cancer or Neuroblastoma

Berenson RJ, Bensinger WI, Hill RS, Andrews RG, Garcia-Lopez J, Kalamasz DF, Still BJ, Spitzer G, Buckner CD, Bernstein ID, Thomas ED (Univ of Washington, Seattle; M D Anderson Cancer Ctr, Houston; Hospital de Sant Pau, Barcelona)
Blood 77:1717–1722, 1991   18–5

Introduction.—The CD34 antigen is expressed on up to 4% of human marrow cells, but not on mature peripheral blood cells. It also is found on nearly all colony-forming cells and blast colony-forming cells. Marrow cells expressing CD34 can engraft lethally irradiated baboons. The antigen is not found on tumor cells from most patients having solid tumors. Positive selection of CD34⁺ cells therefore may provide marrow cells capable of engraftment but not associated with tumor.

Methods.—In 7 patients with stage IV breast cancer and 2 with stage IV neuroblastoma, marrow cells were separated by immunoabsorption with the anti-CD34 antibody 12–8. Of positively selected cells, 64% were CD34⁺. After marrow ablation, the patients received $1-5 \times 10^6$ CD34-enriched cells per kilogram.

Results.—Evidence of engraftment was found in 6 of the 9 patients. Granulocyte counts exceeded 500/mm³ in these patients, and platelets exceeded 20,000/mm³, 30–45 days after transplantation. Engraftment was durable in 5 of the patients; 3 patients, 2 of whom had early engraftment, died within 3 weeks of marrow transplantation.

Conclusion.—Marrow preparations highly enriched in CD34⁺ cells can reconstitute hemopoiesis after myeloablation in patients with metastatic breast cancer or neuroblastoma. More effective conditioning regimens may be needed to eradicate residual tumor and prevent relapse after autologous marrow transplantation.

Flow Cytometry for Clinical Estimation of Circulating Hematopoietic Progenitors for Autologous Transplantation in Cancer Patients

Siena S, Bregni M, Brando B, Belli N, Ravagnani F, Gandola L, Stern AC, Lansdorp PM, Bonadonna G, Gianni AM (Istituto Nazionale Tumori, Milan, Italy; Ospedale Niguarda, Milan; Sandoz Clinical Research, Basel, Switzerland; Cancer Control Agency of British Columbia, Vancouver, Canada; Università degli Studi, Milan)
Blood 77:400–409, 1991   18–6

Background.—The best method for harvesting circulating hematopoietic progenitors for autologous transplantation to support myeloablative cancer therapy remains unknown. This is mainly because of the lack of an assay for marrow-repopulating stem cells. The most commonly used assay, the granulocyte-macrophage colony-forming unit (CFU-GM) assay, is not well standardized and can be assessed only retrospectively. It is known that hematopoietic progenitors express CD34 and CD33 differentiation antigens. A dual-color direct immunofluorescence flow cytometry assay based on this principle was developed.

Methods.—Both the flow cytometry assay and the CFU-GM assay were used to test 157 blood samples from 20 patients. All patients were recovering from pancytopenia induced by high-dose cyclophosphamide or etoposide cancer therapy. Most received recombinant human GM colony-stimulating factor (rhGM-CSF). When CD34$^+$ cells appeared in the circulation, hematopoietic progenitors had increased to over 500 CFU-GM/mL, which is sufficient for large-scale harvest by leukapheresis.

Results.—There was a good correlation between total numbers of CD34$^+$ cells and CFU-GM. The data could be fitted by a linear regression line according to the equation:

$$y = 388.3 + 64.0x$$

where y is CFU-GM/mL and x is CD34$^+$ cells/μL. In 6 patients who received myeloablative chemoradiotherapy, the number of transplanted CD34$^+$/CD33$^+$ cells was a better predictor of functional recovery than either total nucleated cells, CFU-GM, CD34$^+$/CD33$^-$ cells, or CD34$^-$/CD33$^+$ cells.

Conclusions.—The CD34/CD33 flow cytometry technique may be a useful clinical guide to harvesting circulating hematopoietic progenitors for autologous transplantation. It may also help in determining the role of the various types of progenitor cells in achieving marrow recovery.

The Evolving Role of Autologous Peripheral Stem Cell Transplantation Following High-Dose Therapy for Malignancies

Kessinger A, Armitage JO (Univ of Nebraska, Omaha)
Blood 77:211–213, 1991   18–7

Background.—Transplantation of circulating autologous hematopoietic stem cells after high-dose ablative anticancer therapy is becoming widely used. Indications for peripheral stem cell transplantation (PSCT) have been expanding as well. Issues related to the use of this technique, especially the mobilization of stem cells, were reviewed.

Mobilization, Collection, and Transplantation.—The advantage of restoring bone marrow function more rapidly is achieved only if the cells are collected when their numbers are expanded. The only methods applied clinically are chemotherapy-induced mobilization and, more recently, use of recombinant human growth factor granulocyte-macrophage colony-stimulating factor (rhGM-CSF). A problem with any technique is determining the best time to collect cells. Stem cell assays may take 2 weeks to complete, and collections are made long before the results are known. Morbidity and even mortality are major problems with the chemotherapy approach, and some patients do not exhibit mobilization. The need for apheresis is a problem as well. Fewer studies have been done with rhGM-CSF than with chemotherapy, but PSCT with this technique appears to yield rapid recovery and sustained hematopoiesis. The technique is less predictable than chemotherapy, and it may or may not avoid its difficulties. Both methods used together may increase the number of circulating progenitors more than either method alone. Siena et al. have described a flow cytometric technique for estimating progenitors that can detect a meaningful expansion on the day of occurrence, based on collection of a specific number of CD34+ cells. This may offer a major advantage.

Other Uses of PSCT.—Use of PSCT has been proposed for patients who are candidates for high-dose therapy but have no suitable donor or suitable marrow for transplantation. The goal in these situations is the opportunity to administer high-dose therapy. Mobilization is not attempted. This procedure generally has recovery rates comparable to those in patients who have autologous transplantation. Until $CD34^+$ cells can be detected in nonmobilized collections, adequate collection must be defined by CFU-GM content or mononuclear cell content.

Discussion.—In the future, use of a combination of growth factors may mobilize sufficient cells to collect a transplant product with a single apheresis procedure. Also, PSCT might be used as an alternative to purging for patients with malignant involvement of the marrow.

▶ The search for the hematopoietic stem cell (HSC) has long been an important quest among experimental and clinical hematologists. Recognition of CD34 as a potential marker for HSC represents a major breakthrough (1, 2).

Combined with new technologies for separation and cell sorting of marrow and peripheral blood cells, the CD34 marker provides new opportunities for studying the properties of stem cells as described below by Caux et al. (Abstract 18–4). The effect of cytokines on hematopoiesis involves complex interactions among stem cells, committed progenitor cells, adherent cells, and lymphoid cells. Advances in identifying early progenitor cells has made possible the separation of purified populations and allowed a more critical analysis of the effects of growth factors on cellular proliferation, differentiation, and studies of the regulation of transcription and translation of specific genes. Ultimately, these experiments will identify the conditions and growth factors essential for optimizing the sustained function in vitro and in vivo of hematopoietic stem cells.

Clinical applications of CD34 selection may include marrow purging as demonstrated by Berenson et al. (Abstract 18–5) and the collection of HSC from peripheral blood for autologous transplantation as discussed by Sienna et al. (Abstract 18–6) and Kessinger and Armitage (Abstract 18–7).—J.A. Hansen, M.D.

References

1. Civin CI, et al: *J Immunol* 133:157, 1984.
2. Andrews RG, et al: *Blood* 67:842, 1986.

The Role of Donor Lymphoid Cells in Allogeneic Marrow Engraftment
Martin PJ (Univ of Washington)
Bone Marrow Transplant 6:283–289, 1990   18–8

Background.—There is no satisfactory method of prophylaxis against graft-vs.-host disease (GVHD) currently available for patients who receive unmodified marrow from an unrelated donor or from a related donor who is mismatched for more than 1 HLA antigen. The effect of donor lymphoid cells in allogeneic marrow engraftment was evaluated.

Discussion.—When disparity exists for major histocompatibility complex (MHC) class I antigens or minor histocompatibility antigens presented by MHC-class I molecules, CD8 cells appear to cause GVHD. If there is disparity for MHC-class II antigens or minor antigens presented by MHC class II molecules, CD4 cells cause the disease. In both HLA-identical and HLA-nonidentical transplantation, T-cell depletion of the donor marrow can avoid posttransplant immunosuppression and reduce risk of GVHD; however, it also increases the risk of graft failure. The donor T cells appear to eliminate or inactivate host lymphocytes that survive the preparative regimen and remain capable of causing rejection. However, it remains unclear whether the T cells that facilitate engraftment are the same as the T cells that cause GVHD. According to the few applicable animal models, cells which do not initiate GVHD can mediate a marrow graft-enhancing effect. In addition, GVHD itself does not necessarily enhance engraftment. Donor T cells could have "veto activity," by which they can specifically prevent a "host-vs.-graft" immune response when they are recognized by host T cells. Donor T cells may also produce lymphokines or cytokines to promote the growth and differentiation of hematopoietic stem cells; this could also facilitate engraftment without causing GVHD. There might also be a graft-vs.-host effect specific for host lymphoid cells, thus preventing rejection without necessarily, causing GVHD if the mediating donor cells recognize host alloantigens that are not expressed in the skin, liver, or gut.

Conclusions.—The possible mechanisms of donor lymphoid cells in promoting marrow graft enhancement are examined. Studies of the relative importance of these mechanisms are essential, as the results will have important implications in trials of GVHD prevention by T-cell depletion.

▶ This is a timely and comprehensive review of clinical and experimental data describing the role of donor lymphoid cells in facilitating sustained allogeneic hematopoietic engraftment. Graft-vs.-host disease (GVHD) remains a significant clinical problem, especially in HLA-mismatched and unrelated donor transplants. However, graft failure also occurs after HLA-mismatched transplants. T-cell depletion of donor marrow is effective in preventing GVHD, but has been associated with a relatively high graft failure rate. Graft failure appears to be mediated by host lymphoid cells, which may be more likely to survive transplantation if the donor marrow has been T-cell depleted. Persistence of host cells or split chimerism is less likely to occur after transplantation of unmodified marrow grafts that contain immunologically competent donor T cells. Unfortunately, little is known about the mechanisms by which residual host lymphoid cells interact with donor T cells and hematopoietic stem cells. Understanding the critical events in the early stages of engraftment may provide rationale for more selective cellular manipulations or the use of growth factors to abrogate GVHD without compromising engraftment.—J.A. Hansen, M.D.

Syngeneic and Allogeneic Bone Marrow Engraftment After Total Body Irradiation: Dependence on Dose, Dose Rate, and Fractionation
Down JD, Tarbell NJ, Thames HD, Mauch PM (State University of Groningen, The Netherlands; Harvard Med School, Boston; M.D. Anderson Hosp and Tumor Inst, Houston)
Blood 77:661–669, 1991   18–9

Background.—Graft failure or rejection of T-cell-depleted allogeneic marrow is a current problem in bone marrow transplantation (BMT). It remains unknown how the routine colony-forming unit (CFU) assay reflects ablation of more primitive stem cells or suppression of host immunity. Representative bone marrow chimera models of syngeneic and allogeneic BMT were established in mice to address these issues.

Methods.—The recipient animals were standard B6 mice. Male B6-Hbb^d congenic mice were used as donors of syngeneic marrow, and LP, H-2 compatible mice were used as donors of allogeneic marrow. Host total body irradiation (TBI) was given at varying doses, dose rates, and fractionation schemes. Gel electrophoresis was done on host and donor stem-cell–derived hemoglobin phenotypes (Hbb^s and Hbb^d 3 months after transplantation to determine stable marrow chimerism.

Results.—In the syngeneic model, partial engraftment was seen at doses as low as 2 Gy. The donor component increased with TBI dose to 100% at 7 Gy. The hosts' immunologic resistance prevented allogeneic engraftment up to a dose of 5.5 Gy; at 6 Gy and above, there was a very steep radiation dose response, such that the level of chimerism was comparable with syngeneic engraftment. In both models, a low dose rate and fractionated TBI required higher total doses for equivalent engraftment; this displacement was noted with interfraction intervals of 3 and 6 hours. When the interval was extended to 18 and 24 hours, any further dose-sparing effect was limited to the allogeneic model. It was difficult to apply the linear-quadratic model for radiation cell survival because multiple target cell populations were involved in determining allogeneic engraftment.

Conclusions.—In both syngeneic and allogeneic models of BMT, the recovery with a low TBI dose rate and 6-hour interfraction intervals is consistent with significant sublethal damage repair in the host's primitive self-renewing stem cell population. This is in contrast to the poor repair capability of 11-day spleen CFUs after fractionated irradiation, and it lends credence to the idea that ablation of early stem cells in the pre-CFU compartment is essential for long-term marrow engraftment.

▶ This study examines dose rate, fractionation, and total dose of TBI on the engraftment of syngeneic and allogeneic bone marrow cells in mice. These results illustrate the variable radiation sensitivity of 2 relevant populations of host cells, hematopoietic stem cells, and the cells responsible for immune-mediate graft resistance. Analysis of the radiation dose response of 2 endpoints, the level of sustained chimerism and spleen CFUs, suggests that the elimination of stem cells as well as suppression of host immunity is required to achieve full donor engraftment.—J.A. Hansen, M.D.

Impact of Pretransplant Conditioning and Donor T Cells on Chimerism, Graft-Versus-Host Disease, Graft-Versus-Leukemia Reactivity, and Tolerance After Bone Marrow Transplantation
Truitt RL, Atasoylu AA (Med College of Wisconsin, Milwaukee)
Blood 77:2515–2523, 1991   18–10

Introduction.—Immunologic reactivity between donor and recipient cells, in all its manifestations, significantly influence survival after allogeneic bone marrow transplantation. A murine model of major histocompatibility complex (MHC) compatible marrow transplantation was used to examine relationships between pretransplant conditioning and the T-cell content of donor marrow on the one hand, and graft-vs.-host disease and T-cell chimerism on the other.

Methods.—Host AKR mice received total body irradiation at an optimal or suboptimal level and then were given marrow cells from B10.BR donor mice, with or without spleen cells added as a source of T lymphocytes. A supralethal dose of AKR leukemia cells was administered to marrow recipients 20 and 45 days after transplantation.

Observations.—The occurrence of graft-vs.-leukemia (GVL) reactivity depended on the receipt of mature donor T cells, and was noted only in complete chimeras. Transplantation of T cell-deficient marrow led to the persistence of host T cells even after lethal total body irradiation. Mixed chimerism correlated with a lack of GVL reactivity. Provision of a moderate number of donor T cells enhanced T-cell engraftment, provided a significant GVL effect, and produced only mild graft-vs.-host disease. Severe and even fatal graft-vs.-host disease developed with a higher dose of irradiation.

Conclusion.—The presence of mature T cells in transplanted bone marrow appears to be the most significant factor determining survival in leukemic hosts.

▶ Truitt and Atasoylu address a question similar to that discussed in the study by Down et al. (Abstract 18–9). Truitt and Atasoylu examine an additional variable by analyzing the effect of donor T cells on engraftment. An essential relationship is demonstrated between the total dose of TBI and the number of donor T cells present in the graft with the level of posttransplant donor chimerism. These 3 factors interact to determine the incidence and severity of GVHD and GVL activity. This study does not address the key issue of whether the effector cells causing GVHD and GVL are the same, but it does clearly demonstrate that immunologically competent donor T cells must be present in the graft and apparently must persist for some time in the recipient before a GVL effect can occur.—J.A. Hansen, M.D.

Total Lymphoid Irradiation to Prevent Graft Rejection in Recipients of HLA Non-Identical T Cell-Depleted Allogeneic Marrow
Soiffer RJ, Mauch P, Tarbell NJ, Anderson KC, Freedman AS, Rabinowe SN, Takvorian T, Murrey CI, Coral F, Bosserman L, Dear K, Nadler LM, Ritz J (Harvard Med School)
Bone Marrow Transplant 7:23–33, 1991   18–11

Background.—In patients undergoing bone marrow transplantation (BMT) using nonidentical T cell-depleted bone marrow, graft failure may occur in up to 30% to 60%. The process of rejection is an active one, mediated by $CD3^+$ $CD8^+$ host T cells that are specifically cytotoxic for donor hematopoietic cells. A pilot study of total lymphoid irradiation (TLI), as an adjunct to total body irradiation, was performed to suppress the activity of residual host-derived alloreactive lymphocytes.

Methods.—The patients were 10 adults, median age 29 years, who underwent allogeneic BMT using marrow from non-HLA identical siblings. All received a preparative regimen of cyclophosphamide, 60 mg/kg/day × 2, followed by total body irradiation, up to 1,400 cGy. Before hospitalization, the patients received TLI; in most cases, 750 cGy delivered to 2 complementary radiation ports in five 150 cGy fractions. Marrow infusion was done 30–38 days later.

Results.—Nine patients achieved full hematologic engraftment, defined as an absolute neutrophil count of .5 × 10^9/L and platelet count of 40 × 10^9/L. By comparison, none of 4 patients who did not receive TLI achieved engraftment. Median time to reach the target neutrophil count was 19 days, and median time to reach the target platelet count was 23 days. Patients undergoing TLI had significant lymphopenia before transfusion, but there were no suppressive effects on reconstitution of donor lymphocytes.

Conclusions.—Total lymphoid irradiation, as an adjunct to T cell depletion, may decrease graft rejection in patients who undergo BMT with imperfectly HLA-matched donors. The treatment is well tolerated and can be done on an outpatient basis. Further study of this treatment for patients at high risk of rejection is ongoing.

► Although these investigators were able to show a beneficial effect of TLI on engraftment of HLA nondentical T cell-depleted marrow grafts, others have failed to show a positive effect for TLI (1, 2). These differences are likely because of variations in the way T cell depletion is done, differences in HLA matching, and differences in the TLI procedure. Although the preliminary results reported here are encouraging, a large clinical trial will be necessary to gauge more fully the acute and long-term toxicity of adding TLI, and eventually patient survival.—J.A. Hansen, M.D.

References

1. Ganem G, et al: *Transplantation* 45:244, 1988.
2. Champlin RE, et al: *Transplant Proc* 19:2616, 1987.

The Effect of Combining Cyclophosphamide With Total-Body Irradiation on Donor Bone Marrow Engraftment

Down JD, Mauch PM (University of Groningen, The Netherlands; Harvard Med School, Boston)
Transplantation 51:1309–1311, 1991

18–12

Background.—The combination of cyclophosphamide (CY) and total-body irradiation (TBI) should improve engraftment by preventing graft-vs.-host reaction. There are few data on the optimal combination of these 2 conditioning regimens, however. The combination of CY and TBI was studied in mouse models of syngeneic and allogeneic bone marrow transplantation (BMT).

Methods.—Recipient animals received CY, in a single bolus of 200 mg/kg, either 3 days or 3 hours before irradiation at 4 to 8 Gy, followed by allogeneic transplantation. At TBI doses of 5 and 7 Gy, CY was given at greater intervals. The same CY pretreatment intervals were observed for mice undergoing syngeneic transplantation, but TBI was limited to a single 4-Gy dose.

Results.—There was a severe dose-dependent increase in allogeneic engraftment with irradiation, and at higher TBI doses engraftment was comparable to syngeneic engraftment. Cyclophosphamide was completely ineffective when given as a sole conditioning agent. It did, however, enhance engraftment when added 3 hours before TBI, as reflected by partial chimerism at 4 and 5 Gy. Giving CY 3 days before TBI inhibited engraftment, allowing partial chimerism at 7 and 8 Gy.

Conclusions.—Use of CY for immune suppression before BMT can remove hose resistance of H-2–identical allogeneic marrow engraftment when given 24 and 3 hours before, but not when given 3 days after TBI. A key to the success of BMT is the sequencing and timing of this regimen; the current use of CY in clinical conditioning regimens may need reevaluation.

▶ In the model studied here, cyclophosphamide used as a single agent was not sufficient for achieving sustained engraftment of MHC identical marrow allografts, but was effective in combination with TBI. The authors hypothesize that sustained engraftment depends not only on the immunosuppressive properties of cyclophosphamide and TBI, but also on the ablation of host hematopoietic stem cells, which presumably must be eliminated to avoid recovery of host hematopoiesis and mixed chimerism.—J.A. Hansen, M.D.

Anti-Asialo GM1 Antiserum Treatment of Lethally Irradiated Recipients Before Bone Marrow Transplantation: Evidence That Recipient Natural Killer Depletion Enhances Survival, Engraftment, and Hematopoietic Recovery

Tiberghien P, Longo DL, Wine JW, Alvord WG, Reynolds CW (Natl Cancer Inst, Frederick, Md)
Blood 76:1419–1430, 1990   18–13

Introduction.—Previous studies suggested that natural killer (NK) cells play an important role in the resistance of lethally irradiated recipients to bone marrow transplantation (BMT). One possible mechanism for the detrimental effect of NK cells was noted in a patient with aplastic anemia who had repeated syngeneic graft failure. In vitro studies showed that NK cells from the recipient inhibited the growth of donor bone marrow (BM) granulocyte progenitor cells. The effects of recipient NK depletion on survival, chimerism, and hematopoietic reconstitution after lethal irradiation and the transplantation of limiting amounts of T cell-deficient BM were investigated.

Method.—Experiments were carried out in male, 8- to 12-week-old mice. Several short- and long-term effects of depleting recipient NK activity were investigated in lethally irradiated mice before BMT. Long-term survival and chimerism after transplantation were first measured. To quantify more sensitively the effect of recipient NK depletion, limited amounts of BM were infused. T cell-deficient BM was selected to eliminate graft-vs.-host disease and allow for the correlation of survival with immunohematopoietic reconstitution.

Results.—Anti-asialo GM1 (ASGM1) antiserum treatment, when administered before BMT, was associated with a marked increase in survival in 3 of 3 allogeneic combinations (BALB/c into C3H/HeN, C57Bl/6, or C3B6F1). Anti-ASGM1 treatment also increased survival in recipients of syngeneic BM, suggesting that NK cells can adversely affect engraftment independent of genetically controlled polymorphic cell surface determinants. Overall, depletion of NK activity by anti-ASGM1 had a favorable influence on hematopoietic events after transplantation.

Conclusion.—Human patients might benefit from pretransplant regimens designed to deplete NK cells. Depletion of NK cells also affected peripheral cell counts, with significantly enhanced platelet and red blood cell recovery and a moderate increase in granulocyte recovery.

▶ The kinetics of hematopoietic engraftment in mice after lethal doses of total body irradiation (1,000–1,200 rads) and treatment with anti-ASGM1 antiserum is reported in detail. A new finding of interest was the observation that NK cells can adversely affect hematopoietic stem cell engraftment independent of genetic disparity. Anti-ASGM1 treatment was effective in enhancing the rate of engraftment and increasing survival in recipients of both allogeneic and syngeneic marrow. It is unclear whether this occurs simply because of the depletion of NK cells or as the result of some other unrecognized effect of the anti-ASGM1 antiserum.—J.A. Hansen, M.D.

Improvement of Allogeneic Marrow Engraftment by Treatment With Anti-LFA-1 (CD11a) Monoclonal Antibodies

▶ ↓ The review by Martin summarized earlier (Abstract 18–8) discussed the pathogenesis of graft failure and the potential importance of residual host immune cells in suppressing or rejecting donor hematopoietic stem cells. The following 2 papers describe an experimental model (Abstract 18–14) and results of a multicenter clinical trial (Abstract 18–5) using monoclonal antibodies specific for the CD11a component of the LFA-1 complex to facilitate engraftment of T cell-depleted donor marrow. These are very encouraging data and provide an important alternative to the approaches described earlier that are based on intensification of pretransplant cytotoxic therapy. Increasing the dose or dose rate of TBI increases both immunosuppression and stem cell depletion in the recipient, but the margin of safety between the desired beneficial effects and excessive regimen-related toxicity (including the potentiation of GVHD) is limited.—J.A. Hansen, M.D.

Evidence That Anti-LFA-1 In Vivo Improves Engraftment and Survival After Allogeneic Bone Marrow Transplantation
van Dijken PJ, Ghayur T, Mauch P, Down J, Burakoff SJ, Ferrara JLM (Dana-Farber Cancer Inst, Boston; Joint Ctr for Radiation Therapy, Boston; Wilhemina Children's Hospital, Utrecht, The Netherlands)
Transplantation 49:882–886, 1990   18–14

Introduction.—Rejection of allogeneic bone marrow can be lethal, especially when T cells have been depleted to reduce the chance of graft-vs.-host disease. An anti-LFA-1 (Cd11a) monoclonal antibody (MAb) was developed for use as a preventative treatment of graft rejection. The LFA-1 molecule was used in mice to increase hematologic and immunologic reconstitution and survival of transplant recipients.

Methods.—After T cells were depleted, they were injected into C57BL/6 (B6→B6) or A/J (B6→A/J) mice, some of which were preconditioned with 1,100 cGy of total body irradiation. An IgG2b rat antimouse LFA-1 MAb, M7/15, was injected intraperitoneally for the first 5 days after bone marrow transplantation. At 1 month and 6 months after transplantation, 4 animals from each group were killed and analyzed. Cell surface phenotyping was performed with pooled cells.

Findings.—Hematopoiesis increased by fourfold when measured by peripheral hematocrit and by almost sixfold when assayed by the frequency of colony-forming units in serum in animals receiving anti-LFA-1. Immunologic reconstitution was also significantly improved in these animals. Both hematopoiesis and lymphopoiesis increased within 1 month after marrow transplantation. Long-term survival and lymphohematopoietic reconstruction were enhanced in A/J recipients of allogeneic T-cell-depleted C57BL/6 bone marrow, demonstrating that anti-LFA-1 given in vivo prevents graft failure. Six months after bone marrow transplantation, hematologic and immunologic reconstitution approached normal levels in the B6→A/J chimeras for antibody rejection. Lymphocytes from these animals were found to contain lower pPTL frequencies when compared to normal or B6→B6 BMT controls.

Conclusions.—These findings indicate that animals receiving anti-LFA-1 treatment had significantly improved long-term survival with no loss of lymphohematopoietic reconstitution. These results establish the ability of the single MAb anti-CD11a to provide a broad target cell range to improve engraftment of T cell-depleted bone marrow when given with 1,100 cGy of total body irradiation to precondition the host.

Reduction of Graft Failure by a Monoclonal Antibody (Anti–LFA-1 CD11a) After HLA Nonidentical Bone Marrow Transplantation in Children With Immunodeficiencies, Osteopetrosis, and Fanconi's Anemia: A European Group for Immunodeficiency/European Group for Bone Marrow Transplantation Report

Fischer A, Friedrich W, Fasth A, Blanche S, Le Deist F, Girault D, Veber F, Vossen J, Lopez M, Griscelli C, Hirn M (Hôpital des Enfants-Malades, Paris; Dept of Pediatrics, Ulm, Germany; Dept of Pediatrics, Goteborg, Sweden; Dept of Pediatrics, Leiden, The Netherlands; CTS, Saint-Antoine, Paris)
Blood 77:249–256, 1991   18–15

Background.—Several approaches have been successful in allowing sustained engraftment of major histocompatibility complex (MHC)-incompatible bone marrow, but many cannot be used in humans because of their potential toxicity. A series of children was treated with an anti-CD11a-lymphocyte function-associated antigen 1 (LFA-1) monoclonal antibody (MoAb) to prevent graft failure.

Patients.—The study was comprised of 46 infants and children, 25 with inherited immunodeficiency disorders, 17 with malignant osteopetrosis, and 4 with Fanconi's anemia. All received from a related donor HLA-nonidentical bone marrow that was T cell-depleted to reduce the risk of graft-vs.-host disease. The mouse CD11a-LFA-1 MoAb was administered in 5 infusions of .1 mg/kg on alternate days from 3 days before to 5 days after BMT in 11 patients. In the remaining 35 patients, the MoAb was given in a dose of .2 mg/kg/day from 3 days before to 6 days after BMT.

Outcome.—The children achieved a 72% rate of sustained engraftment, compared to 26.1% in a group of 24 historical controls. There was no late rejection, and the E-rosetting T cell-depletion method improved the rate of engraftment. The degree of HLA incompatibility also affected engraftment to some extent. There was a 35.5% rate of acute GVHD and a 12.9% rate of chronic GVHD. At a mean follow-up of 28 months, the rate of survival with a functional graft was 47.3% for patients with immunodeficiency and osteopetrosis. None of the patients with Fanconi's anemia survived. The average time to full T-cell function was 6 months, and that to full B-cell function was 10 months. Most patients had serious infectious problems after BMT, including B-cell proliferative syndrome induced by the Epstein-Barr virus.

Conclusions.—In patients with life-threatening immunodeficiency and osteopetrosis, anti-CD11a-LFA-1 Moab immunosuppressive therapy in HLA-nonidentical T cell-depletion BMT may promote engraftment, survival, and correction of the primary disease. The treatment has not been successful in patients with Fanconi's anemia.

Measuring the Degree of Donor Chimerism After Allogeneic Marrow Transplantation

Amplification by the Polymerase Chain Reaction of Hypervariable Regions of the Human Genome for Evaluation of Chimerism After Bone Marrow Transplantation

Ugozzoli L, Yam P, Petz LD, Ferrara GB, Champlin RE, Forman SJ, Koyal D, Wallace RB (City of Hope Natl Med Ctr, Duarte, Calif; Univ of California, Los Angeles; Instituto Nazionale per la Ricerca sul Cancro, Genoa, Italy)
Blood 77:1607–1615, 1991   18–16

Background.—Hypervariable regions of the human genome are polymorphic because of variation in the number of tandemly repeated sequences in different alleles: the so-called variable number of tandem repeats (VNTR) loci. These markers are inherited in a Mendelian manner and, when a locus has multiple alleles, they may be very informative. Synthetic oligonucleotide probes complementary to VNTR repeat units can detect mixed hematopoietic chimerism when the recipient DNA constitutes 1% to 2% of total leukocyte DNA.

Objective.—The polymerase chain reaction (PCR) was combined with oligonucleotide hybridization to assess posttransplant chimerism in 13 patients having marrow transplantation.

Methods.—Specific oligonucleotides for use in hybridization were synthesized homologous to tandemly repetitive core sequences of regions with VNTRs. Primers flanking the repeat region of each corresponding VNTR were used for amplification. Conventional restriction fragment length polymorphism analysis also was carried out.

Findings.—Mixed chimerism was discovered in 4 patients and complete chimerism was found in 5. Two patients had recurrent leukemia, and 2 exhibited endogenous repopulation of hematopoiesis after marrow transplantation. In all patients but 2, the PCR data correlated with restriction fragment length polymorphism data; in these exceptional patients, PCR was more sensitive. The limit of detection of the minor component in a given mixture was .1%.

Conclusions.—This is a significant improvement over previous methods of analyzing postmarrow transplant chimerism. It is very sensitive, uses only 250 ng of DNA, and precludes the need for restriction enzymes. Studies may be completed in 2 days.

▶ The polymerase chain reaction has had a broad impact on biological and medical sciences. As reported in the previous 2 papers, PCR amplification of the highly polymorphic tandem repeated sequences provides an overall more sensitive assay for detecting minimal numbers of chimeric cells (to approximately .1%), and substantially smaller quantities of cells or DNA are required compared to conventional RFLP assays. Future studies of mixed chimerism, GVHD, GVL, and tolerance will gain substantially from the availability of this new method.—J.A. Hansen, M.D.

Evaluation of Mixed Chimerism by In Vitro Amplification of Dinucleotide Repeat Sequences Using the Polymerase Chain Reaction
Lawler M, Humphries P, McCann SR (St James' Hospital and Trinity College, Dublin, Ireland)
Blood 77:2504–2514, 1991   18–17

Background.—Allogeneic marrow transplantation now is an effective approach to many patients having leukemia or aplastic anemia, but the influence of mixed hematopoietic chimerism (MC) after transplantation remains uncertain. Mixed chimerism does appear to be a frequent sequel. Polymerase chain reaction (PCR) to analyze fragment length polymorphisms (PCR-FLP) is a very sensitive means of evaluating chimerism after marrow transplantation.

Study Plan.—Simple dinucleotide repeat sequences, so-called microsatellites, vary in their repeat number among individuals. This variation was used to type 30 allogeneic and 2 syngeneic donor-recipient pairs after marrow transplantation. A panel of 7 microsatellites served to distinguish between donor and recipient cells, and informative microsatellites then were used to assess MC. Seventeen transplants involved an opposite-sexed donor, allowing cytogenetics and Y chromosome-specific PCR to indicate chimerism.

Findings.—Mixed chimerism was detected in 56% of patients by PCR. Analysis of microsatellites or Y chromosome material was effectively carried out using stored slide material. Mixed chimerism was detected cytogenetically in 3 of the 17 assessable patients; it was more frequent in patients given T cell-depleted marrow but also occurred in 44% of those who received unaltered bone marrow. Recipient cells tended to increase relatively suddenly in patients who later had relapse, and patients who had relapse had a higher proportion of recipient cells than those exhibiting stable MC.

Conclusions.—Although MC does not in itself indicate a poor outlook after marrow transplantation, a sudden rise in the proportion of recipient cells may precede marrow graft rejection or relapse. Further studies will show whether different conditioning regimens influence the incidence of stable MC.

Analysis of Factors Predicting Speed of Hematologic Recovery After Transplantation With 4-Hydroperoxycyclophosphamide-Purged Autologous Bone Marrow Grafts
Rowley SD, Piantadosi S, Marcellus DC, Jones RJ, Davidson NE, Davis JM, Kennedy J, Wiley JM, Wingard JR, Yeager AM, Santos GW (Johns Hopkins Oncology Ctr, Baltimore)
Bone Marrow Transplant 7:183–191, 1991   18–18

Background.—Previous research has indicated the predictive value of graft colony-forming units granulocyte macrophage (CFU-GM) content after 4-hydroperoxycyclophosphamide (4-HC) purging for the duration of aplasia after autologous bone marrow transplantation. Despite uniform 4-HC concentrations, there was heterogeneity in CFU-GM survival and engraftment kinetics. The variability in speed of engraftment after autologous bone marrow transplantation with 4-HC purged grafts was further studied.

Methods and Results.—Patient and graft characteristics of 154 patients undergoing autologous transplantation with 4-HC purged grafts were analyzed. Those patients with transplants for the treatment of malignant lymphoma reached a peripheral blood granulocyte count of more than $.5 \times 10^9$/L and platelet transfusion independence significantly more quickly than those with acute non-lymphoblastic leukemia; differences were independent of graft CFU-GM content. Many other patient and graft factors also predicted the kinetics of engraftment in univariate and multivariate analysis. These factors included patient age, peripheral blood counts on the day of harvest, and amounts of other hematopoietic progenitors. Cytomegalovirus infection occurring in the aplastic period predicted delayed granulocyte recovery but not platelet recovery.

Conclusions.—Many patient, graft, and posttransplant factors predict the engraftment ability of autografts and the kinetics of engraftment with 4-HC purged grafts. These multiple factors can account for a significant portion of the variability in engraftment kinetics seen after transplantation with 4-HC purged autografts.

▶ Factors affecting engraftment of allogeneic hematopoietic stem cells (HSC) are complex even when donor and recipient are HLA genotypically identical. This report evaluates the engraftment of autologous HSC after treatment in vitro with an alkylating agent for purging of malignant cells. A critical issue in studies such as this has been the need for in vitro assays for measuring the proliferative and differentiation capacity of marrow progenitor cells. Unfortunately, there is no assay system for assessing the quantity and activity of HSC. This group has previously shown that the granulocyte macrophage colony-forming unit (CFU-GM) assay predicts the kinetics of engraftment of purged marrow autografts (1), however, the engraftment of individual cases can be highly variable. The current report identifies clinical and treatment dependent variables that significantly affect the kinetics and quality of engraftment of autologous marrow. These variables should also affect the kinetics of allogeneic HSC engraftment, in addition to the genetic and immunological problems that are so important to allografts.—J.A. Hansen, M.D.

Reference

1. Rowley SD, et al: *Blood* 70:271–275, 1987.

19 The Experimental and Clinical Use of Recombinant Hematopoietic Growth Factors

▶ ↓ The major rationale underlying the use of marrow transplantation for treatment of hematologic malignancies is the ability to use high doses of marrow ablative chemoradiotherapy followed by the infusion of autologous cryopreserved or normal donor hematopoietic stem cells to allow the rescue of marrow function. Studies of hematopoietic colony-stimulating factors (G-CSF and GM-CSF) have shown accelerated recovery of granulocytes after both conventional chemotherapy and autologous marrow transplantation after high-dose chemotherapy (1–3).—John A. Hansen, M.D.

References

1. Brandt SJ, et al: *N Engl J Med* 318:869, 1988.
2. Nemunaitis J, et al: *Blood* 72:834, 1988.
3. Sheridan WP, et al: *Lancet* 2:891, 1989.

Acceleration of the Hemopoietic Reconstitution in Mice Undergoing Bone Marrow Transplantation by Recombinant Human Granulocyte Colony-Stimulating Factor

Tamura M, Yoshino T, Hattori K, Kawamura A, Nomura H, Imai N, Ono M
(Chugai Pharmaceutical Co, Shizuoka, Japan)
Transplantation 51:1166–1170, 1991   19–1

Background.—Human granulocyte and human granulocyte macrophage colony-stimulating factors (CSFs) appear to enhance recovery of peripheral blood neutrophils and shorten the leukopenic period after bone marrow transplantation (BMT) in both humans and animals. The effects of recombinant human granulocyte CSF (rG-CSF) were investigated in a mouse model of BMT.

Methods.—The animals were 8-week-old male C57BL/6N mice. All animals received 900 cGy of irradiation and then infusion of 1×10^6 bone marrow cells from syngeneic mice. From days 1 to 21 after this procedure, the mice received rG-CSF, 10 µg/kg/day, or control vehicle. Peripheral blood cells were measured at intervals up to 39 days after BMT, after which bone marrow and spleen cell suspensions were prepared for assays of stem cells and committed progenitor cells.

Results.—In mice treated with rG-CSF, in both bone marrow and spleen, increased numbers of spleen colony-forming units (CFUs), granulocyte-macrophage CFUs, megakaryocyte CFUs, and erythroid burst-forming units were found. These values increased approximately twofold (1.12 to 2.53 times) during the administration period. Although progenitor cell numbers increased, the peripheral blood showed accelerated recovery of neutrophils only, not of erythrocytes or platelets.

Conclusions.—In a model of BMT in mice, rG-CSF appears to accelerate granulopoietic recovery. Recovery of stem cells and the progenitors for erythrocytes and megakaryocytes is enhanced. In humans, rG-CSF could be useful in enhancing hemopoietic reconstitution after BMT.

Recombinant Granulocyte-Macrophage Colony-Stimulating Factor After Autologous Bone Marrow Transplantation for Relapsed Non-Hodgkin's Lymphoma: Blood and Bone Marrow Progenitor Growth Studies. A Phase II Eastern Cooperative Oncology Group Trial
Lazarus HM, Andersen J, Chen MG, Variakojis D, Mansour EG, Oette D, Arce CA, Oken MM, Gerson SL (Eastern Cooperative Oncology Group; Case Western Reserve Univ, Cleveland; Dana-Farber Cancer Inst, Boston; Mayo Clinic, Rochester, Minn; Northwestern Univ, Chicago, et al)
Blood 78:830–837, 1991   19–2

Introduction.—To evaluate the safety and efficacy of infusions of a mammalian-expressed recombinant human hematopoietic growth factor granulocyte-macrophage colony-stimulating factor (rhGM-CSF) during a total body irradiation-containing regimen, 16 patients with non-Hodgkin's lymphoma were studied. Specific effects on bone marrow (BM) and blood progenitors were examined.

Methods.—All 16 patients had either relapsed lymphoma or tumor resistant to cytotoxic drug therapy. Treatment consisted of involved-field radiotherapy, cyclophosphamide, 60 mg/kg/day administered intravenously for 2 days, and fractionated total-body irradiation, 1,200 cGy. The patients received a median of 26 days rhGM-CSF therapy after autologous bone marrow transplantation.

Results.—Only mild toxicities such as fever, chills, rash, myalgias, and synovial effusions occurred. Neutrophil recovery greater than 500/μL occurred at a median of 14 days after marrow infusion, significantly (6 days) earlier than the median time in historic controls. The median time to self-sustaining platelet counts greater than 20,000/μL was comparable to that of controls (23.5 days). As early as 7 days after marrow reinfusion, stem-cell progenitors and burst-forming unit-erythroid were detected in bone marrow; at 30–60 days, however, these values remained much lower than before transplant. And within 24–72 hours of discontinuing rhGM-CSF infusions, neutrophils transiently decreased in most (13) patients.

Conclusion.—Hematopoietic growth factor infusions have appeared to reduce morbidity in some patients undergoing transplantation. These findings suggest that rhGM-CSF therapy enhances neutrophil recovery by forcing stem cells to produce mature elements at an enhanced rate. However, marrow stem cells and early progenitor population sizes may not be affected by this therapy.

▶ The previous 2 reports describe the effects of recombinant growth factors on hematopoietic recovery in mice after syngeneic marrow transplantation and in humans after autologous transplantation. Tamura et al. (Abstract 19–1) describe the effects of G-CSF in syngenic transplants, and demonstrate that in addition to accelerating the rate of granulocyte recovery, G-CSF also increases the activity of progenitors for erythrocytes and megakaryocytes in bone marrow and spleen of mice. Lazarus et al. (Abstract 19–2) report additional phase II clinical data showing the safety, relatively low toxicity, and apparent efficacy of GM-CSF administered from day 1 to 26 after transplantation in accelerating granulocyte recovery. The activity of BFU-E and CFU-GM in bone marrow and blood were increased during GM-CSF therapy, but fell after completing the GM-CSF infusions, suggesting that the rate of progenitor maturation was increased without significant expansion of the stem cell pool.—J.A. Hansen, M.D.

Long-Term Follow-Up of Patients Who Received Recombinant Human Granulocyte-Macrophage Colony Stimulating Factor After Autologous Bone Marrow Transplantation for Lymphoid Malignancy
Nemunaitis J, Singer JW, Buckner CD, Mori T, Laponi J, Hill R, Storb R, Sullivan KM, Hansen JA, Appelbaum FR (Fred Hutchinson Cancer Research Ctr; VA Med Ctr; Immunex Corp, Seattle)
Bone Marrow Transplant 7:49–52, 1991   19–3

Background.—In patients undergoing autologous bone marrow transplantation (BMT), treatment with recombinant human granulocyte-macrophage colony-stimulating factor (rhGM-CSF) appears to reduce sepsis and shorten hospital stay. No studies have addressed the long-term consequences of rhGM-CSF. A long-term follow-up analysis of 27 patients treated with rhGM-CSF after autologous BMT was studied.

Patients.—The patients all received rhGM-CSF in phase I, II trials of autologous BMT for lymphoid malignancies, most commonly non-Hodgkin's lymphoma. There were 16 males and 11 females, median age 28 years. Twenty-four patients received rhGM-CSF, 15–240 $\mu g/m^2$/day either in a 2-hour or continuous infusion for 14 or 21 days after marrow remission.

Findings.—By the day of last contact, 13 of 26 evaluable patients had relapsed (median time 98 days after BMT). Thirteen patients were alive and 11 were disease-free at a median of 774 days. Marrow graft function was stable in all surviving patients who remained in remission.

Conclusions.—In patients undergoing autologous BMT, rhGM-CSF treatment does not appear to have any serious adverse long-term consequences. The small size and nonprospective nature of the reported trial are emphasized. If rhGM-CSF therapy has significant early benefits, randomized trials of larger size are indicated.

▶ This paper addresses 3 potential concerns about treatment with GM-CSF: late toxicity, failure to achieve long-term stem cell engraftment because of growth factor-driven depletion of the stem cell compartment during the early posttransplant period, and stimulation of residual malignant cells causing increased relapse. Within the limits of this phase II study, no significant adverse effects were detected. A definitive analysis will await the outcome of larger randomized trials.—J.A. Hansen, M.D.

The Use of Recombinant Human Granulocyte–Macrophage Colony Stimulating Factor for the Treatment of Delayed Engraftment Following High Dose Therapy and Autologous Hematopoietic Stem Cell Transplantation for Lymphoid Malignancies
Vose JM, Bierman PJ, Kessinger A, Coccia PF, Anderson J, Oldham FB, Epstein C, Armitage JO (Univ of Nebraska, Omaha; Hoechst-Roussel Pharmaceutical, Somerville; Immunex, Seattle)
Bone Marrow Transplant 7:139–143, 1991   19–4

Background.—Granulocyte-macrophage colony-stimulating factor (GM-CSF) accelerates hematopoietic recovery in primates subjected to total-body irradiation (TBI) and infusion of autologous bone marrow. Clinical trials of hematopoietic growth factors used to accelerate bone marrow recovery in humans treated with conventional chemotherapy or high-dose chemo-radiotherapy followed by autologous bone marrow transplantation have yielded encouraging results. The value of recombinant human GM-CSF was assessed in the treatment of delayed engraftment after high-dose therapy and autologous hematopoietic stem cell transplantation.

Methods.—Twelve patients with recurrent non-Hodgkin's lymphoma or Hodgkin's disease participated. The patients had an absolute granulocyte count of less than $150 \times 10^6/L$ on day 30 after autologous hematopoietic stem cell infusion. The study design was open-label and nonrandomized. The 12 patients were compared with 21 patients who served as historical controls.

Results.—Overall, patients treated with GM-CSF had a mean absolute granulocyte count of $705 \times 10^6/L$ on day 44 after stem cell infusion. The historical controls had a mean of $408 \times 10^6/L$. The GM-CSF–treated patients had significantly fewer documented bacterial and fungal infections after day 30. The toxicity associated with GM-CSF treatment was minimal. Only 1 patient had chills.

Conclusions.—Recombinant human GM-CSF appears to be effective in the treatment of delayed engraftment after high-dose therapy and autologous hematopoietic transplantation for lymphoid malignancies.

Most patients have accelerated granulocytic recovery and a decreased incidence of infections.

▶ This nonrandomized phase II study provides strong, although preliminary, evidence that GM-CSF can increase granulocyte production and decrease the incidence of clinical infection in patients who have failed to achieve adequate hematopoietic stem cell function after autologous marrow transplantation. Although these are encouraging results, the data available do not demonstrate substantial overall improvement in graft function. Overall, the treated patients had persistent marrow hypocellularity, continued to require platelet transfusions, and remained significantly neutropenic. Thus this therapy may be useful, but it does not seem to be a remedy for delayed engraftment.—J.A. Hansen, M.D.

In Vivo Administration of Granulocyte Colony-Stimulating Factor (G-CSF), Granulocyte-Macrophage CSF, Interleukin-1 (IL-1), and IL-4, Alone and in Combination, After Allogeneic Murine Hematopoietic Stem Cell Transplantation
Atkinson K, Matias C, Guiffre A, Seymour R, Cooley M, Biggs J, Munro V, Gillis S (St Vincent's Hospital, Sydney, Australia; Immunex Corp, Seattle)
Blood 77:1376–1382, 1991   19–5

Objective.—The use of various cytokines, alone and in combination, was explored in a murine model of allogeneic hematopoietic stem-cell transplantation to see whether they accelerate hematopoietic reconstitution.

Methods.—BALB/c mice received 10 Gy of total-body irradiation, followed by 10^7 marrow cells and 10^6 spleen cells from C57BL/6 donor mice. Recombinant cytokines were administered intraperitoneally twice daily.

Observations.—Circulating neutrophils were increased most effectively at 1 week by a combination of granulocyte colony-stimulating factor (G-CSF) and interleukin-1, followed by G-CSF alone, granulocyte macrophage colony stimulating factor (GM-CSF) plus interleukin-1, and G-CSF plus GM-CSF. At 10 days, neutrophil counts were highest in animals given G-CSF plus (GM-CSF). Neither G-CSF nor GM-CSF made graft-vs.-host disease more frequent or more severe. Animals given GM-CSF had improved survival. Administration of interleukin-1 in doses of 100 ng or more twice daily caused considerable early mortality. Doses of 500 ng of interleukin-4 twice daily may have increased late mortality through exacerbating graft-vs.-host disease.

Conclusions.—Certain combinations of cytokines can increase circulating neutrophils in mice given allogeneic bone marrow transplants. Studies of interleukins 3 and 6 would be of interest.

▶ Previous studies in syngeneic and autologous transplants have firmly established the efficacy of G-CSF and GM-CSF in accelerating granulocyte recovery, but additional studies were needed to demonstrate the effect of these growth factors in allografts and to determine whether or not they might adversely affect graft rejection and GVHD. The model described by Atkinson et al. should be useful for screening new growth factors and combinations of growth factors that might add to the activity of G-CSF or GM-CSF as single agents. Unfortunately, there still is no growth factor available that will facilitate engraftment and function of megakaryocytes.—J.A. Hansen, M.D.

Phase I/II Trial of Recombinant Human Granulocyte-Macrophage Colony-Stimulating Factor Following Allogeneic Bone Marrow Transplantation
Nemunaitis J, Buckner CD, Appelbaum FR, Higano CS, Mori M, Bianco J, Epstein C, Lipani J, Hansen J, Storb R, Thomas ED, Singer JW (Fred Hutchinson Cancer Res Ctr, Seattle; Univ of Washington, Seattle; Dept of VA Med Ctr, Seattle; Immunex Corp, Seattle; Hoechst Roussel Pharm Inc, Sommerville, NJ)
Blood 77:2,065–2,071, 1991   19–6

Background.—The use of recombinant human granulocyte-macrophage colony-stimulating factor (rhGM-CSF) in patients after autologous bone marrow transplantation (BMT) has produced encouraging results. The safety and efficacy of rhGM-CSF in patients who receive allogeneic BMT from HLA-matched, sibling donors were studied. Because of concern that concurrent rhGM-CSF might adversely affect hematopoietic reconstitution, 2 independent rhGM-CSF dose escalations were performed.

Methods.—Dose escalations of rhGM-CSF were performed in patients undergoing HLA-identical sibling BMT. One group of 27 patients was treated without methotrexate (MTX) and a group of 18 patients received MTX-containing graft-vs.-host disease (GVHD) prophylactic regimens.

Results.—Group 1, without MTX, reached an absolute neutrophil count of 1,000/μL by a median of day 14 and had fewer febrile days and shorter initial hospitalizations than group 2. The patients treated with GVHD prophylactic regimens containing MTX reached the same absolute neutrophil count on a median of day 20. There were no differences in the incidence or severity of GVHD between the 2 groups, and the overall incidence was similar to that of "good risk" patients who did not receive rhGM-CSF. A dose of 250 μg/m²/day of rhGM-CSF was well tolerated.

Conclusions.—The incidence or severity of GVHD in HLA-identical sibling donor transplants is not likely to increase with rhGM-CSF. Hematopoietic reconstitution was not adversely effected by rhGM-CSF even in patients receiving concurrent MTX. Further trials may determine whether rhGM-CSF affects transplant-related toxicities and whether survival can be improved while decreasing the BMT-associated morbidity.

▶ In this study of patients receiving allogeneic marrow transplantation, the ability of GM-CSF to accelerate myeloid engraftment was more apparent in patients receiving cyclosporine and prednisone for GVHD prophylaxis compared to patients receiving cyclosporine and methotrexate. More importantly, GM-

CSF did not cause an apparent increase in the incidence or severity of GVHD. The data also suggested that GM-CSF administered to allografts may be beneficial in reducing regimen related toxicity, fever, and clinical infection even in the absence of a significant shortening of the duration of neutropenia. The ultimate usefulness of GM-CSF in marrow allografts however is yet to be determined by appropriate randomized trials.—J.A. Hansen, M.D.

Regulation of Cytokine and Growth Factor Gene Expression in Human Bone Marrow Stromal Cells Transformed With Simian Virus 40

Slack JL, Nemunaitis J, Andrews DF III, Singer JW (Univ of Washington; VA Med Ctr, Seattle)
Blood 75 2319–2327, 1990   19–7

Background.—Differentiation and self-renewal of hematopoietic progenitor cells in long-term bone marrow culture depends on a supportive population of adherent cells (microenvironment or marrow stroma). Previous studies have suggested a model in which colony-stimulating factors (CSFs) aid in this process. The mechanisms of CSF and cytokine gene regulation were investigated in human marrow stromal cells. Also examined were the molecular mechanisms by which interleukin-1α (IL-1α) and tumor necrosis factor-α (TNF-α) alter growth factor and cytokine expression in simian virus 40-transformed marrow stromal cell lines (SV-MSCs).

Methods.—Normal donors contributed marrow aspirates for study. Cells were harvested by trypsinization, and total cellular RNA was isolated using acid guanidium thiocyanate-phenol-chloroform extraction. Isolated nuclei were subjected to run-on analysis.

Results.—The SV-MSCs constitutively expressed mRNA for macrophage (M)-CSF and tumor growth factor-β. Some cell lines also expressed small amounts of steady-state message for IL-6 and IL-1β. When treated with recombinant human IL-1α, SV-MCSs had a rapid and significant increase in steady-state mRNA for IL-6, IL-1β, and granulocyte/macrophage (GM)-CSF. Message induction occurred within 1 hour (8 hours for maximal effect) after the addition of IL-1α, whereas G-CSF mRNA was induced more slowly. The nuclear run-on assays indicated that IL-1α activated the genes for IL-6, GM-CSF, and IL-1β via transcription, but TNF-α induced expression of the IL-6 and IL-1β genes through transcription. The mRNA for IL-6 and IL-1β became "superinduced" by applying both TNF-α and cycloheximide. When the SV-MSC cells were cultured in the semisolid medium, they appeared as blastlike cells and formed colonies; these, when applied to the plastic medium, began adherent growth again. These SV-MSC colony-derived cells constitutively expressed colony-stimulating activity and mRNA for IL-6, IL-1β, GM-CSF, and G-CSF.

Implications.—These results suggest that the specific cytokine effects were not regulated by intermediate alterations in the viral protein expression of SV-MSCs. It would appear that SV-MCSs provide a reasonable model system for studying the molecular mechanisms of gene regulation of the cytokines and growth factors in human blood cells.

▶ Growth differentiation and self-renewal of hematopoietic stem cells requires interaction with a group of cells referred to collectively as the marrow stroma or hematopoietic microenvironment (1). Marrow stromal cells have the capacity to produce hematopoietic CSF as well as other cytokines. The finding that IL-1 and TNF can induce CSF activity and the molecular analysis of how the CSF genes are regulated are important not only to understanding the physiologic control of these growth factors, but also suggest possible mechanisms by which infection and immunologic reactions such as GVHD may affect stem cell function and hematopoiesis.—J.A. Hansen, M.D.

Reference

1. Dexter TM, et al: *J Cell Physiol* 91:335, 1977.

20 Graft-Versus-Host Disease (GVHD): Pathogenesis, Prevention, and Treatment

Conditioning-Related Toxicity and Acute Graft-Versus-Host Disease in Patients Given Methotrexate/Cyclosporine Prophylaxis
Deeg HJ, Spitzer TR, Cottler-Fox M, Cahill R, Pickle LW (Lombardi Cancer Research Ctr, Georgetown Univ Med Center, Washington DC; Naval Med Research Ctr, Bethesda, Md)
Bone Marrow Translant 7:193–198, 1991   20–1

Background.—Significant morbidity and mortality accompany intensive chemoradiotherapy conditioning regimens and acute graft-vs.-host-disease (GVHD) after bone marrow transplantation. Whether the conditioning regimen affects the development of acute GVHD was assessed in 30 patients with a lymphohematopoietic malignancy and 4 with severe aplastic anemia.

*Methods.*The patients were prepared for transplantation with cyclophosphamide (CY) alone, with CY combined with total body irradiation, or with CY combined with etoposide and total body irradiation or busfulfan. Prophylaxis of GVHD consisted of methotrexate, 10 mg/m^2, on days 1, 3 and 6, and daily cyclosporine begun the day before bone marrow transplantation and lasting to day 180.

Results.—Acute GHVD occurred in 36% of the patients. When assessed by severity of conditioning regimen-related toxicity, the incidence of GVHD grades II–IV was 0% for patients with mild toxicity, 37% for those with moderate toxicity, and 50% for those with severe toxicity. Compliance with GHVD prophylaxis decreased as the intensity and toxicity of the conditioning regimen increased.

Conclusions.—A GHVD prophylaxis regimen of continued infusion of cyclosporine and a shortened schedule of methotrexate is effective in preventing acute GVHD. The incidence of GHVD appears to correlate with the intensity of the transplant conditiong regimen, although the precise mechanism for this is not clear.

▶ High doses of marrow-ablative chemotherapy and radiation are given for maximum antitumor effect to patients with hematologic malignancy before marrow transplantation. However, these high-dose regimens can cause extensive mucositis and significantly compromise the function of the liver, lungs, kidneys, and myocardium (1). As reported by Deeg et al., the incidence and severity of acute GVHD appear to correlate with regimen-related toxicity (RRT). However, it is not clear whether RRT is directly involved in the pathogenesis of GVHD or whether it affects GVHD indirectly by interfering with the administration of the prescribed doses of immunosuppressive drugs. Both cyclosporine and methotrexate, 2 drugs commonly used for GVHD prophylaxis, are themselves potentially toxic, and are difficult to administer, especially in patients with RRT causing hepatic and renal dysfunction. Data were presented in an earlier review by Truitt and Atasoylu (2) that demonstrated an increased GVHD in allografted mice given higher doses of TBI. The latter observation was not correlated with RRT, but was associated with a diminished number of residual host cells posttransplant, suggesting that mixed chimerism may reduce the incidence or intensity of GVHD. A similar finding and hypothesis has been suggested by Hill et al. (3) based on studies of GVHD and mixed chimerism in patients receiving marrow transplants for treatment of aplastic anemia.—J.A. Hansen, M.D.

References

1. Bearman SI, et al: *J Clin Oncol* 6:1562, 1988.
2. Truitt RL, Atasoylu AA: *Blood* 77:2515, 1991.
3. Hill RS, et al: *Blood* 67:811, 1986.

Risk Factors for Acute Graft-Versus-Host Disease in Histocompatible Donor Bone Marrow Transplantation
Weisdorf D, Hakke R, Blazar B, Miller W, McGlave P, Ramsay N, Kersey J, Filipovich A (Univ of Minnesota, Minneapolis)
Transplantation 51:1197–1203, 1991   20–2

Introduction.—Allogeneic bone marrow transplantation (BMT) from histocompatible sibling donors often results in acute and chronic graft-vs.-host disease (GVHD), which is a significant cause of post-BMT morbidity and mortality. Previous studies have suggested various risk factors associated with acute GVHD. To design improved risk-directed prophylactic measures, the incidence, clinical risk factors, and posttransplant techniques associated with differing hazards of acute GVHD in patients with allogeneic BMT from matched sibling donors were defined.

Patients.—During a 9-year study period, 469 patients received allogeneic marrow transplants from HLA-matched sibling donors, of whom 238 had acute GVHD at a median of 32 days after BMT. Forty-one patients had maximum clinical grade I acute GVHD.

Results.—After univariate analysis, patient or donor age 18 years or older was significantly associated with increased risk of acute GVHD. Only 23% of patients younger than age 10 years and 34% of patients aged 10–20 years had acute GVHD. The risk of acute GVHD did not increase with age in older adults. Neither recipient sex nor donor sex predicted differing rates of GVHD. However, donor:recipient sex mismatch significantly increased GVHD risk. Female:female transplants were associated with the lowest incidence of GVHD. Increased risk of GVHD was associated with chronic myelogenous leukemia, cytomegalovirus seropositivity, and pre-existing donor alloimmunity from pregnancy or transfusion. The allele HLA-A26 was associated with increased risk of GVHD, whereas HLA-DR3 was associated with decreased GVHD risk. Stepwise multivariate analysis confirmed the significance of patient age and the presence of HLA-A26 as independent GVHD risk factors, and of female-to-female sex matching as predictive of lower GVHD.

Conclusion.—Older age is the predominant clinical risk factor for GVHD after allogeneic BMT from HLA-matched sibling donors. Donor-to-recipient sex matching, particularly in female to female combinations, is significantly and independently associated with lower GVHD risk.

▶ This paper reports findings generally concordant with other studies of GVHD risk factors, especially the increased risk of acute GVHD in older patients and in sex-mismatched transplants, especially when the donor is an alloimmunized female (1–5). Infection with CMV has been previously reported in some but not all studies to increase the incidence of GVHD. The current study found significantly less GVHD when patient and donor were CMV seronegative in a univariate analysis; however, in a subsequent multivariate analysis CMV status was no longer a significant factor.—J.A. Hansen, M.D.

References

1. Storb R, et al: *N Engl J Med* 308:302, 1983.
2. Bross DS, et al: *Blood* 63:1265, 1984.
3. Atkinson K, et al: *Br J Haematol* 63:231, 1986.
4. Klingemann H-G, et al: *Blood* 67:770, 1986.
5. Gale RP, et al: *Br J Haematol* 67:397, 1987.

Risk Factors for Chronic Graft-Versus-Host Disease After HLA-Identical Sibling Bone Marrow Transplantation
Atkinson K, Horowitz MM, Gale RP, van Bekkum DW, Gluckman E, Good RA, Jacobsen N, Kolb H-J, Rimm AA, Ringdén O, Rozman C, Sobocinski KA, Zwaan FE, Bortin MM (Med College of Wisconsin; St Vincent's Hospital, Sydney, Australia; Univ of California, Los Angeles; Radiobiological Inst TNO, Rijswijk, The Netherlands; Hôpital Saint-Louis, Paris; et al)
Blood 75:2459–2464, 1990   20–3

Background.—Several clinical features of chronic graft-vs.-host disease (GVHD) resemble those of autoimmune disorders. The relationship between acute and chronic GVHD is not completely understood. Risk factors for chronic GVHD were examined in 2,534 patients given HLA-identical sibling bone marrow transplants and in a special subset of 217 patients who had chronic GVHD without an acute phase.

Findings.—The probability of chronic GVHD developing within 3 years of marrow transplantation was 46% in this series. Acute GVHD was the chief risk factor. Among patients without significant acute GVHD, the most important risk factors for chronic disease were age older than 20 years, use of bone marrow non–T cell-depleted donor marrow, and an alloimmune female donor for a male recipient.

Discussion.—Acute and chronic GVHD may have the same cause—alloreactive T cells in donor bone marrow—and therefore may share risk factors for their clinical expression. Whether acute GVHD develops may depend on the type of prophylaxis used and the number of T cells administered. The onset of chronic GVHD may depend on a reduction in immunosuppressive medication and on the development of suppressor and autoreactive T cells.

▶ This study convincingly showed that the risk of chronic GVHD increased progressively with increasing severity of acute GVHD (see Figure 1 in the original article). The association between clinically significant grade II–IV acute and probability of chronic GVHD was not significantly affected by other variables that predict chronic GVHD in patients with no or minimal grade I gut GVHD such as patient age ≥20 years, non–T cell-depleted grafts and a multiparous (i.e., alloimmunized) female donor for a male recipient. These data suggest a cause and effect relationship and support the hypothesis that clinically significant acute GVHD may be responsible for inducing a progressive immune dysfunction that eventually manifests itself as cutaneous fibrosis, sicca syndrome, and chronic active hepatitis (1–3), as well as immune deficiency and susceptibility to infection (4). Data from Parkman (5) have provided insight to the mechanism by which successive and distinct populations of alloreactive donor T cells may be responsible for the distinct lesions seen in acute and chronic GVHD. Cytotoxic T cell clones reactive with the recipient are observed during acute but not chronic GVHD, and autoreactive T cell clones are observed in chronic but not acute GVHD (4).—J.A. Hansen, M.D.

References

1. Shulman HM, et al: *Am J Pathol* 91:545, 1978.
2. Graze PR, Gale RP: *Am J Med* 66:611, 1979.
3. Sullivan KM, et al: *Blood* 57:267, 1981.
4. Atkinson K, et al: *Blood* 60:714, 1982.
5. Parkman R: *J Immunol* 136:3543, 1986.

Prevention of Graft-Versus-Host Disease With T Cell Depletion or Cyclosporin and Methotrexate. A Randomized Trial in Adult Leukemic Marrow Recipients

Ringdén O, Pihlstedt P, Markling L, Aschan J, Båryd I, Ljungman P, Lönnqvist B, Tollemar J, Janossy G, Sundberg B (Karolinska Institute, Stockholm; Royal Free Hospital, London)

Bone Marrow Transplant 7:221–226, 1991   20–4

Background.—Animal and human studies show that T cell depletion of the transplanted marrow is an effective way to prevent GVHD. However, most of these studies also show that T cell depletion of the marrow results in an increased incidence of graft failure and leukemic relapse. T cell depletion was compared with effective pharmacologic immunosuppression using a combination of methotrexate and cyclosporine A.

Methods.—Fifty adult leukemic marrow recipients of HLA-identical sibling marrow participated. Twenty-three randomized to T cell depletion and 25 to cyclosporine A and 4 doses of methotrexate were evaluated.

Findings.—Anti-CD8 and anti-CD6 antibodies plus complement depleted a mean of 95.3% of CD3 cells. All but 1 patient, who died early, had engraftment. In those given T-cell–depleted marrow, the time to reach $.2 \times 10^9$ white blood cells per liter was shorter, but they needed more erythrocyte units. The 2 treatment groups were comparable with regard to platelet transfusions, infections, and length of time in the hospital. The incidence of grades II–III acute GVHD was 23% in the T-cell–depletion group and 12% in the drug-treated patients. Chronic GVHD developed in 51% and 23%, respectively. Patients receiving T-cell-depleted marrow who had grades I–III acute GVHD received more T cells than those without acute GVHD. In both groups the major cause of death was relapse, with a 4-year cumulative incidence of 39% in the T-cell–depleted marrow recipients and 54% in the drug-treated recipients. The 3-year actuarial leukemia-free survival in the 2 groups was 42% and 44%, respectively.

Conclusions.—Four doses of cyclosporine A combined with methotrexate appears to be as effective as T cell depletion in preventing acute GHVD in recipients of marrow from HLA-identical siblings. In both treatment groups, the level of GVHD was reduced to such a degree that it no longer represented a major clinical problem. This was achieved without an increased risk of graft failures.

▶ Prevention of GVHD is one of the major issues today in clinical marrow transplantation, especially for patients receiving HLA-incompatible or unrelated donor grafts. The focus of attention and effort divides along 2 strategies: T cell depletion of donor marrow and prophylactic immunosuppressive therapy. Ringden et al. meet this issue head on in patients with leukemia who underwent transplantation from an HLA-identical sibling. They did a randomized study comparing T cell depletion performed with anti-CD6 and anti-CD8 monoclonal antibody plus rabbit complement according to the method of Prentice et al. (1) versus prophylaxis with methotrexate (MTX) and cyclosporine (CSP) (2). To overcome the graft failure that might occur after T cell depletion, patients in the T-cell–depletion group received a combination of total body irradiation and total lymph node irradiation, while patients in the MTX + CSP group received TBI alone. Engraftment was not a problem in either group, but GVHD occurred in the T-cell–depletion group, indicating that T cell depletion was not complete. Leukemia-free survival was equivalent in the 2 groups, and thus overall there was no apparent advantage to either approach. Unfortunately, the primary question addressed by this study remains unanswered. Successful T cell depletion must allow sustained engraftment and prevent GVHD without loss of the GVL effect. In HLA-incompatible and unrelated donor transplants, situations where alternate therapy for preventing GVHD is most needed, successful T cell depletion may be even more challenging because clinical variables and risk factors such as HLA matching and risk of graft failure and GVHD may require differen degrees of T cell depletion to optimize the final clinical outcome.—J.A. Hansen, M.D.

References

1. Prentice HG, et al: *Lancet* i:472, 1984.
2. Storb R, et al: *N Engl J Med* 314:729–735, 1986.

Increased Risk of Leukemia Relapse With High-Dose Cyclosporine A After Allogeneic Marrow Transplantation for Acute Leukemia
Bacigalupo A, Van Lint MT, Occhini D, Gualandi F, Lamparelli T, Sogno G, Tedone E, Frassoni F, Tong J, Marmont AM (Ospedale San Martino Genvoa, Genova, Italy)
Blood 77:1423–1428, 1991   20–5

Introduction.—The most widely used agent for prophylaxis of graft-vs.-host disease (GVHD) after allogeneic bone marrow transplantation is cyclosporine A. Two different doses of intravenously administered Cya were compared in patients with acute leukemia undergoing allogeneic marrow transplantation, from an HLA-identical sibling.

Methods.—The 44 patients with acute myeloid leukemia and 37 with acute lymphoblastic leukemia were randomly assigned to receive cyclosporine A 1 mg/kg/day (group A) or 5 mg/kg/day (group B) from day -1 to $+20$ after bone marrow transplantation. Thereafter, all patients took cyclosporine A orally at the same dose. The patients were prepared with cyclophosphamide 120 mg/kg and fractionated total-body irradiation. All patients received unfractionated bone marrow from an HLA-identical sibling.

Results.—The median follow-up for survivors was 983 days in group A and 632 days in group B. Patients in the first group had lower serum levels of cyclosporine A, lower bilirubin levels, lower creatinine levels, and a lower proportion of $CD8^+$ cells in peripheral blood within 21 days. First day to $.5 \times 10^9/L$ neutrophils in the 2 groups was comparable. According to a Cox model, the actuarial risk of GVHD grade II+ after stratification for age was significantly lower in the patients in group B. Patients in both groups had a comparable actuarial risk of chronic GVHD developing. Actuarial transplant-related mortality at 240 days was 28% in group A and 26% in group B. The major cause of death was GVHD in group A and multiorgan toxicity in group B. Overall, the actuarial risk of relapse at 2 years was 20% in group A and 52% in group B. For patients in their first remission this risk was 9% in group A and 43%

in group B and for those in a later complete remission 48% in group A and 63% in group B. The actuarial 2-year disease-free survival overall was 58% in group A and in group B; 71% and 35% respectively in first remissions; and 30% and 23% respectively in advanced disease.

Conclusions.—Protection from GVHD-related death with high-dose cyclosporine A is offset by significant organ toxicity and leukemia relapse. Long-term disease-free survival is clearly better in patients given low doses of cyclosporine A after cyclophosphamide and fractionated total-body irradiation.

▶ A greater incidence of leukemia relapse was observed in this randomized study in the patient group receiving the higher dose of cyclosporine during the first 20 days after transplantation. The study was designed to compare a high dose and low dose cyclosporine regimen administered from day −1 to day +20. All patients were to receive the same dose of cyclosporine after day 20. The actual doses administered differed most during the first 10 days, because the percent of prescribed dose given to patients in the high dose arm declined after day +10 because of cyclosporine-associated toxicity. As described above, the higher dose regimen was successful in reducing the incidence of GVHD, but survival was not improved because the relapse rate was significantly greater in the high-dose group. These results dramatically demonstrate how the antileukemic or graft-vs.-leukemia (GVL) effect of a marrow allograft can be compromised by potent immunosuppression, and they emphasize the importance of immune-mediated reactions in eliminating residual leukemic cells after high-dose marrow ablative chemoradiotherapy. The effector mechanism responsible for the latter is unknown.—J.A. Hansen, M.D.

Methotrexate Combined With Cyclosporin A Decreases Graft-Versus-Host Disease, But Increases Leukemic Relapse Compared to Monotherapy
Aschan J, Ringdén O, Sundberg B, Gahrton G, Ljungman P, Winiarski J (Huddinge Hospital, Stockholm)
Bone Marrow Transplant 7:113–119, 1991   20–6

Background.—Methotrexate and cyclosporine A, the 2 most commonly used immunosuppressive drugs in bone marrow transplantation, are equally effective in preventing acute and chronic graft-vs.-host disease (GVHD). However, the role of these immunosuppressive drugs in relapse has not been established. The results of methotrexate combined with cyclosporine A were evaluated in the prevention of acute GVHD after bone marrow transplantation in leukemic patients with HLA-identical sibling donors.

Methods.—Forty patients were treated with 4 doses of methotrexate combined with cyclosporine. The results were then compared with those in 57 historical controls treated with methotrexate alone and 30 treated with cyclosporine alone. Patients were followed for more than 2 to almost 7 years.

Findings.—Engraftment was slowest in the group given the combined drugs and fastest in those given cyclosporine A alone. Moderate-to-severe acute GVHD occurred in 8% of patients treated with the combined drugs in 26% given methotrexate, and in 47% given cyclosporine A. Chronic GVHD developed in 25%, 42%, and 40%, respectively, a nonsignificant difference. None of the patients treated with combination therapy had cytomegalovirus-caused interstitial pneumonia, compared with 23% given methotrexate and 11% given cyclosporine. The actuarial 3-year survival was 56% in the combined drug group and 53% in the mono-therapy groups. The 3-year probability of relapse in the combination therapy group was significantly higher at 45% than that in the group given methotrexate (14%), but not significantly higher than that in the cyclosporine-treated group (27%). After 3 years, patients given combined treatment had a leukemia-free survival of 46%. This rate was 51% for patients given methotrexate and 50% for those given cyclosporine.

Conclusions.—Methotrexate combined with cyclosporine A is more effective in preventing GVHD than either drug alone used in historical control groups. Combination treatment is associated with a higher incidence of relapse, however, thus the rate of leukemia-free survival is unchanged.

▶ As shown previously, the combination of methotrexate (MTX) and cyclosporine (CSP) is more effective than either alone in preventing GVHD in patients with leukemia receiving marrow allografts from HLA-identical sibling donors (1, 2). However, Storb et al. (3) have reported that the improved immunosuppression and decreased incidence of GVHD achieved with MTX + CSP may be offset clinically by an increased relapse rate for patients with acute myeloblastic leukemia (AML) but not chronic myeloid leukemia (CML), compared with the use of CSP alone for GVHD prophylaxis. In this report, Aschan et al. compared MTX + CSP treated patients with AML, acute lymphoblastic leukemia (ALL), and CML to historical controls treated with either MTX or CSP alone. Although the actual 3-year survival for the 3 groups was equivalent, the probability of relapse by 3 years was higher in the MTX + CSP group (56%) compared to MTX or CSP alone (14% and 27%). Although a larger and randomized study would be required to determine more precisely the degree to which relapse may increase in specific diseases (ALL, AML, CML, and lymphoma), these results further emphasize the profound interrelationship of increased immunosuppression for GVHD prevention (or T cell depletion of donor marrow), decreased GVHD, and increased relapse, which is evidence of loss of the allograft GVL affect (4). Because risk of GVHD is age-dependent and strongly influenced by HLA matching, and risk of relapse is disease-and disease stage-dependent, the selection of the most appropriate GVHD prophylaxis may to be different for different patient groups.—J.A. Hansen, M.D.

References

1. Storb R, et al: *N Engl J Med* 314:729, 1986.
2. Morishima Y, et al: *Blood* 6:2252, 1989.
3. Storb R, et al: *Blood* 60:1729, 1989.
4. Horowitz MM: *Blood* 75:555, 1990.

What Role for Prednisone in Prevention of Acute Graft-Versus-Host Disease in Patients Undergoing Marrow Transplants?

Storb R, Pepe M, Anasetti C, Appelbaum FR, Beatty P, Doney K, Martin P, Stewart P, Sullivan KM, Witherspoon R, Bensinger W, Buckner CD, Clift R, Hansen J, Longton G, Loughran T, Petersen FP, Singer J, Sanders J, Thomas ED (Univ of Washington, Seattle)

Blood 76:1037–1045, 1990   20–7

Introduction.—Acute graft-vs.-host disease (GVHD) still develops in about one fourth of bone marrow recipients given methotrexate and cyclosporine, and the risk of death is significantly increased as a result. Prednisone is of established value in treating acute GVHD. Prednisone, given in addition to cyclosporine and methotrexate, was evaluated in 147 consecutive patients given marrow grafts from HLA-identical siblings or HLA-haploidentical relatives with no more than 1 HLA locus mismatched.

Methods.—Cyclophosphamide was given intravenously before marrow transplantation to patients with leukemia, followed by total body irradiation. Patients with myelodysplasia and aplastic anemia also received cyclophosphamide in conjunction with irradiation. After transplantation, the patients received methotrexate and cyclosporine. Half of the patients were randomized to receive methylprednisolone, starting the day of marrow transplantation and continuing for 35 days. The maximum dose was 1 mg/kg.

Results.—Both acute and chronic GVHD were more prevalent in HLA-identical recipients given prednisone, but the resultant increase in transplant-related mortality was offset by an increase in leukemic relapse in patients not given prednisone. The overall disease-free survival was similar in the 2 groups; more than half of the patients were alive 2 years after marrow transplantation. In a pilot study, administration of steroids starting on day 15 did not alter the occurrence of GVHD.

Conclusion.—The prophylactic use of prednisone in marrow transplant recipients given methotrexate and cyclosporine is not beneficial, at least in patients given HLA-identical marrow grafts.

▶ As shown in this randomized study, the addition of prednisone to a combined GVHD prophylaxis including methotrexate and cyclosporine has a significant but unexpected effect on the incidence of both acute and chronic GVHD. The potential complexity of interaction therapy in marrow allograft patients was further demonstrated by the finding of an increased graft-vs.-leukemia (GVL) effect in the prednisone group, presumably a consequence of increased GVHD. The mechanism of this effect is unknown, but it is likely that prednisone in combination with methotrexate and cyclosporine inhibited the negative selection of donor T cells reactive with host alloantigen, a phenomenon that may require induction of apotosis in the thymus or peripheral anergy.—J.A. Hansen, M.D.

Prophylaxis of Graft-Versus-Host Disease by Administration of the Murine Anti-IL-2 Receptor Antibody 2A3

Anasetti C, Martin PJ, Storb R, Appelbaum FR, Beatty PG, Calori E, Davis J, Doney K, Reichert T, Stewart P, Sullivan KM, Thomas ED, Witherspoon RP, Hansen JA (Fred Hutchinson Cancer Research Ctr, Univ of Washington, Seattle; Becton-Dickinson Monoclonal Ctr, San Jose)

Bone Marrow Transplant 7:375–381, 1991   20–8

Background.— More than 70% of potential marrow transplant recipients have no HLA-identical sibling. Thus, any potential donor is likely to be partially mismatched, and the risk of graft-vs.-host disease will be increased substantially. The efficacy of murine monoclonal IgG1 antibody 2A3 specific for the 55 kD chain of the human IL-2 receptor was assessed for prophylaxis of acute (GVHD) in patients undergoing transplantation with unmodified non T-cell depleted marrow from related HLA-haploidentical donors incompatible for 2 or 3 HLA loci of the nonshared haplotype.

Methods.— All patients had advanced leukemia. Thirty-six patients comprised the control group and received standard cyclosporine and methotrexate as GVHD prophylaxis. In addition to this standard treatment, 11 patients were also given antibody 2A3, 1 mg/kg on day −1 and .5 mg/kg daily from day 0 through day 19.

Results.— Antibody administration did not produce appreciable toxicity or adversely affect engraftment. Circulating CD25+ cells appeared to be saturated by the infused antibody during treatment, and "hyperacute GVHD" appeared to be suppressed in antibody-treated patients. Patients given antibody 2A3 tolerated more cyclosporine than those in the control group, with lower increase in serum creatinine in the first month. Seventy percent of the 10 assessable patients in the experimental group had acute GVHD grade II–IV, with a median onset of 20 days. Eighty-seven percent of the 31 assessable controls had acute GVHD grade II–IV, with a median onset of 13 days. Trough serum levels of antibody 2A3 ranged from 7.2 mg/L to 68.8 mg/L. Lower levels were correlated with the occurrence of acute GVHD. Four patients had a human antimouse immunoglobulin antibody response, which was not associated with lower levels of antibody 2A3 in the serum. Two patients in the experimental group and 2 in the control group have survived for more than 1 year.

Conclusions.— Administration of antibody 2A3 appears to suppress and delay activation of alloantigen-specific T cells, although it does not eliminate them. Antibody 2A3 may ameliorate "hyperacute GVHD" in high-risk patients. Its administration was safe and did not impair engraftment in this series.

▶ Prophylaxis for GVHD with methotrexate and cyclosporine is effective in patients who undergo transplantation from an HLA-identical sibling, but this 2-drug therapy does not adequately control GVHD in HLA-incompatible transplants (1). Anti-IL-2 receptor antibody therapy has been shown to be active in suppressing GVHD in mice (2, 3). The goal of this phase I–II trial was to show the safety and feasibility of administering the murine IgG1 anti-IL-2 receptor (CD25) antibody 2A3 in the immediate postransplant period as prophylaxis for GVHD in patients at high risk of developing clinically severe disease. The overall incidence of GVHD was not affected by 2A3 treatment; however, there was a delay in the onset of GVHD, an apparent suppression of the "hyperacute GVHD" syndrome, a lower maximum serum creatinine level, and a greater percentage of the prescribed dose of cyclosporine was administered to patients receiving the anti-IL-2R antibody. Further evidence suggesting the efficacy of anti-IL-2R antibody as treatment for GVHD comes from Herve et al. who gave antibody B-B10 to patients with steroid-resistant GVHD (4).

Advances in recombinant technology have made it possible to genetically engineer humanized versions of murine monoclonal antibodies. This has been done with the murine anti-IL-2R Tac antibody. The new humanized Tac, designated HAT, is a recombinant Ig molecule incorporating the antigen binding portion of the IgG2 Tac antibody with a human IgG1 antibody (2). Hat has a much better half-life and biodistribution in primates than Tac, and HAT but not Tac is capable of mediating antibody-dependent cellular cytotoxicity (ADCC) (5). Brown et al. reported prolongation of primate cardiac allografts with HAT (6). These preliminary data are a strong impetus for new clinical trials aimed at determining the efficacy of this humanized anti-IL-2R antibody as an immunosuppressive agent in humans.—J.A. Hansen, M.D.

References

1. Anasetti C, et al: *Human Immunol* 29:79, 1990.
2. Ferrara J, et al: *J Immunol* 137:1874, 1986.
3. Kupiec-Weglinski JW, et al: *Proc Natl Acad Sci USA* 83:2624, 1986.
4. Herve P, et al: *Lancet* ii:1072, 1988 (letter).
5. Junghans RP, et al: *Cancer Res* 50:1495, 1990.
6. Brown PS Jr, et al: *Proc Natl Acad Sci USA* 88:2663, 1991.

▶ ↓ The following 2 papers by Martin et al. (Abstracts 20–9 and 20–10) represent unique retrospective studies of GVHD treatment involving a relatively large number of patients from a single transplant center. The data base analyzed is comprehensive and allows assessment by multivariate analysis of relevant patient and disease characteristics. Overall the results indicate that the staging of acute GVHD and the evaluation of treatment outcome are complex issues that are influenced by multiple variables, and unfortunately there is no treatment that shows a high degree of safety and durable effectiveness.—J.A. Hansen, M.D.

A Retrospective Analysis of Therapy for Acute Graft-Versus-Host Disease: Initial Treatment
Martin PJ, Schoch G, Fisher L, Byers V, Anasetti C, Appelbaum FR, Beatty PG, Doney K, McDonald GB, Sanders JE, Sullivan KM, Storb R, Thomas ED, Witherspoon RP, Lomen P, Hannigan J, Hansen JA (Fred Hutchinson Cancer Research Ctr, Univ of Washington, Seattle; Xoma Corp, Berkeley, Calif)
Blood 76:1464–1472, 1990   20–9

---

264 / Transplantation

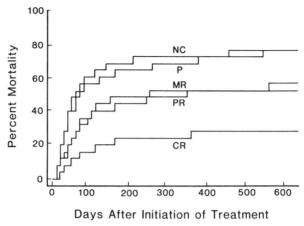

Days After Initiation of Treatment

Fig 20–1.—Nonrelapse mortality of patients categorized according to treatment outcome. *Abbreviations: CR,* complete response; *PR,* partial response; *MR,* mixed response; *NC,* no change; *P,* progression (*P* < .0001 for equality among groups). (Courtesy of Martin PJ, Schoch G, Fisher L, et al: *Blood* 76:1464–1472, 1990.)

Introduction.—Acute graft-vs.-host disease (GVHD) is an important cause of morbidity and mortality in patients receiving allogeneic marrow transplantation. The results of therapy for acute GVHD were analyzed retrospectively in 1 patient series.

Patients.—Seven hundred forty patients with grades II–IV GVHD after allogeneic marrow transplantation were treated. At the beginning of treatment, 81% of the patients had rash, 50% had liver dysfunction, and 54% had gut dysfunction.

Management.—Initial treatment was with glucocorticoids in 531 patients, cyclosporine in 170, antithymocyte globulin in 156, and monoclonal antibody either singly in 633 or in combination in 107.

Results.—Improvement rates were 43% for skin disease, 35% for

Overall Response to Treatment

				Outcome		
Agent † (n)	Evaluable	CR	CR + PR	CR + PR + MR	NC	P
ATG (61)	56	6 (11)	13 (23)	19 (34)	14 (25)	23 (41)
Cyclosporine (78)	75	16 (21)	32 (43)	42 (56)	18 (24)	15 (20)
Glucocorticoids (491)	456	92 (20)	216 (47)	271 (59)	82 (18)	103 (23)
Single Agents (633)	590	114 (19)	262 (44)	334 (57)	114 (19)	142 (24)
Combined Agents (107)	94	17 (18)	42 (45)	58 (62)	10 (11)	26 (28)
Overall (740)	684	123 (18)	304 (44)	392 (57)	124 (18)	168 (25)

Abbreviations: CR, complete response; *PR,* partial response; *MR,* mixed response; *NC,* no change; *P,* progression; *NE,* not evaluable; *ATG,* antithymocyte globulin. Data indicate numbers of patients in each category. Numbers in parentheses indicate the percent of evaluable patients in each category. The difference in outcome distribution between ATG and other treatments is statistically significant (*P* < .01).

†Results are shown for single agent treatment with ATG, cyclosporine, or glucocorticoids; 95 patients received ATG as part of a combined regimen, 92 patients received cyclosporine as part of a combined regimen, and 40 patients received glucocorticoids as part of a combined regimen.

(Courtesy of Martin PJ, Schoch G, Fisher L, et al: *Blood* 76:1464–1472, 1990.)

evaluable liver disease, and 50% for evaluable gut diseae. Overall, 44% of the patients had complete or partial responses. Nonrelapse mortality for patients in each response category was analyzed (Fig 20–1). According to 3 models of analysis, GVHD prophylaxis using cyclosporine combined with methotrexate was associated with favorable GVHD treatment outcome compared with prophylaxis with either agent alone. Treatment with glucocorticoids or cyclosporine was more successful than with antithymocyte globulin (table). Other factors associated with unfavorable outcomes were recipient HLA disparity with the donor, the presence of a liver complication other than GVHD, and early onset of GVHD.

Conclusions.—The treatment of acute GVHD remains unsatisfactory. Glucocorticoids represent the best initial treatment available, although there is much room for improvement.

A Retrospective Analysis of Therapy for Acute Graft-Versus-Host Disease: Secondary Treatment

Martin PJ, Schoch G, Fisher L, Byers V, Appelbaum FR, McDonald GB, Storb R, Hansen JA (Fred Hutchinson Cancer Research Ctr; Univ of Washington; Seattle; Xoma Corp, Berkeley, Calif)
Blood 77:1821–1828, 1991   20–10

Introduction.—The risk of acute graft-vs.-host disease (GVHD) remains high in patients transplanted with HLA-nonidentical marrow or with marrow from an unrelated donor.

Methods.—Data were reviewed on 427 patients with acute GVHD to define the natural history of the disease, to determine patient and disease characteristics that influence therapeutic response and survival, to assess treatment factors relevant to outcome, and to evaluate methods for analysis of future treatment trials.

Results.—None of the patients had a durable satisfactory response after primary treatment for GVHD. At the beginning of primary treatment, 83% of patients had a rash, 51% had liver dysfunction, and 57% had gut dysfunction. Secondary treatment consisted of glucocorticoids, cyclosporine, antithymocyte globulin, or monoclonal antibody, either singly or in combination. Improvement or resolution was seen in 45% of those with skin disease, 25% with evaluable liver disease, and 35% with evaluable gut disease. Overall, 40% of the patients had complete or total responses. A factor associated with both a decreased likelihood of complete response and an increased treatment failure rate was severe dysfunction in the skin, liver, and gut at the beginning of treatment. The highest complete response rate with secondary therapy (23%) was found when GVHD recurred during the taper phase of primary glucocorticoid treatment and was managed with an increased dose of glucocorticoids.

Conclusion.—If the patients in this highest response group are excluded from analysis, responses to secondary treatment were less favorable than those after primary treatment. These findings suggest that assessment of the benefits of new immunosuppressive agents for patients with acute GVHD should take into account the influence of disease severity at the start of treatment.

8-Methoxypsoralen and Ultraviolet A Therapy for Cutaneous Manifestations of Graft-Versus-Host Disease

Eppinger T, Ehninger G, Steinert M, Niethammer D, Dopfer R (University Children's Hospital, Tübingen; Medical Hospital, Tübingen; University Hospital, Tübingen, Germany)
Transplantation 50:807–811, 1990
20–11

Introduction.—Preliminary studies reported a potential benefit of 8-methoxypsoralen plus ultraviolet A irradiation (PUVA) in the treatment of patients with graft-vs.-host disease (GVHD) after allogeneic bone marrow transplantation (BMT). The potential role for PUVA therapy was further investigated in a larger series of patients with GVHD after allogeneic BMT.

Patients.—Eleven patients aged 8–35 years with histologically confirmed acute or chronic cutaneous GVHD that had not responded to combination immunosuppressive therapy were treated with PUVA for 2–24 weeks. All patients received cyclosporine A for GVHD prophylaxis after BMT. Five patients with mismatched grafts also received methotrexate or monoclonal antibody campath-1 after BMT. At the start of PUVA therapy, 10 of the 11 patients were receiving immunosuppressive treatment. The PUVA treatment was initially given 4 times a week. After resolution of the cutaneous lesions, the frequency of treatment was reduced to twice a week and later to once a week.

Results.—Five patients had a complete response to PUVA therapy with disappearance of all symptoms. Six patients had a partial response with remission periods lasting from 12 days to 6 months. After initiation of PUVA treatment, immunosuppressive drugs could be withdrawn in 2 patients and reduced in 8. Ultraviolet A-induced exacerbation of GVHD did not occur. No cutaneous neoplasms or preneoplastic lesions have been observed after a follow-up of up to 1½ years. The only side effect was mild, tolerable nausea.

Conclusion.—Psoralen plus ultraviolet A irradiation is a promising therapeutic adjunct to conventional therapy in the treatment of acute or chronic cutaneous GVHD after BMT.

▶ In several studies, PUVA has been shown to provide effective salvage therapy for patients with clinically significant acute GVHD refractory to primary treatment with corticosteroids, and the complete response rate reported by Eppinger et al. of approximately 45% is encouraging. There is now ample preliminary evidence that PUVA can be an effective GVHD therapy; however, it is unclear how PUVA fits into the overall strategy for treating GVHD and whether it should be considered as first line therapy for acute GVHD. These questions can only be addressed in an appropriately designed randomized study, which must include a long-term follow-up component to fully evaluate the potential delayed toxicities of this treatment, especially the carcinogenic risk, which may be most pertinent for patients with chronic GVHD and persistent prolonged immune deficiency.—J.A. Hansen, M.D.

Cyclosporin A and Chronic Graft Versus Host Disease
Bacigalupo A, Maiolino A, Van Lint MT, Occhini D, Gualandi F, Clavio M, Lamparelli T, Tong J, Marmont AM (Ospedale San Martino, Genova, Italy)
Bone Marrow Transplant 6:341–344, 1990   20–12

Background.—Cyclosporine A (CSA) is widely used to prevent graft-vs.-host disease (GVHD) in patients undergoing bone marrow transplantation (BMT). However, the optimal dose and length of treatment after BMT are unknown. The incidence and severity of chronic GVHD, occurring before or after discontinuation of CSA, were analyzed in a series of 117 patients treated with BMT.

Patients.—All patients underwent allogeneic BMT, 99 for leukemia and 18 for severe aplastic anemia, and were alive more than 180 days after the graft. Cyclosporine A was given from the day before BMT to 20 days after at a dose of 1–5 mg/kg/day intravenously, after which it was given 12/mg/kg/day by mouth for 94 to more than 988 days. T cell depletion was done in 19 patients.

Findings.—Seventy-four patients, or 63%, had chronic GVHD before discontinuation of CSA. In 12 patients, chronic GVHD occurred de novo, 20 had occurrence after resolution of acute GVHD, and 42 had progression from the acute disease. One hundred twelve patients had discontinuation of CSA—80 elected to do so, 24 had relapse of leukemia, and 8 had toxicity. Cyclosporine A treatment was never halted in 5 patients. Chronic GVHD occurred in 25 patients who discontinued CSA. Eight percent of those treated for more than 150 days had the disease compared to 41% of those treated for less than 150 days. Cyclosporine A was restarted in 15 patients and could be discontinued a second time in 14 of these patients. Ninety-four percent of patients finally discontinued CSA treatment.

Conclusions.—A study of CSA treatment in BMT patients suggests that treatment should continue for at least 5 months because the incidence of chronic GVHD is much higher in those treated for less than 5 months. In most cases, the patient can eventually achieve independence from CSA.

▶ This paper addresses an important question. The conclusions should be considered tentative, however, because this was a retrospective study. All patients were initially placed on a 5-month treatment schedule, which was modified according to clinical events. The duration of cyclosporine treatment may affect the incidence and severity of chronic GVHD, but this could only be proven by a randomized trial.—J.A. Hansen, M.D.

The Presence of Infectious Virus but not Conventional Antigen Can Exacerbate Graft-Versus-Host Reactions

Cray C, Levy RB (Univ of Miami, Fla)
Scand J Immunol 32:177–182, 1990

20–13

Introduction.—There is considerable evidence that pathogens, especially the DNA viruses, cytomegalovirus (CMV) and herpes simplex virus (HSV) are associated with an increased risk of severe graft-versus-host disease (GVHD) in marrow transplant recipients. A study was done to show whether infectious pathogens are unique in their ability to exacerbate GVH reactions.

Findings.—Mice given donor lymphoid cells and dinitrophenyl–bovine serum albumin, a T-dependent antigen, did not exhibit an exaggerated GVH reaction. Phenotypic changes were not noted, and there was no donor antihost cytotoxic activity or elevated natural killer activity. The recipients produced normal levels of IgM and IgG anti-dinitrophenyl antibodies. Mice given ultraviolet light-inactivated murine cytomegalovirus also failed to exhibit an exaggerated GVH reaction.

Discussion.—Apparently, infectious viruses can uniquely exacerbate GVH reactions. Viral-induced immune responses therefore may be critical in the ability of a pathogen to produce a severe GVH reaction.

▶ Murine CMV infection can exacerbate the severity of experimental GVH reactions (1, 2). As shown in this study, however, in vivo stimulation with conventional antigen or attenuated noninfectious virus did not potentiate GVHR. These results demonstrate that T cell-dependent antigens are not inherently capable of enhancing an alloimmune response. The mechanism by which a viral infection affects the GVH reaction is unknown, but it presumably involves activation of some component of the alloimmune response and associated inflammation. Our strategies for GVHD prevention and treatment might be greatly improved if we had better understanding of the pathogenesis of GVHD.—J.A. Hansen, M.D.

References

1. Cray C, Levy RB: *Transplantation* 1990.
2. Grundy JE, Shanley JD, Shearer GM: *Transplantation* 39:548, 1985.

Hyper IgE in Stimulatory Graft-*Versus*-Host Disease: Role of Interleukin-4

Doutrelepont JM, Moser M, Leo O, Abramowicz D, Vanderhaegen ML, Urbain J, Goldman M (Hôpital Erasme; Université Libre de Bruxelles, Brussels)
Clin Exp Immunol 83:133–136, 1991

20–14

Introduction.—The role of donor B and T cells and the involvement of interleukin-4 (IL-4) in hypersecretion of IgE associated with stimulatory graft-vs.-host disease was analyzed in hybrid mice.

Methods and Results.—Injection of DBA/2 spleen cells into adult

(C57BP/6 × DBA/2)F1 mice resulted in a stimulatory graft-vs-host reaction (GVHR) linked to the recognition by donor CD4$^+$ T cells of Ia alloantigens on host B cells. Stimulatory GVHR was associated with a significant increase in serum IgE levels. Host B cells appear responsible for the enhanced secretion of IgE seen in this model. This effect was dependent on the presence of donor CD4$^+$ T cells. Interleukin-4 (IL-4) administered during the first 12 days after induction of stimulatory GVHR prevented the development of hyper IgE.

Conclusions.—Stimulatory GVHR in mice was associated with a major increase in serum IgE, which was mediated by IL-4. The similarities of murine and human IgE regulation may mean that the hyper IgE observed in human graft-vs.-host disease could also be related to an enhanced production of IL-4.

▶ This report underscores the importance of cytokines as effector molecules in graft-vs.-host reactions. Although the hyper IgE observed in this "parent into F1" model for GVHD was dependent on both host B cells and donor-derived CD4$^+$ T cells, IL-4 was identified as the specific mediator molecule. The response of donor T cells to host alloantigen in this experiment was responsible for an inflammatory reaction that involved the recruitment of residual host B cells as the eventual effector cell. These results emphasize the protean pathophysiology and manifestations of GVHD. They also suggest a rationale for the management of GVHD by blocking of specific cytokine pathways rather than relying only on broad nonspecific immunosuppression.—J.A. Hansen, M.D.

Inflammatory Cells in Graft-Versus-Host Disease on the Rectum: Immunopathologic Analysis
Weisdorf SA, Roy J, Snover D, Platt JL, Weisdorf DJ (Univ of Minnesota, Minneapolis)
Bone Marrow Transplant 7:297–301, 1991   20–15

Background.—Increasing attention has recently been focused on the immunopathogenesis of graft-vs.-host disease (GVHD) after allogeneic bone marrow transplantation. However, little is known about the cellular constituents of the inflammatory reaction in intestinal GHVD.

Methods.—Twenty biopsy specimens from 11 allogeneic bone marrow transplant recipients were assessed in 4 groups. Biopsy specimens were taken before transplantation, after transplantation from patients without GVHD, from patients with extraintestinal GVHD only, and from patients with intestinal GVHD. Indirect immunofluorescence was used to study the inflammatory infiltrate in GVHD.

Results.—Few differences were found in total T cell number in the lamina propria in the 4 groups. The CD4$^+$ lymphocytes seemed to be reduced in GVHD whereas CD8$^+$ lymphocytes were significantly elevated. Thus, the CD4/CD8 ratio was significantly lowered. In patients before transplantation and in patients without GVHD, this ratio was comparable to that in normal peripheral blood, but was significantly lower in extraintestinal and intestinal GVHD. Acute intestinal GVHD was characterized by a four-fold rise in CD57$^+$ lymphoid cells in the epithelium and lamina propria.

Conclusions.—The composition of lymphoid infiltrates in the rectum in patients with GVHD may resemble the current findings observed in GVHD of the small intestinal mucosa. The presence of CD57$^+$ cells, which may include natural killer-like cells, in rectal lymphoid infiltrates suggests that non-HLA restricted effector cells may play a role in GVHD of the rectum.

▶ Although T cells play a critical role in the initiation of acute GVHD, the pathogenesis of GVH in different organs is not clearly understood. Lymphoid infiltrates are most intense in the acute phase; however, the content of these infiltrates may be modified by endotoxin and infection and variably affected by different immunosuppressive therapies. Cellular infiltrates are usually much less prominent in chronic GVHD. Cytokines, especially IL-1 and tumor necrosis factor, may play a significant role as mediators of cellular activation and inflammation. Once a cytokine cascade has been induced, cells other than T cells may become involved in the sustained production of cytokines. The presence of CD57$^+$ cells in the epithelium and lamina propria of the rectum suggests that nonspecific effector cells such as natural killer cells may play a role in the inflammatory lesions associated with GVHD.—J.A. Hansen, M.D.

An Immunohistological Study of γ/δ Lymphocytes in Human Cutaneous Graft-Versus-Host Disease

Norton J, Al-Saffar N, Sloane JP (Royal Marsden Hospital, Sutton, England)
Bone Marrow Transplant 7:205–208, 1991   20–16

Background.—Human T lymphocytes express 1 of 2 types of heterodimeric receptor for antigen α/β or γ/δ. Each of these is associated with a complex of invariant polypeptides known collectively as CD3. Acute graft-vs.-host disease (GVHD) after allogeneic bone marrow transplantation (BMT) in patients with leukemia is characterized by damaged epithelium in the skin, intestine, and bile ducts. An immunohistologic study was made of human cutaneous GVHD using antibodies to the β and δ chains of the T cell receptor and CD3 to determine the relative proportion of α/β and γ/δ lymphocytes in normal skin and GVHD in the early post-BMT period.

Methods and Findings.—Punch biopsies of skin were performed in 9 marrow allograft recipients in whom rashes developed at different times after BMT. Six control biopsy specimens were obtained from donors from the posterior iliac crest. Eight biopsy specimens were also obtained from BMT recipients without rashes. The proportion of γ/δ cells was very low in GVHD—4.3%. However, it was significantly higher than in skin from normal donors and recipients without GVHD, at proportions of .8% and 0%, respectively. There was no apparent localization of γ/δ cells to the epidermis. All were identified in the dermis, particularly in the perivascular zone.

Conclusions.—This study suggests that γ/δ cells do not play an important role in producing the epidermal damage characteristic of GVHD. The significance of these cells in GVHD is not clear. Whether this phenomenon represents selective localization of these cells to the skin, or simply reflects peripheral blood values in the early posttransplant period in some GVHD patients, is not known.

▶ In mice, T lymphocytes expressing the γ/δ T cell receptor (TCR) are found preferentially in the epidermis and epithelium of the intestine (1, 2). In humans, however, the γ/δ TCR is found only infrequently among T cells in normal skin, intestine, and blood (3). A small number of δ$^+$ cells in the current study were observed in the dermis, but not the epidermis of patients with cutaneous disease, indicating that these interesting but poorly understood T cells probably do not play a significant or unique role in human GVHD. These results suggest that the alloantigens responsible for cutaneous GVHD are not preferentially recognized by the γ/δ TCR repertoire.—J.A. Hansen, M.D.

References

1. Koning F, et al: *Science* 236:834, 1987.
2. Goodman T, Lefrancois L: *Nature* 333:855, 1988.
3. Groh V, et al: *J Exp Med* 169:1277, 1989.

ICAM-1 Expression on Epidermal Keratinocytes in Cutaneous Graft-Versus-Host Disease
Norton J, Sloane JP (Royal Marsden Hospital, Sutton, England)
Transplantation 51:1203–1206, 1991   20–17

Background.—The authors previously demonstrated that some patients with cutaneous graft-vs.-host disease (GVHD) show no diagnostic changes on skin biopsy. In GVHD, keratinocytes show increased expression of HLA-DR. An immunohistologic study was made of epidermal keratinocytes for ICAM-1, the intracellular adhesion molecule.

Methods.—Thirty-one biopsies from 27 allogeneic bone marrow recipients were investigated. All patients developed a skin rash between 12 and 48 days after transplantation. Recipients' mean age was 29 years, and more than half had acute myeloid leukemia. Biopsy specimens from normal donors and from the patients before transplantation were studied as controls.

Results.—Control specimens stained weakly for ICAM-1, with relatively few cells staining. Posttransplant, the number of positive cells and their staining intensity increased significantly in specimens with histologic evidence of GVHD. However, no increase was seen in normal-appearing specimens or those with possible cytotoxic or radiation-related epidermal abnormalities. The ICAM-1 was strongly and positively correlated with HLA-DR expression by keratinocytes, with all samples showing increased ICAM-1 also showing increased HLA-DR antigens. On the other hand, there were 6 HLA-DR–positive biopsies that showed no detectable increases in ICAM-1

Conclusions.—Immunostaining with ICAM-1 appears to be of little help in the early diagnosis of cutaneous GVHD. A more detailed study of inflammation-associated molecules, including ICAM-1, is underway. In the early posttransplant period, local cytokine release may stimulate both ICAM-1 and HLA-DR.

Vessel Associated Adhesion Molecules in Normal Skin and Acute Graft-Versus-Host Disease
Norton J, Sloane JP, Al-Saffar N, Haskard DO (Royal Marsden Hospital, Institute of Cancer Research, Sutton, England; Royal Postgraduate Medical School, London)
J Clin Pathol 44:586–591, 1991   20–18

Background.—Earlier studies found that biopsy specimens from patients with rashes who had graft vs.-host disease (GVHD), or in whom it subsequently developed, lacked the diagnostic leukocytic infiltrate. The increased HLA-DR expression on epidermal keratinocytes in these "negative" specimens was strongly associated with the subsequent development of systemic GVHD. The expression of the endothelial leukocyte adhesion molecule-1 (ELAM-1) and the vascular adhesion molecule-1 (VCAM-1) in the skin of allogeneic marrow recipients was investigated to detect a possible role of adhesion molecules in acute GVHD and in the early diagnosis of GVHD.

Methods.—Punch biopsy specimens were obtained from 24 allogeneic bone marrow recipients after transplantation. Group 1 specimens exhibited unequivocal histologic evidence of GVHD with leukocytic infiltration of the upper dermis and lower epidermis; group 2 specimens lacked a leukocytic infiltrate but exhibited keratinocyte HLA-DR positivity.

Results.—In normal skin, ELAM-1 staining was restricted to a variable but small number of endothelial cells that were significantly increased in GVHD but only when the fully developed histologic picture of epidermal basal damage and leukocytic infiltration was present. Specimens with histologic evidence of GVHD had increased positive perivascular dendritic cells and large numbers of similar cells throughout the upper dermis. When a rash was present after transplantation, an increase in VCAM-1 positive cells was seen in some specimens that lacked the leukocytic infiltrate diagnostic of GVHD.

Conclusions.—In marrow recipients, VCAM-1 positive cells were found in biopsy specimens without detectable lymphocytic infiltration obtained soon after the onset of rash. Identification of VCAM-1 positive cells may be useful in the early diagnosis of GVHD.

▶ Studies aimed at identifying early events in cutaneous GVHD are helpful in understanding pathogenesis, especially the roles played by endothelial cells and the dendritic cells that surround small vessels and extend into the upper dermis. Leukocyte infiltration into tissues, which is the hallmark of GVHD, must be preceded by interactions with specific adhesion molecule, the activity of which are regulated by cytokines (1). In earlier studies these investigators showed that HLA-DR expression is increased on epidermal keratinocytes before the appearance of diagnostic leucocyte infiltrates (2). In the first study (Abstract 20–17), the expression of the intercellular adhesion molecule ICAM-1 (CD54) was increased on keratinocytes during GVHD. However, when ICAM-1 was increased, DR was also increased. Thus ICAM-1 did not add to the early diagnosis of GVHD. In the second study (Abstract 20–18), the same investigators showed a significant increase in ELAM-1 on endothelial cells, but only after a fully developed leucocytic infiltrate was present. However, there was a relatively early increase in VCAM-1 on dendritic cells before any detectable leucocytic infiltration, suggesting that VCAM-1 expression might be diagnostic in early GVHD.—J.A. Hansen, M.D.

References

1. Springer TA: *Nature* 346:3025, 1990.
2. Sloan JP, Elliott CJ, Powles R: *Transplantation* 46:840, 1988.

Endothelial Changes in Cutaneous Graft-Versus-Host Disease: A Comparison Between HLA Matched and Mismatched Recipients of Bone Marrow Transplantation
Sviland L, Sale GE, Myerson D (Royal Victoria Infirmary, Newcastle Upon Tyne, England; Univ of Washington, Seattle)
Bone Marrow Transplant 7:35–38, 1991   20–19

Background.—Bone marrow transplant (BMT) recipients with acute graft-vs.-host disease (GVHD) appear to have significantly more endothelial cell injury than those without GVHD and may have a primary immunologic injury to the vasculature. The DR antigens are expressed on endothelial cells in response to certain cytokines. The HLA-mismatched and matched BMT recipients with grade 3 GVHD of the skin were studied to determine whether the mismatched recipients showed more endothelial damage.

Methods.—Skin biopsy specimens from 44 HLA-matched and-mismatched BMT recipients were evaluated. The histologic features of endothelial and vascular changes seen in cell-mediated immune reactions were assessed. Of the 24 mismatched patients, 14 were classified as being 11D-mismatched" and 10 were "AB-mismatched." Graft-vs.-host disease—clinical grade III and histologic grade II—occurred in all patients. Biopsy specimens from 10 patients without GVHD were also studied for comparison.

Results.—All BMT patients had evidence of a nonspecific vascular response. The main manifestation of this response was a perivascular lymphocytic infiltrate, perivascular edema, and factor VI-related antigen extravasation. Scattered perivascular nuclear dust was seen mainly in mismatched recipients, suggesting that these patients had a greater degree of endothelial cell damage.

Conclusions.—Most allogeneic BMT recipients have a mild, nonspecific vascular reaction. Mismatched BMT recipients who have acute GVHD appear to have a greater degree of endothelial damage as evidenced by the presence of perivascular nuclear dust. The role of the endothelial cell in acute GVHD requires further study.

▶ The established changes described here appear to correlate with severity of GVHD, and they suggest that HLA-incompatible recipients with GVHD may suffer more extensive damage to tissues than HLA-matched recipients. The incidence of acute GVHD, both clinically significant grade II–IV and grade III–IV, is increased in HLA-incompatible patients (although all HLA-incompatible patients do not develop clinically severe GVHD) and there is a well-established clinical impression that GVHD in the latter is more refractory to treatment. Therefore these pathologic changes may predict a subset of patients for whom the most intensive immunosuppression therapy should be used early in the course of disease.—J.A. Hansen, M.D.

Deoxyspergualin in Lethal Murine Graft-Versus-Host Disease
Nemoto K, Hayashi M, Ito J, Sugawara Y, Mae T, Fujii H, Abe F, Fujii A, Takeuchi T (Nippon Kayaku Co, Ltd; Institute of Microbial Chemistry, Tokyo)
Transplantation 51:712–715, 1991   20–20

Background.—Deoxyspergualin (DSG) is a spergualin derivative that suppresses rejection of various allografts in animal models. Its benefits in lethal graft-vs.-host disease (GVHD) were studied in a major histo incompatible donor-recipient combination.

Methods.—Lethal GVHD was elicited in CBA mice receiving marrow transplantation from C58BL/6 mice. The cytotoxicity of cells recovered from host spleens was examined, and the effect of DSG on the inhibition of the generation and proliferation of these effector cells was studied.

Results.—Deoxyspergualin appeared to have a marked potential for the treatment of animals with lethal GVHD. In animals that received both DSG and methotrexate, survival was longer than in those that received either agent alone. When mice who survived for long periods received DSG treatment, they became stable chimeras, as reflected by cell-surface analysis of their spleen cells. Animals with lethal GVHD had high H-2-reactive cytotoxic T lymphocyte levels in their spleens; natural killer cell activity was increased only slightly. Cytotoxic T lymphocyte activity was also inhibited by DSG, not only in the induction but also in the advanced stage of GVHD.

Conclusions.—Deoxyspergualin may have beneficial effects in bone marrow transplantation, either alone or combined with methotrexate. In the current animal study, it prolongs survival in a dose-dependent fashion when given for 10 days after transplantation. It also appears to prolong survival when treatment is started during GVHD crisis.

▶ As noted previously, the available therapies for preventing and treating acute and chronic GVHD in high-risk marrow transplant patients (older patients), patients who are HLA-mismatched with their donor, and unrelated donor transplants) are inadequate. Results reported here suggest that deoxyspergualin in combination with other immunosuppressive agents may contribute to the control of GVHD.—J.A. Hansen, M.D.

Simultaneous Upper and Lower Endoscopic Biopsy in the Diagnosis of Intestinal Graft-Versus-Host Disease
Roy J, Snover D, Weisdorf S, Mulvahill A, Filipovich A, Weisdorf D (Univ of Minnesota, Minneapolis)
Transplantation 51:642–646, 1991   20–21

Introduction.—The symptoms of acute graft-vs.-host disease (GVHD) involving primarily the upper gastrointestinal (GI) tract are not specific. In patients with upper GI symptoms but no lower GI complaints, the differential diagnosis of GVHD can be confirmed by histologic confirmation. The usefulness of upper endoscopy in the diagnosis of upper GI GVHD has not yet been examined. The purpose of this retrospective study was to assess how upper and lower GI endoscopy with biopsy might influence patient management.

Patients.—Seventy-seven symptomatic patients who had received an allogeneic marrow transplant underwent both upper GI endoscopy and sigmoidoscopy with biopsy within a 7-day interval. Only 9 patients were younger than age 18 years. Sixty-five patients had received a marrow transplant from an HLA-MLC-compatible sibling, and 12 had received a transplant from unrelated donors.

Results.—Thirty-four patients had histologically confirmed upper GI GVHD and 43 had negative upper GI biopsy specimens. Twenty of the 34 patients with upper GI GVHD also had a positive rectal biopsy specimen. Thirty-five patients had negative findings on both biopsies. Of 51 patients with either no or limited skin GVHD at the time of GI biopsy, 18 had histologically confirmed upper GI GVHD. The association between clinically apparent skin GVHD and upper GI GVHD was statistically significant. Of 58 patients with normal liver function when upper GI biopsy was performed, 27 had upper GI GVHD at biopsy. Seven of the 19 patients with clinical liver GVHD had a positive upper GI biopsy specimen and 12 patients had no upper GI GVHD. There was a trend toward statistical significance for the association between upper GI GVHD and overall clinical GVHD grade. Upper GI endoscopy yielded a histologic diagnosis of GVHD in 44% of symptomatic patients and indicated the need for a change in GVHD treatment from local to systemic therapy in 16% of patients. Furthermore, 71% of patients had other enteric pathology identified that required specific therapy.

Conclusion.—Upper GI endoscopy with biopsy is an important tool in the diagnosis of intestinal GVHD. It should be performed in all patients who are symptomatic after undergoing allogeneic bone marrow transplantation.

▶ This reports adds to previous studies demonstrating the importance of upper GI endoscopy and appropriate diagnostic procedures for patients who complain of significant or persistent upper GI symptoms with or without other evidence of GVHD (1–3).—J.A. Hansen, M.D.

References

1. McDonald GB, et al: *Transplantation* 42:460, 770, 1986.
2. Spencer GD, et al: *Transplantation* 42:602, 1986.
3. Weisdorf DJ, et al: *Blood* 76:624, 1990.

Toxicity and Efficacy of Anti– T-Cell Ricin Toxin A Chain Immunotoxins in a Murine Model of Established Graft-Versus-Host Disease Induced Across the Major Histocompatibility Barrier

Vallera DA, Carroll SF, Snover DC, Carlson GJ, Blazar BR (Univ of Minnesota; Fairview Southdale Hosp, Minneapolis; XOMA Corp, Berkeley, Calif)
Blood 77:182–194, 1991   20–22

Background.—T-cell depletion of donor bone marrow can reduce graft-vs.-host disease (GVHD) in patients undergoing bone marrow transplantation (BMT), but it also increases problems with engraftment. The value of anti-T-cell ricin toxin A chain immunotoxin (IT) therapy was assessed in a murine model of GVHD.

Methods.—Graft-vs.-host disease was induced across the major histocompatibility complex (MHC) by injection of marrow and splenocytes into lethally irradiated mice. The recipients were treated with anti-Ly1, the murine equivalent of anti-CD5, conjugated to ricin toxin A chain (anti-Ly1-RTA). Control animals received phosphate-buffered saline or an irrelevant RTA IT.

Results.—The IT inhibited T-cell proliferation in vivo, even in the absence of progenitors. In mice with GVHD, treatment reduced numbers of splenic Thyl.2$^+$ T cells and improved survival. When this treatment ceased, however, GVHD and weight loss occurred. Neutrophils rose substantially with anti-Ly1-RTA treatment, and mild hepatotoxicity occurred with higher doses. Treatment with anti-Thy1.2-RTA decreased numbers of lymphocytes but not of neutrophils, caused sudden weight gain, decreased total plasma protein, and increased pleural and peritoneal effusions, as in vascular leak syndrome (VLS). Its toxic effects precluded any survival advantage, but histopathologic studies demonstrated a definite anti-GVHD effect. The greatest decline in GVHD was seen in the skin, followed by the liver and lung. When anti-Thy1.2-RTA was given intraperitoneally to syngeneic BMT recipients to investigate the cause of IT toxicity, the same weight gain, hypoproteinuria, and VLS seen in the

GVHD model occurred. Animals that received higher doses died. The effect on renal function was negligible, but there was patchy dropout of renal tubules. Pulmonary vascular congestion was seen, but liver, brain, and colon toxicity were not. Irradiation enhanced weight gain. Comparable doses of anti-Ly1-RTA did not kill the recipients, but the mice lost weight and had significant increases in neutrophil numbers, as in the GVHD model. There was no effect on plasma protein levels, liver, kidney, or lung.

Conclusions.—$Ly1^+$ cells appear to have at least some role in the effector phase of GVHD. Radiation enhances the toxicity of IT, and the toxicities noted in mice are similar to those observed in humans. Immunotoxin made with a monoclonal antibody that recognizes different determinants may have different toxicities that are dictated to some extent by the monoclonal antibody moiety of the IT.

▶ The experimental GVHD model described here can be useful not only for screening new immunotoxins for therapeutic efficacy in preventing or treating GVHD, but it also provides opportunity for more detailed and analytical studies of problems encountered in the treatment of human GVHD. The data pertaining to the anti-CD5 Ricin Toxin A (RTA) chain immunotoxin are especially pertinent, because an anti-human CD5-RTA has already entered clinical trials (1).—J.A. Hansen, M.D.

Reference

1. Byers VS, et al: *Blood* 75:1426, 1990.

▶ ↓ The following 2 papers address the question of how cyclosporine induces "syngenic GVHD" following syngeneic marrow transplantation, a phenomena that has been observed experimentally in rats and mice (1–3). Most attention has focused on the ability of cyclosporine to inhibit T cell differentiation and block intrathymic clonal depletion (4–8). Syngeneic GVHD does not actually appear until cyclosporine treatment is discontinued, suggesting that the cells responsible are allowed to develop but not manifest themselves in the presence of cyclosporine. The papers that follow demonstrate that the alterations of T cell differentiation observed in syngeneic radiation chimeras exposed to cyclosporine are complex. Bryson et al. (Abstract 20–24) demonstrate that autoreactive cells are generated early in certain strains of mice, and furthermore their presence does not correlate with GVHD.—J.A. Hansen, M.D.

References

1. Glazier A, et al: *J Exp Med* 158:1, 1983.
2. Hess AD, et al: *J Exp Med* 161:718, 1985.
3. Bryson JS, et al: *Transplantation* 48:1042, 1989.
4. Sorokin R, et al: *J Exp Med* 164:1615, 1986.
5. Jenkins MK, Schwartz RN, Pardoll DM: *Science* 241:1655, 1988.
6. Gao EK, et al: *Nature* 336:176, 1988.
7. Shi Y, Sahai BM, Green DR: *Nature* 339:625, 1989.
8. Kosugi A, Sharrow SO, Shearer GM: *J Immunol* 142:3026, 1989.

Effect of Cyclosporine on T Lymphocyte Development: Relationship to Syngeneic Graft-Versus-Host Disease

Fischer AC, Laulis MK, Horwitz L, Hess AD (Johns Hopkins Univ Hosp, Baltimore)
Transplantation 51:252–259, 1991
20–23

Background.—Cyclosporine (CsA) appears to markedly change the thymic dependent lymphopoiesis in mice. This leads to release of autoreactive T cells in the periphery and manifestation of graft-vs.-host disease (GVHD) only when the autoregulatory system is absent. An attempt was made to correlate phenotypic and functional T-cell development with induction of syngeneic GVHD in rats.

Methods.—Syngeneic bone-marrow transplantation was performed in Lewis rats, after which the effects of CsA on reconstitution of T lymphocytes were investigated. This analysis included its role in the development of syngeneic GVHD. The investigators correlated the maturation of $CD4^+$ and $CD8^+$ T cells with the onset of syngeneic GVHD.

Results.—After administration of CsA, developmental arrest of both $CD4^+$ and $CD8^+$ T lymphocytes in the thymus was noted, as well as marked reduction in cells expressing the $\alpha\beta$ T-cell receptor. The CD4/CD8 ratio in the peripheral lymphoid compartment was also altered. The $CD8^+$ cells responded normally to mitogenic signaling, but only marginal proliferative responses were seen by $CD4^+$ cells. Syngeneic B lymphoblasts caused a reaction in both subsets, comparable to that of T lymphocytes from non–CsA-treated syngeneic marrow recipients. This suggests that autoreactive cells were produced despite treatment with CsA. Thymic T-cell differentiation was rapidly restored to normal when CsA was discontinued. A compensatory insurgence of $CD4^+$ T helper cells was observed concurrent with the onset of syngeneic GVHD.

Conclusions.—T-cell differentiation in the thymus is markedly affected by CsA, with the production of mature lymphocytes inhibited to a great extent. Self-reactive lymphocytes are allowed to develop in the presence of CsA. This process appears to result in immunologic homeostatic failure to maintain self-tolerance.

Relationship of Cyclosporine A-Mediated Inhibition of Clonal Deletion and Development of Syngeneic Graft-Versus-Host Disease

Bryson JS, Caywood BE, Kaplan AM (Univ of Kentucky Med Ctr, Lexington)
J Immunol 147:391–397, 1991
20–24

Background.—A strain-specific form of graft-vs.-host disease (GVHD) is described in syngeneic mouse radiation chimeras given cyclosporine A (CsA) treatment. It has been hypothesized that autoreactive T cells consequent to CsA treatment might develop when clonal deletion is inhibited, and might be responsible for GVHD in this setting.

Objective.—Induction of tolerance was examined by estimating expression of T-cell receptors (TCR) in syngeneic radiation chimeras, some of which received CsA treatment. Clonal deletion was evaluated using anti-TCR Vβ-chain monoclonal antibody.

Observations.—Clonal deletion proceeded normally in mouse strains inducible for syngeneic GVHD. In contrast, mice exhibiting T cells bearing self-reactive TCR did not develop GVHD. The difference could not be ascribed to a generalized difference in the effects of CsA in various strains of mice.

Interpretation.—Mechanisms other than the generation of autoreactive T cells apparently are involved in the development of this strain-specific form of GVHD. The pathogenesis of syngeneic GVHD clearly is a multifactorial process.

21 The Graft-Versus-Leukemia Effect (GVL)

▶ ↓ Marrow allografts in patients with leukemia are associated with a lower relapse rate compared to autologous and syngeneic marrow transplants. This phenomenon is known as the graft-vs.-leukemia effect (GVL). Graft-vs.-leukemia effect is associated with GVHD (1–5). As discussed throughout Chapter 20, the prevention of GVHD with either potent combination immunosuppression therapy or T-cell depletion of donor marrow is associated with an increase in posttransplant relapse. Although GVL presumably involves an immunologic response of donor-derived T cells to residual leukemic cells, the specificity of GVL is unknown. It is possible that the GVL effect cannot be disassociated from GVHD; however, both the GVL and GVHD responses may be heterozygous, and certain clonally derived effector cells may exist that are specific for one or the other. Ideally GVL effector cells exist that are specific for malignant cells.—J.A. Hansen, M.D.

References

1. Weiden PL, et al: *N Engl J Med* 300:1068, 1979.
2. Weiden PL, et al: *N Engl J Med* 304:1529, 1981.
3. Kersey JH, et al: *N Engl J Med* 317:461, 1987.
4. Sullivan KM, et al: *Blood* 73:1720, 1989.
5. Horowitz MM, et al: *Blood* 75:555, 1990.

Contribution of CD4+ and CD3+ T Cells to Graft-Versus-Host Disease and Graft-Versus-Leukemia Reactivity After Transplantation of MHC-Compatible Bone Marrow

Truitt RL, Atasoylu AA (Med College of Wisconsin, Milwaukee)

Bone Marrow Transplant 8:51–58, 1991
21–1

Background.—T cell depletion in bone marrow transplantation (BMT) decreases graft-vs.-host disease (GVHD), but its effect on disease-free survival is controversial. In preliminary clinical trials, selective depletion of $CD8^+$ or partial depletion of $CD5^+$ or $CD3^+$ T cells with preservation of NK/LAK precursor cells has shown promise. A murine model of allogeneic BMT was used to determine the importance of $CD4^+$ and $CD8^+$ T cells in establishing donor T-cell chimerism and in the development of GVHD and graft-vs.-leukemia (GVL) reactivity.

Methods.—Host AKR ($H-2^k$) mice were given 9 Gy of total body irradiation as pretransplant immunosuppression and transplanted with allogeneic marrow from B10.BR (H-2k) mice. To deplete spleen cell suspensions of CD4$^+$ or CD8$^+$ T cells ex vivo, 2 cycles of antibody plus complement-mediated lysis were used. Two-color immunofluorescence was used to establish chimerism.

Results.—When the host mice were conditioned with suboptimal irradiation, the addition of mature donor T cells from spleen were essential for complete chimerism. Mixed chimerism resulted when donor marrow only was transplanted; however, when marrow containing additional T cells was given, the mice developed into stable and complete chimeras. Mixed chimerism increased when T-cell subsets were depleted. Lethal GVHD increased with the number of T cells added to marrow; GVHD mortality was eliminated with ex vivo depletion of CD4$^+$ T cells. Survival was unaffected by removal of CD8$^+$ cells. Graft-vs.-leukemia reactivity was compromised by removal of either CD4$^+$ or CD8$^+$ cells, and this suggests that both types of T cells are required for an optimal GVL response. In those chimeras, depletion of T-cell subsets did not interfere with induction of donor-host tolerance and may have even facilitated it.

Conclusions.—In major histocompatability complex-compatible BMT, CD4$^+$ donor T cells appear to be essential for development of GVHD. The GVHD and GVL reactivity may be prevented or suppressed by a synergistic action of the loss of GVHD/GVL effector cells because of T-cell depletion and the development of donor-host tolerance.

▶ There has been great interest in the potential use of T-cell depletion of donor marrow for prevention of GVHD in humans. However, T-cell depletion can lead to mixed chimerism even after HLA identical transplantation, a condition associated with an increased risk of both graft rejection and leukemia relapse. Partial T-cell depletion or depletion of certain T-cell subsets have been proposed as alternative means for ameliorating GVHD without compromising engraftment and GVL; however, efforts at doing so have been empiric, and standard preferred methods have not been established. Further work in experimental animals will be necessary to define the role of T cells and cytokines in hematopoietic engraftment, GVHD, and GVL. It is likely that different T-cell subsets may be involved in GVHD and GVL depending on the degree of donor and recipient matching. Disparity for class I or class II appears to be another important variable. In the model reported here, Truitt and Atasoylu show that the elimination of CD4$^+$ cell but not CD8$^+$ cells from donor allografts prevented GVHD in H-2^k-compatible transplants, and the elimination of either CD4$^+$ or CD8$^+$ cells allowed a greater degree of mixed chimerism over time (CD4 depletion > CD8 depletion). Unfortunately, removal of either CD4$^+$ or CD8$^+$ cells also compromised GVL, indicating in this model that optimal GVL activity requires both CD4$^+$ and CD8$^+$ T cells. Previous studies analyzing GVHD and GVL activity in certain strains of mice at the clonal level have suggested that distinct effector cells may be specific for either GVHD or GVL targets, and in some cases they may react with both (1). This is an encouraging observation, suggesting that it may be possible to disassociate GVL and GVHD and to prevent GVHD without diminishing GVL.—J.A. Hansen, M.D.

Reference

1. Truitt RL, et al: Graft-versus-leukemia effect, in Burakoff SJ, Deeg HJ, Ferrara J, Atkinson K (eds): *Graft-vs-Host Disease: Immunology, Pathophysiology, and Treatment.* New York, Marcel Dekker, 1990, pp 177–204.

Evidence of a Graft-Versus-Lymphoma Effect Associated With Allogeneic Bone Marrow Transplantation

Jones RJ, Ambinder RF, Piantadosi S, Santos GW (Johns Hopkins Med Institutions, Baltimore)
Blood 77:649–653, 1991   21–2

Background.—Allogeneic bone marrow transplantation (BMT) is associated with an immunologic antileukemia reaction. No such graft-vs.-tumor effect has been shown against lymphomas, however. To find evidence of this type of effect, 118 patients undergoing BMT for relapsed Hodgkin's disease or aggressive non-Hodgkin's lymphoma were reviewed.

Patients.—The patients, 85 males and 33 females, were treated over nearly 8 years. Sixty-three had non-Hodgkin's lymphoma and 55 had Hodgkin's disease. Fifty-two patients had had 2 or more relapses. Most patients received a preoperative regimen of cyclophosphamide and total body irradiation. Thirty-eight patients were younger than age 50 and had HLA-matched donors; they underwent allogeneic BMT. The remaining 80 patients received purged autologous grafts. In both groups, the median age was 26 years.

Results.—The overall probability of event-free survival was 29% at 4 years. The only factor influencing event-free survival was the patient's response to conventional salvage therapy before BMT. The probability of relapse was significantly affected by both the response to pretreatment salvage therapy and the type of graft. Patients who did respond to salvage therapy had a 46% probability of relapse after autologous BMT, compared with only 18% after allogeneic BMT. The difference in event-free survival at 4 years among patients with responsive lymphomas—47% for allogeneic transplants and 41% for autologous transplants—was not significant. The higher mortality of allogeneic BMT, largely caused by graft-vs.-host disease, offset its beneficial antitumor effect.

Conclusions.—There appears to be a significant graft-vs.-lymphoma effect in patients undergoing BMT, and its magnitude is similar to that seen in leukemias. Although the benefits of this effect are offset by increased mortality, allogeneic BMT continues to be an important approach for study in patients with lymphoma.

▶ The GVL effect is well established in acute leukemias and chronic myelogenous leukemia (CML). This report by Jones et al. demonstrates a lower relapse rate and thus a significant GVL effect in patients receiving marrow allografts for treatment of lymphoma compared to a similar group of patients receiving marrow allografts. Unfortunately, the most important measure of clinical outcome, the probability of disease-free survival, was not different between the 2 groups, because the benefits of GVL were offset by the complications of GVHD. Once again, the need to better understand and control GVHD without interfering with the GVL effect is clearly demonstrated.—J.A. Hansen, M.D.

Induction of In Vitro Graft-Versus-Leukemia Activity Following Bone Marrow Transplantation for Chronic Myeloid Leukemia

Mackinnon S, Hows JM, Goldman JM (Royal Postgraduate Medical School, London)
Blood 76:2037–2045, 1990   21–3

Objective.—Donor bone marrow now only allows recovery of marrow function, but it may mediate a significant antileukemia or graft-vs.-leukemia effect. Whether graft-vs.-leukemia activity can be induced in vitro after marrow transplantation for chronic myeloid leukemia (CML) was determined.

Methods.—Lymphokine-activated killer (LAK) cells were generated by incubating blood mononuclear cells taken after bone marrow transplantation with recombinant interleukin-2. The cells were phenotyped and tested for activity in a ^{51}Cr release assay and a CFU-GM assay.

Findings.—Lymphokine-activated killer cells were mainly activated natural killer cells, but some were $CD3^+$ T cells. Lymphokine-activated killer cells from 20 to 33 allogeneic marrow recipients and 2 of 4 syngeneic marrow recipients killed recipient CML cells. In most instances, HLA-disparate leukemic cells also were killed. Colony growth usually was inhibited when LAK cells were incubated with CML cells before plating. The proliferation of donor marrow CFU-GM was largely unaffected. A graft-vs.-leukemia effect was demonstrable after LAK effectors were depleted of $CD3^+$ T cells. It was seen in marrow recipients with and those without graft-vs.-host disease.

Implications.—The fact that donor marrow is less susceptible than recipient CML progenitors to LAK cells means that interleukin-2/LAK cell treatment after marrow transplantation might enhance antileukemic activity without impeding engraftment. The risk of inducing or enhancing graft-vs.-host disease might be reduced by depleting donor marrow of T cells.

▶ Mackinnon et al. address the question of whether in vivo interleukin (IL)-2–generated LAK can discriminate between leukemic cells and normal hematopoietic precursor cells. Their results demonstrate that LAK-mediated lytic activity against CML target cells appears to be greater than the ability of LAK cells to suppress in vitro progenitors of CFU-GM. These are encouraging results that are relevant to patients undergoing autologous transplantation. However, as mentioned by the authors, the use of IL-2–induced LAK cell therapy in vivo may not be feasible for patients undergoing allogeneic marrow transplantation if IL-2 administration potentiates GVHD. The optimal use of

IL-2–induced LAK cell therapy would presumably require treatment early after transplantation, when residual disease should be minimal, but this may be the time when IL-2 is most likely to activate donor cells capable of causing GVHD. Later, as tolerance in established and host-reactive donor T cells have been eliminated or a state of stable "anergy" has been induced, IL-2–induced LAK therapy and the infusion of IL-2 should be safer.—J.A. Hansen, M.D.

Donor Leukocyte Transfusions for Treatment of Recurrent Chronic Myelogenous Leukemia in Marrow Transplant Patients
Kolb HJ, Mittermüller J, Clemm Ch, Holler E, Ledderose G, Brehm G, Heim M, Wilmanns W (University of Munich, Germany)
Blood 76:2462–2465, 1990   21–4

Introduction.—Patients with chronic myelogenous leukemia who relapse after bone marrow transplantation rarely enter cytogenetic remission unless a second transplant is performed. Hematologic relapse of chronic myelogenous leukemia has been successfully treated with interferon-α and transfusion of buffy coat cells from marrow donor.

Experience.—Three patients who relapsed after bone marrow transplantation were given interferon α 2b in a daily dose of 5×10^6 units/m^2 subcutaneously without suppression of Philadelphia chromosome-positive host cells. Three to 5 buffy coat transfusions were given within 5–9 days. The patients received no additional chemotherapy or radiotherapy. All 3 patients entered complete hematologic and cytogenetic remission, lasting 32–91 weeks. In 2 patients, acute GVHD developed after buffy coat transfusions, which required immunosuppressive therapy.

Conclusion.—These cases represent successful adoptive immunotherapy. Interferon alone was not sufficient to induce remission, but the transfusion of donor buffy coat cells in these climeric patients was followed by the elimination of the leukemia host cells.

▶ The experience reported by Kolb et al. in this series of 3 patients is remarkable and compelling. The induction of clinical and cytogenetic remission after the infusion of donor-derived buffy coat cells suggests that GVL may be effectively manipulated in patients with otherwise stable engraftment. Acute GVHD developed in 2 of the 3 patients, further emphasizing the close association between these 2 phenomena. It is not clear whether the mechanism responsible for GVL is distinct from GVHD, and this conundrum raises the potential concern that active GVL immunotherapy involving the infusion of immunologically competent donor T cells may inevitably place the patient at risk of developing clinically significant GVHD. Nevertheless, the prognosis for posttransplant relapse is grim, and there are no alternatives other than a second transplant. The inherent hazards of continuing these clinical trials in well informed patients are justified given the dramatic results achieved in these 3 patients.—J.A. Hansen, M.D.

Amplification of the Graft-Versus-Leukemia Effect in Man by Interleukin-2

Verdonck LF, van Heugten HG, Giltay J, Franks CR (University of Utrecht, The Netherlands)
Transplantation 51:1120–1123, 1991

21–5

Introduction.—Incubating mononuclear cells with interleukin-2 (IL-2) in vitro generates effector cells that can lyse tumor-cell targets. Some patients with refractory malignancies have exhibited substantial tumor regression when given recombinant IL-2.

Case Report.—Woman, 45, was seen with acute myeloid leukemia and bone marrow necrosis. A hypodiploid karyotype was documented. Remission occurred on initial chemotherapy but the patient had extensive cutaneous relapse when readmitted for bone marrow transplantation. A second skin relapse occurred 5 months after bone marrow transplantation. It responded well to electron beam irradiation, but multiple relapses ensued. Two 5-day courses of recombinant IL-2 infusion followed. The patient became febrile and had bronchospasm and some fluid retention, as well as hyperbilirubinemia. Tumor was reduced by more than 80%. Pneumonia of probable fungal origin occurred shortly after IL-2 treatment ended, and the patient requested that no treatment be given for the pneumonia.

Discussion.—Interleukin-2 can activate cell-mediated cytotoxicity directly and also can generate the release of other lymphokines (e.g., γ-interferon and tumor necrosis factor). Further studies of IL-2 appear warranted in recipients of allogeneic marrow transplants who are at high risk of relapsing. Production of IL-2 is quite low for the first 2 years after bone marrow transplantation.

▶ This is an interesting and unique case report demonstrating induction of a GVL effect in a woman 5 months after she received a T-cell–depleted marrow graft from an HLA-identical sister. Mild grade I GVHD developed, but resolved after treatment with steroids. The relapse involved leukemic skin lesions, but these responded to rIL-2 therapy by decreasing size and number without any evidence of GVHD. This is a very important observation. Induction of GVHD could limit the use of IL-2 for inducing GVL in allograft patients. In this particular case, the fact that this patient received a T-cell–depleted transplant may have significantly facilitated a durable graft-vs.-host tolerance that could not be affected by the IL-2 infusion. Patients receiving unmodified marrow grafts and still requiring immunosuppression for control of GVHD may be more susceptible to the GVHD-inducing potential of IL-2.—J.A. Hansen, M.D.

22 Cytomegalovirus

▶ ↓ Cytomegalovirus (CMV) has been the scourge of marrow transplantation, especially in patients receiving allografts. In a large single-center series of 525 marrow transplant patients studied over a period of 10 years, the overall incidence of CMV pneumonia was 17% with a mortality rate of 85% (1). Activation and CMV infection occur in almost all seropositive patients, however, the risk of CMV pneumonia is greatest in patients developing GVHD. Cytomegalovirus pneumonia can also occur in patients receiving autografts, although at a much lower incidence (2, 3). Primary CMV infection in patients occurs by the transfusion of blood products or transplantation of marrow cells from CMV seropositive donors. Primary CMV infection can be prevented by the transfusion of blood products from SMV seronegative donors (4–6).—J.A. Hansen, M.D.

References

1. Meyers JD, Flournoy N, Thomas ED: *Rev Infect Dis.* 4:1119, 1982.
2. Pecego R, et al: *Transplantation* 42:515, 1986.
3. Wingaard JR, et al: *Blood* 71:1432, 1988.
4. Yeager AS, et al: *J Pediatr* 98:281, 1981.
5. Preiksaitis JK, et al: *J Infect Dis* 147:974, 1983.
6. Bowden RA, et al: *N Engl J Med* 314:1006, 1986.

Prevention of Cytomegalovirus Infection Following Bone Marrow Transplantation: A Randomized Trial of Blood Product Screening
Miller WJ, McCullough J, Balfour HH Jr, Haake RJ, Ramsay NKC, Goldman A, Bowman R, Kersey J (Univ of Minnesota)
Bone Marrow Transplant 7:227–234, 1991   22–1

Background.—Cytomegalovirus (CMV) infects 40% to 50% of patients undergoing bone marrow transplantation (BMT). The results of a controlled, blinded trial of blood product screening for preventing CMV infection in seronegative recipients after BMT were assessed.

Methods.—From 1983 to 1987, CMV-seronegative allogeneic BMT recipients were randomly assigned to receive screened CMV-seronegative or unscreened blood products. Data were available for analysis on 125 patients.

Results.—Cytomegalovirus infection developed in 18% of the patients receiving screened products and in 38% of those receiving unscreened products. Only 2 of 64 patients in the first group and 7 of 61 in the second, however, had culture or biopsy-proved CMV infections. Bone marrow donor CMV seropositivity was associated with an increased risk of acquiring CMV infection. Also, CMV infection was not prevented by blood product screening if the bone marrow donor was seropositive. The

1-year survival censored for relapse was 52% and 68% in the screened and unscreened groups, respectively. Gram-negative bacteremia complicated BMT in 35% and 15%, respectively. The 2 groups had comparable rates of relapse. According to multivariate analysis, high-risk disease, CMV infection, screened blood products group membership, recipient age of more than 17 years, chronic GVHD, and gram-negative bacteremia had independent negative effects on survival.

Conclusions.—Blood product screening appears to be effective in preventing CMV infections after BMT if both recipient and donor are CMV seronegative. The use of seronegative blood products, however, was associated with increased gram-negative bacteremia and did not improve survival, despite the decreased rate of CMV infection.

▶ This study confirms previous reports demonstrating a lower incidence of CMV infection in seronegative allograft recipients who are transfused with blood products from seronegative donors compared to unscreened donors. However, in this group of patients the lower incidence of CMV infection (18% vs. 38%) did not result in an improved 1-year survival (censored for relapse) as expected.—J.A. Hansen, M.D.

Use of Leukocyte-Depleted Platelets and Cytomegalovirus-Seronegative Red Blood Cells for Prevention of Primary Cytomegalovirus Infection After Marrow Transplant

Bowden RA, Slichter SJ, Sayers MH, Mori M, Cays MJ, Meyers JD (Fred Hutchinson Cancer Research Ctr; Univ of Washington; Puget Sound Blood Ctr, Seattle)
Blood 78:246–250, 1991   22–2

Introduction.—Cytomegalovirus (CMV) pneumonia remains a significant cause of infectious death after marrow transplantation. The fact that CMV-seronegative blood is not universally available suggests a need for alternative ways of protecting against primary CMV infection.

Objective.—A prospective study was carried out in 77 CMV-senonegative marrow transplant recipients. Those given standard unscreened blood products were compared with patients who received both leukocyte-depleted platelets and CMV-seronegative red blood cells. Leukocyte-depleted platelets were prepared by centrifugation. Most patients (n = 65) received autologous transplants (n = 60) because of hematologic malignancy.

Outcome.—There were 7 CMV infections in the control group and none in patients given leukocyte-depleted platelets, a significant difference. One patient in the control group contracted CMV pneumonia. Comparable amounts of red blood cells and platelets were given to patients in the 2 study groups.

Conclusions.—Leukocyte-depleted platelets are an effective means of preventing transfusion-associated CMV infection in autologous marrow transplant recipients.

▶ The availability of CMV-seronegative blood depends on the prevalence of CMV in the community, and in some areas, adequate quantities of CMV-seronegative platelets or red blood cells may not be available. Alternate methods for preventing exposure of susceptible patients to CMV are needed. This report demonstrates the efficacy of leukocyte depletion of platelet concentrates by centrifugation in significantly diminishing the probability of primary infection in a group of predominantly autologous transplant recipients. A similar protection has been reported for filtered blood products (1). In addition to leukocyte depletion, another option for increasing the supply of CMV-seronegative blood products is the expansion of platelet pheresis programs using selected CMV-seronegative donors. The latter is occurring in some blood centers, especially in programs where there is a very high relative need for platelets compared to red blood cells.—J.A. Hansen, M.D.

Reference

1. Bowden RA, et al: *Transplantation* 29:5205, 1989.

Cytomegalovirus Infection Causes Delayed Platelet Recovery After Bone Marrow Transplantation

Verdonck LF, de Gast GC, van Heugten HG, Nieuwenhuis HK, Dekker AW (University Hospital Utrecht, The Netherlands)
Blood 78:844–848, 1991   22–3

Background.—Cytomegalovirus (CMV) infection after bone marrow transplantation (BMT) can cause pneumonia enteritis, hematologic abnormalities, or graft failure. The effect of CMV infection on the hematopoietic recovery after marrow transplant was studied retrospectively in 87 recipients of autologous BMT and 56 recipients of allogeneic BMT.

Methods.—Patients were divided into 2 groups based on CMV-positive or -negative status before transplant. The CMV-negative patients were kept negative by transfusion of leukocyte-poor red blood cells and platelets from CMV-negative clones.

Results.—Platelet recovery in the patients receiving allogeneic transplants was significantly slower in CMV-positive patients than in CMV-negative patients. This difference was apparent in patients with and without clinically significant acute graft-vs.-host disease. In patients undergoing autologous BMT for lymphoma, a delayed recovery of platelets is apparent in CMV-positive patients. Patients undergoing autologous BMT for acute leukemias, however, had a delayed recovery of both platelets and granulocytes irrespective of CMV status. Cytomegalovirus status had no effect on the recovery of granulocytes in autologous or allogeneic BMT.

Conclusions.—Cytomegalovirus infection caused delayed platelet recovery in patients after both autologous and allogeneic BMT. In recipients of autologous BMT, however, the primary disease, for example acute leukemia, may have a dominant effect on posttransplant hematopoiesis and obscure any effect of CMV infections. A transfusion policy that prevents transmission of CMV to CMV-negative BMT recipients may have a major impact on morbidity and mortality.

▶ This report demonstrates an interesting biological consequence of CMV infection that may contribute significantly to morbidity and cost of transplant. Prolongation of thrombocytopenia increases the risk of hemorrhagic complications and requires the transfusion of additional blood products. The mechanisms by which CMV infection can delay platelet recovery is unclear, but suppression of megakaryocytes and platelet consumption caused by a shortened platelet half-life may contribute.—J.A. Hansen, M.D.

Adoptive Transfer of Anti-Cytomegalovirus Effect of Interleukin-2–Activated Bone Marrow: Potential Application in Transplantation

Agah R, Charak BS, Chen V, Mazumder A (Univ of Southern California, Los Angeles)

Blood 78:720–727, 1991

22–4

Objective.—Cytomegalovirus (CMV) infection and CMV-caused pneumonia can occur in both autologous and allogeneic bone marrow transplantation. The most significant risk factor for CMV infection is positive pretransplant CMV serology. Earlier studies have shown that interleukin-2 (IL-2)–activated murine bone marrow (ABM) cells have cytotoxic activity against murine CMV (MCMV)-infected target cells in vitro, with a reconstituting ability comparable to that of fresh bone marrow cells. The use of ABM cells in bone marrow transplantation to prevent CMV infection was further explored in an animal model.

Results.—The ABM cells lysed the MCMV-infected cells in vitro at both acute and chronic stages of infection. The ABM cells supplemented with IL-2 therapy virtually eradicated the viral infection and prolonged the survival of MCMV-infected mice in both a preventive or therapeutic setting, even in mice immunocompromised by irradiation. Combination therapy also prevented reactivation of chronic MCMV infection after irradiation. The Thy-1$^+$ and asialo GM1$^+$ cells limited MCMV proliferation by approximately 30% and 80%, respectively. Bone marrow macrophages limited the proliferation of MCMV by 100%.

Conclusions.—In this animal study, bone marrow transplantation with ABM cells followed by IL-2 therapy improved host resistance against CMV disease in the posttransplant period. Bone marrow macrophages and Thy-1$^+$ cells in the presence of IL-2 are also important agents in controlling MCMV. Interleukin-2 appears to have a beneficial effect in allogeneic bone marrow transplantation and should be explored in combination with ABM for an anti-CMV effect.

▶ Significant CMV disease is more likely to occur when there is a profound and prolonged deficiency in cell-mediated immunity. Immune T cells are a prerequisite for establishing effective control of CMV infection, but other effector cells also play important roles in different disease models (1). This report demonstrates that the nonspecific amplification of effector cells in immunosuppressed and CMV-infected mice by infusion of bone marrow cells activated in vitro with IL-2 and supplemented with IL-2 therapy in vivo has a protective effect by suppressing active infection, preventing reactivation of chronic infection and improving survival. Natural killer cells, T cells, and macrophages all appeared to have anti-CMV activity, and these protective effects of IL-2 may be further amplified by the release of other cytokines such as γ-interferon and tumor necrosis factor (TNF). These observations further illuminate the importance of immune deficiency in contributing to transplant-associated complications such as CMV infection. Given the availability of alternate approaches to the prevention and treatment of CMV disease (see Abstract 23–1), IL-2 therapy as tested in this model may not be feasible in allografts, where the administration of IL-2 at critical times in the posttransplant period may counteract GVHD prophylaxis and potentiate GVHD. Therapy with IL-2 initiated later in the post-transplant period, however, may play a significant role in preventing tumor relapse, and in the absence of GVHD may also provide protection from reactivation of CMV latent infection.—J.A. Hansen, M.D.

Reference

1. Rapp F: The biology of cytomegalovirus, in Roizman B (ed): *The Herpes Viruses.* New York, Plenum, 1983, p 1.

Cytomegalovirus Pneumonia in Allogeneic Bone Marrow Transplantation: An Immunopathologic Process?

Chien J, Chan CK, Chamberlain D, Patterson B, Fyles G, Minden M, Meharch-and J, Messner H (University of Toronto, Canada)
Chest 98:1034–1037, 1990   22–5

Introduction.—Cytomegalovirus (CMV) produces a pneumonia in bone marrow transplant (BMT) patients that is a major cause of death in this population, with the mortality rate at about 85%. The clinical course of a BMT patient with CMV pneumonia, who successfully responded to combined therapy of gamma immune globulin (GIG) and dihydroxy-2-propoxymethyl-guanine (DHPG), but who had continuous immune system activation that resulted in bronchiolitis obliterans organizing pneumonia (BOOP).

Case Report.—Man, 31, had acute myeloblastic leukemia in remission and received a BMT from his mother. Both subjects were CMV-negative before the transplant. On the 25th day after transplant, the patient developed diarrhea, low-grade fever, and a generalized skin rash. On the 64th day after BMT, his clinical symptoms and BAL fluid were positive for CMV. The patient responded to DHPB and GIG treatment. Six months after BMT, he had a general illness and chest x-ray showed bilateral infiltrates. Open lung biopsy demonstrated the presence of BOOP, which responded to intravenous methylprednisolone treatment.

Findings.—The patient recovered from the acute CMV pneumonia episode after treatment with both GIG and DHPG. Although CMV was not found in the BAL fluid after this therapy, the lymphocytosis in the BAL fluid after this acute infection continued after the CMV could not be detected.

Conclusions.—This case report proposes that BMT patients with CMV pneumonia should be observed for a 2-phase disease development: an acute episode and a later chronic episode. In the first stage, the CMV pneumonia can be managed with GIG and DHPG treatment, while the second stage should be monitored for BOOP development. Further studies should determine whether maintenance therapy should be continued in these patients to prevent the occurrence of BOOP.

▶ This case report illustrates the increasing success that has been achieved in using DHPG and intravenous immune globulin (IVIG) to treat CMV pneumonia in marrow transplant patients. The subsequent occurrence of bronchiolitis obliterans in the same patient without recurrent CMV infection is an interesting observation; however, in the absence of any evidence for viral transcription the suggestion that the latter problem had a cause and effect relation to CMV is speculative. The patient received immunosuppression for GVHD, and thus GVHD or prolonged immunodeficiency may have allowed infection with unidentified virus. As suggested by the authors, these patients require careful monitoring, but it is not clear what additional therapy should be administered. High-dose methylprednisolone may be effective therapy for bronchiolitis obliterans, but it would not be prudent to immunosuppress these patients additionally without a specific indication; otherwise, the risk of other opportunistic infections, including recurrence of CMV, will continue to be dangerously high.—J.A. Hansen, M.D.

A Randomized, Controlled Trial of Prophylactic Ganciclovir for Cytomegalovirus Pulmonary Infection in Recipients of Allogeneic Bone Marrow Transplants
Schmidt GM, Horak DA, Niland JC, Duncan SR, Forman SJ, Zaia JA, and the City of Hope-Stanford-Syntex CMV Study Group (City of Hope Nat'l Med Ctr, Duarte, Calif; Stanford Univ, Stanford, Calif)
N Engl J Med 324:1005–1011, 1991   22–6

Introduction.—Cytomegalovirus (CMV)-associated interstitial pneumonia is the most common infectious cause of death after allogeneic bone marrow transplantation (BMT). Combined therapy with ganciclovir and intravenous immune globulin improves survival in patients with CMV pneumonia. A randomized, controlled clinical trial was performed to determine whether prophylactic ganciclovir administration could prevent interstitial pneumonia in allogeneic BMT recipients with asymptomatic pulmonary CMV infection.

Patients.—During a 3-year period, 104 patients with no evidence of respiratory disease after undergoing BMT underwent routine bronchoalveolar lavage on day 35 to determine the presence of pulmonary CMV. Sixty-four patients were CMV-negative. Of the 40 CMV-positive patients, 20 were randomly assigned to prophylactic ganciclovir and 20 to observation only. Intravenous ganciclovir was given twice daily at a dose of 5 mg/kg/body weight for 2 weeks and 5 times per week thereafter until day 120 after BMT.

Results.—Five of the 20 CMV-positive patients (25%) treated with prophylactic ganciclovir died or had CMV pneumonia before day 120, compared with 14 of the 20 untreated, observed CMV-positive patients (70%). None of the patients who received the full course of ganciclovir prophylaxis developed CMV interstitial pneumonia. Twelve (22%) of 55 evaluable CMV-negative patients developed CMV pneumonia. In all, 31 patients had developed CMV interstitial pneumonia by day 120. Cytomegalovirus positivity of lavage-fluid and CMV-positive blood culture obtained on day 35 after BMT were the strongest predictors of CMV interstitial pneumonia.

Conclusions.—Asymptomatic pulmonary CMV infection is a major risk factor for CMV interstitial pneumonia in allogeneic bone marrow recipients. Prophylactic ganciclovir effectively prevents the development of CMV interstitial pneumonia in patients with asymptomatic CMV infection.

▶ The findings by Schmidt et al. represent a major breakthrough. The demonstration that early treatment with ganciclovir is effective in preventing CMV disease clearly emphasizes the importance of blocking viral replication before tissue injury and pathogenic host responses can occur. As pointed out by the authors, the next important questions to address are the identification of patients at risk of infection and the optimal time to initiate ganciclovir therapy. Because of the potential toxicity of this drug, especially in the form of myelosuppression, which could increase the risk of other infections, the priority now is to determine minimal effective doses and dose schedules.—J.A. Hansen, M.D.

Early Occurrence of Human Cytomegalovirus Infection After Bone Marrow Transplantation as Demonstrated by the Polymerase Chain Reaction Technique
Einsele H, Steidle M, Vallbracht A, Saal JG, Ehninger G, Müller CA (University of Tubingen, Germany)
Blood 77:1104–1110, 1991   22–7

Background.—Human cytomegalovirus (HCMV) infection often complicates an allogeneic bone marrow transplantation (BMT). The HCMV episode can lead to sometimes fatal graft-vs.-host disease (GVHD). Recent reports have shown that newer hybridization virus culture techniques may provide a higher sensitivity in detecting HCMS in clinical specimens. The results of tests using polymerase chain reaction (PCR) in diagnosing HCMV infection compared to results from conventional culture testing, the slot-blot assay, and in situ hybridization assay are reported.

Methods.—Twenty-eight BMT patients were followed for possible HCMV infection; the median follow-up period was 10 weeks posttransplant. Five patients died during this period, and only 4 patients were found to be seronegative for CMV. Six percutaneous and postmortem liver biopsy samples and 4 postmortem lung biopsy samples were studied for CMV. All specimens were cryopreserved until tested. The laboratory HCMV strain AD169 and 50 other HCMV clinical isolates were assessed by PCR. Viral DNA probes for the slot-blot and in situ hybridization assays were developed.

Results.—The PCR analysis of the cloned HCMV-DNA segment pCM5018 demonstrated that the 10 fg of the homologous HCMV-DNA was amplified and remained visible after electrophoresis and ethidium bromide staining. The detection limit of 0.1 fg of amplified homologous HCMV-DNA corresponded to a sensitivity of approximately 10 virus copies achievable after 12 hours of exposure. The 4 HCMV seronegative patients were also found to be seronegative using PCR methods. Twenty-four seropositive patients were studied 10 days before hospital discharge or death after MBT using the PCR assay. Of the 30 blood and 28 urine samples from these 24 patients, all were HCMV negative by culture and conventional slot-blot testing, but 3 IgG seropositive patients had HCMV-DNA on PCR amplification. Twenty of the 24 patients had HCMV viremia and viruria 1–6 weeks after BMT as shown by PCR amplification, while 16 of the 24 were found to have HCMV in urine culture and 12 had HCMV using slot-blot DNA hybridization. The most sensitive HCMV detection in lung and liver samples was accomplished by PCR amplification also.

Implications.—These findings indicate that none of the HCMV detection techniques used could predict the development of HCMV infection in any particular patient. However, the high sensitivity of the PCR technique may improve the analysis of different cells and organs affected by latent HCMV infection in BMT patients, which may also aid in excluding blood products or transplant materials contaminated with HCMV.

▶ Early detection of CMV infection has become a more pertinent topic since the demonstration by Schmidt et al. (Abstract 22–6) that early treatment with DHPG can prevent significant CMV disease and pneumonia, a complication that has been associated with a terrifying high rate of mortality (1). Although the PCR assay for CMV DNA was more sensitive than the culture method used in this study, the detection of CMV DNA may not always identify patients with active infection. The serologic assay for anti-CMV antibody has proven to be a very sensitive marker for CMV carriers and a reliable way of identifying individuals at risk for CMV infection. Assays for CMV transcription and infection would have to be based on detection of specific RNA or antigen, or a more sensitive culture method. Currently the gold standard for the diagnosis of CMV infection is the shell vile culture system (2).—J.A. Hansen, M.D.

References

1. Meyers JD, Flournoy N, Thomas ED: *Rev Infect Dis* 4:1119, 1982.
2. Gleaves CA, et al: *Clin Microbiol* 21:217, 1985.

Phase I Study of Safety and Pharmacokinetics of a Human Anticytomegalovirus Monoclonal Antibody in Allogeneic Bone Marrow Transplant Recipients
Drobyski WR, Gottlieb M, Carrigan D, Ostberg L, Grebenau M, Schran H, Magid P, Ehrlich P, Nadler PI, Ash RC (Med College of Wisconsin, Milwaukee; Sandoz Research Inst, East Hanover, NJ)
Transplantation 51:1190–1196, 1991   22–8

Background.—A cell-mediated response is thought to play the main role in the host defense against cytomegalovirus (CMV) infection. A human monoclonal antibody that neutralizes strains of human CMV has been developed to circumvent some of the problems of CMV immunoprophylaxis and therapy with pooled human immunoglobulin. A phase I study was done of the safety and pharmacokinetic profile of 3 dose levels of the monoclonal antibody.

Methods.—The antibody, designated SDZ MSL-109, was studied in a dose-escalation trial in 15 patients undergoing allogeneic bone marrow transplantation. Twelve had chronic myelogenous leukemia and 3 had acute nonlymphocytic leukemia. The patients were separated into 3 groups of 5 and then given the monoclonal antibody in 50-, 250-, and 500-μg/kg doses at intervals of about 3 weeks for 6 months.

Results.—Side effects of the antibody were minimal, and there was no dose-related toxicity. In all dosing groups, the antibody elimination curves were consistent with a 2-compartmental model. The α half-lives were 1.03 days at the low dose, .82 days at the middle dose, and .79 days at the high dose; corresponding β half-lives were 13.9, 14.0, and 16.5 days. Repetitive dosing to approximate plasma volume decreased the volume of distribution. The pharmacokinetic picture was similar to that of human IgG. The monoclonal antibody did not appear to be immunogenic; there was no host antiidiotypic or antiallotypic antibody formation.

Conclusion.—A recently developed human anti-CMV monoclonal antibody appears to be safe for use in patients undergoing allogeneic bone marrow transplantation and may improve and simplify current approaches to preventing and treating CMV infection. The efficacy of this treatment, in both marrow transplant patients and others with immunodeficiency disorders, remains to be studied in controlled trials.

▶ Although animal models of CMV infection and disease suggest a dominant role for T cell-mediated immunity (1, 2) in host defense, the potential for a human monoclonal anti-CMV neutralizing antibody as a therapeutic agent in immunocompromised patients is of great interest. The current phase I study demonstrated safety and established essential pharmacokinetic data for designing a further study of efficacy. Eventually, a randomized study will be necessary to determine whether this approach can prevent recurrent infection or significantly modify disease.—J.A. Hansen, M.D.

References

1. Quinnan G, et al: *N Engl J Med* 307:7, 1982.
2. Bowden R, et al: *Transplantation* 44:504, 1987.

23 Hepatitis and Veno-Occlusive Disease

Hepatic Veno-Occlusive Disease Post-Bone Marrow Transplantation in Children Conditioned With Busulfan and Cyclophosphamide: Incidence, Risk Factors, and Clinical Outcome
Ozkaynak MF, Weinberg K, Kohn D, Sender L, Parkman R, Lenarsky C (Children's Hosp of Los Angeles, Univ of Southern California, Los Angeles
Bone Marrow Transplant 7:467–474, 1991   23–1

Background.—Veno-occlusive disease (VOD) of the liver is a fibrous obliteration of small hepatic venules caused by high-dose chemotherapy, radiation, or bush tea containing pyrrolizidine alkaloids. This syndrome in children with leukemia conditioned for bone marrow transplantation with busulfan-containing regimens has not been studied thoroughly. The incidence, risk factors, and clinical outcome of VOD were documented in 50 such children.

Methods and Results.—The children (median age, 7 years; range, 8 months to 22 years) were prepared for bone marrow transplantation (autologous, n = 24; allogeneic, n = 26) with 16 mg/kg of busulfan and 200 mg/kg of cyclophosphamide. Veno-occlusive disease developed in 14 of the 50 children, or 28%. Half of the children with VOD also had pleural effusion. The incidence of VOD among children who underwent transplantation for leukemia (n = 39) was 36%, whereas none of the patients who underwent transplantation for a genetic disease (n = 11) had VOD. Patient age, sex, remission status, type of graft, history of liver disease, and pretransplant liver functions were not indicators of an increased risk of VOD. Twenty-three children had pretransplant samples that could be tested for antibody to the hepatitis C virus. Three of these were positive.

Conclusions.—Veno-occlusive disease is a common complication of bone marrow transplantation in children with leukemia conditioned with busulfan and cyclophosphamide. However, the syndrome was manageable and nonfatal in this group of young patients.

▶ This study of children undergoing autologous and allogeneic transplants for malignant and genetic diseases underscores the prevalence of VOD as a complication of the busulfan 16 mg and cyclophosphamide 200 mg ("big Bu/Cy") regimen. Fortunately, this was not a fatal complication in this relatively young population. An elevated pretransplant transaminase, an allogeneic transplant and graft-vs.-host disease (GVHD) have been reported to be risk factors for clinically severe VOD (1–3). The reason for the relative resistance of children to severe VOD after Bu/Cy is not known; however, it has been suggested that plasma busulfan levels may be lower in children than in adults (4).—J.A. Hansen, M.D.

References

1. McDonald GB, et al: *Hepatology* 4:116, 1984.
2. Jones JR, et al: *Transplantation* 4:778, 1987.
3. Locasciullia A, et al: *Transplantation* 48:68, 1989.
4. Grochow LB, et al: *Blood* 75:1723, 1990.

Acalculous Cholecystitis After Bone Marrow Transplantation in Adults With Acute Leukaemia: Case Report

Pitkäranta P, Haapiainen R, Taavitsainen M, Elonen E (University Central Hospital, Helsinki)
Eur J Surg 157:361–364, 1991   23–2

Background.—Postoperative complications of bone marrow transplantation for acute leukemia include severe immunodeficiency, transient granulocytopenia, infectious complications, and acute abdominal disorders. Acute acalculous cholecystitis occurred soon after bone marrow transplantation for acute leukemia in 3 patients. Only about 5% of acute cholecystitis cases are acalculous.

Discussion.—The diagnosis was made by ultrasonography in all 3 patients. The ultrasonographic criteria include thickening of the gallbladder wall, enlarged transverse diameter, gallbladder pressure pain, and local hypoechoic areas in the gallbladder wall. Antiemetic and analgesic drugs or epithelial gallbladder damage may be causative factors, but cultures ruled out an infectious cause. Controversy over treatment centers on cholecystectomy versus cholecystostomy, especially in critically ill patients after major surgery.

Conclusions.—Delay in diagnosis and treatment may contribute to the high mortality rate from acute acalculous cholecystitis. Surgical intervention is recommended for progressive acute acalculous leukemia, even in the patient with granulocytopenia, thrombocytopenia, or immunosuppression.

▶ The problems described by these authors are relatively common in marrow transplant patients probably as a result of high-dose chemotherapy and radiation. Enlarged gallbladders with thickened walls and sludge may be detectable in more than 50% of patients by ultrasonography (1). As patients begin to eat, they may develop abdominal pain as the biliary system attempts to empty the sludge. In the absence of abscess or perforation, surgical intervention is probably not necessary.—J.A. Hansen, M.D.

Reference

1. Wolford JL, et al: *J Clin Gastroenterol* 10:419, 1988.

▶ ↓ Liver function abnormalities occur frequently after allogeneic marrow transplantation. High-dose chemotherapy and radiation therapy, sepsis, GVHD, and viral infections may be involved (1). The hepatitis C virus (HCV) has been implicated as a cause of transfusion-associated acute and chronic non-A, non-B hepatitis (2), a disease that is usually mild (3). Non-A, non-B hepatitis after allogeneic marrow transplantation also has been described as a mild disease (4). However, significant numbers of patients who develop posttransplant non-A, non-B hepatitis develop chronic hepatitis, which in some may progress to liver cirrhosis (5, 6). The following 2 articles (Abstracts 23–3 and 23–4) report on the incidence of HCV seropositivity before transplantation, the incidence of seroconversion posttransplantation, and the association of posttransplant liver enzyme abnormalities with seropositivity. The evidence suggests that although acute hepatitis does not appear to be a problem, HCV may play a role in posttransplant chronic liver disease. Further studies of long-term survivors are needed to determine whether HCV will contribute to significant liver disease and cirrhosis.—J.A. Hansen, M.D.

References

1. McDonald GB, et al: *Semin Liver Dis* 7:210, 1987.
2. Alter HJ, et al: *N Engl J Med* 321:1494, 1989.
3. Dienstag J: *Gastroenterology* 85:439, 1983.
4. Myers J, et al: *Ann Intern Med* 87:57, 1977.
5. Mattsson L, Weiland O, Glaumann H: *Liver* 8:184, 1988.
6. Koretz R, et al: *Gastroenterology* 88:1251, 1985.

Hepatitis C Infection in Allogeneic Bone Marrow Transplant Recipients
Ljungman P, Duraj V, Magnius L, Aschan J, Lönnqvist B, Ringdén O, Gahrton G (Huddinge University Hospital, Karolinska Institute, Huddinge, Sweden; National Bacteriological Laboratory, Stockholm)
Clin Transplant 5:283–286, 1991   23–3

Introduction.—Hepatitis C virus (HCV) has recently been identified as the main agent of non-A, non-B hepatitis transmitted by blood transfusions. Infection with HCV is one of the liver function abnormalities detected after allogeneic bone marrow transplantation (BMT).

Methods.—To determine the frequency of HCV infection in long-term survivors after allogeneic BMT, and to compare the frequency of liver function disturbance in patients with and without serologic evidence of HCV infection, antibodies to HCV were determined 2 years after BMT in 83 patients.

Results.—After BMT, 8 patients seroconverted to HCV. There was a significant correlation between seroconversion to HCV and the number of platelet transfusions. The seroconverted patients had more signs of acute hepatitis and persistent liver function abnormalities than the patients who did not seroconvert. Of the 8 patients who seroconverted to HCV, 7 had persistent liver function abnormalities compared with 5 of 61 patients without evidence of HCV infection.

Conclusion.—Infection with HCV appears to be a major cause of persistent liver abnormalities after allogeneic BMT. The patients who seroconverted received more platelet transfusions and had more signs of acute hepatitis than the patients who did not seroconvert.

Hepatitis C Virus Infection in Patients Undergoing Allogeneic Bone Marrow Transplantation
Locasciulli A, Bacigalupo A, Vanlint MT, Tagger A, Uderzo C, Portmann B, Shulman HM, Alberti A (Institute of Hygiene and Virology, Milan; Oespedale Martino, Genoa, Italy; King's College Hospital and Medical School, London; Fred Hutchinson Cancer Research Ctr, Seattle; University of Padua, Padua, Italy)
Transplantation 52:315–318, 1991   23–4

Introduction.—The major causes of liver damage in patients undergoing bone marrow transplantation (BMT) are graft-vs.-host disease and veno-occlusive disease (VOD); viral hepatitis is a less common but severe complication. Viral hepatitis may influence the prognosis of BMT not only by causing posttransplant liver disease, but also by increasing the risk of VOD.

Methods.—Using a recently developed assay, 128 patients undergoing BMT were tested to determine the prevalence of hepatitis C virus (HCV) and its impact on posttransplant liver disease.

Results.—The overall prevalence of anti-HCV in 128 patients tested after BMT was 29.6%. Pretransplant anti-HCV positivity in 35 patients tested was not predictive of more severe liver disease. In addition, posttransplant liver failure caused by VOD or subacute hepatitis and post-BMT increase in tramsaminases occurred regardless of anti-HCV serology. In only 1 anti-HCV$^+$ and 1 anti-HCV$^-$ patients did VOD develop after BMT. The number of patients with liver failure contributing to death was comparable in the anti-HCV$^+$ and anti-HCV$^-$ groups. In 17 patients, there was posttransplant seroconversion from negative to positive. In 9 of 17 patients who seroconverted from negative to positive after BMT, the appearance of anti-HCV was concomitant with hepatitis exacerbation.

Conclusion.—The high prevalence (29%) of anti-HCV positivity in patients undergoing allogeneic bone marrow transplantation supports the role of hepatitis C virus in causing liver disease. The presence of the antibody in serum appears to be a marker of ongoing, rather than past infection. However, the anti-HCV test is of limited accuracy because of low sensitivity and incomplete specificity.

24 Supportive Care and Miscellaneous

Treatment of Marrow Donor Blood Products With Gamma-Irradiation Prevents Transfusion-Induced Sensitization to DLA-Identical Marrow Grafts
Storb R, Bean MA, Appelbaum FR, Schuening FG, Graham TC, Raff RF (Fred Hutchinson Cancer Res Ctr; Univ of Washington; Pacific Northwest Res Found, Seattle)
Transplant Proc 23:1697–1698, 1991   24–1

Background.—In canine littermates genotypically identical for dog leukocyte antigen (DLA) typing, marrow infusions engrafted after a preparation regimen of total body irradiation (TBI) are uniformly successful. However, there was 100% graft rejection after 3 preceding whole blood transfusions from the marrow donor. Treatment of blood by heat did not prevent sensitization to whole blood transfusions. The blood was then exposed to 2,000 cGy gamma radiation in addition to heat-inactivation.

Methods.—Four dogs were transfused with blood treated by exposure to heat alone, 10 dogs were transfused with blood exposed to both heat and radiation, and 10 dogs were transfused with blood treated with radiation alone.

Results.—In this study, 3 of 4 dogs given heat-inactivated blood before TBI rejected and 1 engrafted. Of 10 dogs given blood treated with heat and radiation, 8 engrafted and 1 rejected. In 10 dogs given blood products that were only radiated, 9 engrafted and 1 rejected.

Conclusions.—In this animal study, the treatment of blood products with heat-inactivation alone was not sufficient to prevent sensitization and subsequent marrow graft rejection. Heat-inactivation combined with gamma radiation or gamma radiation alone were sufficient to prevent sensitization. In human patients who are marrow transplant candidates, blood product transfusions should be gamma irradiated to prevent sensitization and reduce risk of marrow graft rejection.

▶ The finding that 2,000 cGy gamma radiation was effective in preventing the sensitizing effect of transfused whole blood from major histocompatibility complex identical donor on subsequent marrow graft rejection was unexpected. The potential application of gamma radiation to induction of tolerance to minor histocompatibility antigens requires additional investigation. These results also suggest a potential change in transfusion practice for patients who are potential marrow transplant candidates.—J.A. Hansen, M.D.

Immunologic Tolerance to Renal Allografts After Bone Marrow Transplants From the Same Donors
Sayegh MH, Fine NA, Smith JL, Rennke HG, Milford EL, Tilney NL (Brigham and Women's Hosp, Boston; Harvard Med School, Boston; Univ of Iowa Hosps and Clinics, Iowa City)
Ann Intern Med 114:954–955, 1991   24–2

Introduction.—Two patients who underwent bone marrow transplantation subsequently received a kidney from the same donor without undergoing immunosuppressive drug therapy.

Case Report 1.—Man, 30, received a successful bone marrow transplant from his HLA-identical brother 6 months after receiving a diagnosis of acute myelomonocytic leukemia. Subsequent pulmonary dysfunction required administration of low-dose prednisone. His renal function gradually deteriorated and chronic ambulatory peritoneal dialysis was initiated. Shortly thereafter he received a renal allograft from the same brother. His transplanted kidney functioned immediately. The patient later had a mild case of graft-vs.-host disease, which resolved within a month without treatment.

Case Report 2.—Girl, 14 years, with acute nonlymphocytic leukemia received a successful bone marrow transplant from her HLA-identical brother. She developed idiopathic pneumonitis that required chronic low-dose administration of prednisone. Her renal function gradually deteriorated and she required institution of peritoneal dialysis. Two weeks later she received a renal allograft from the same HLA identical brother who had donated the bone marrow. Her allograft functioned immediately and she has had no rejection episodes.

Conclusion.—Patients who have received a successful bone marrow transplant and subsequently develop end-stage renal disease may have acquired specific immunologic tolerance and may safely receive a kidney from the same donor without the need for additional immunosuppressive drug therapy.

▶ This is an interesting clinical report of 2 patients successfully transplanted with a kidney from the same HLA-identical sibling who earlier had been the donor for marrow transplantation required for the treatment of leukemia. Although data were not presented, both patients were presumably fully engrafted with hematopoietic cells of donor origin. Immunologic rejection of the renal allografts was not observed. Given full engraftment of donor lymphoid cells, however, rejection of the subsequent renal allografts should not be expected. The absence of rejection of the renal allografts does not represent "immunologic tolerance" as suggested by the title of this paper because the renal allograft and the chimeric immune system of the recipient originate from the same individual and thus are genetically identical. In the absence of ongoing GVHD, tolerance is presumed to exist between the chimeric donor-derived immune system and the transplant recipient. Studies in experimental animals have shown that the donor tolerance of the host can be broken by infusion of presensitized donor lymphocytes but not by normal donor lymphocytes (1). The transient GVHD observed in patient 1 (which was presumably mediated by passenger T cells, as suggested by the authors) suggests that chimeric tolerance may not have been fully established at the time of renal allografting. If it were possible to establish donor chimerism without first subjecting the patient to high-dose marrow ablative therapy to achieve sustained engraftment of donor cells, this form of cellular engineering would be a very attractive approach to inducing donor-specific tolerance before solid organ allografting. Unfortunately, reliable methods do not exist for establishing split chimerism on a permanent basis.—J.A. Hansen, M.D.

Reference

1. Weiden PL, et al: *J Immunol* 116:1212, 1976.

Interstitial Pneumonitis Associated With Human Herpesvirus-6 Infection After Marrow Transplantation
Carrigan DR, Drobyski WR, Russler SK, Tapper MA, Knox KK, Ash RC (Med College of Wisconsin, Milwaukee)
Lancet 338:147–149, 1991   24–3

Objective.—Two adult marrow transplant recipients contracted human herpesvirus-6 (HHV-6) lung infections. Both patients were HHV-6 seropositive before transplantation, and pneumonitis developed within a few weeks of marrow transplantation.

Findings.—Histologic demonstration of virally infected cells in lung tissue, immunohistochemical staining, or in situ hybridization is considered diagnostic of invasive virus-associated lung disease. In patient 1, HHV-6 was isolated from blood and marrow; no other respiratory pathogen was isolated at any time, and large numbers of HHV-6 were observed at autopsy. A lung biopsy specimen from patient 2 contained many HHV-6–infected cells; there were no other respiratory pathogens, and there was repeated isolation of HHV-6 from sputum and bronchoalveolar lavage samples. In both patients' lung tissue, HHV-6 appeared preferentially to infected macrophages and lymphocytes.

Conclusions.—Human herpesvirus-6–infected cells, primarily intra-alveolar macrophages, were found in lung tissue from 2 marrow transplant recipients who had severe pneumonitis. This organism is a potential cause of unexplained lung disease in immunocompromised patients.

▶ Human herpesvirus-6 has only recently been associated with disease (1, 2). Although little is known at this time about the epidemiology or clinical response to therapy, the availability of diagnostic reagents and documentation that this agent can be a cause of infection and pneumonia in immunocompromised patients should provide impetus for new and informative studies.—J.A. Hansen, M.D.

References

1. Huang LM, et al: *Lancet* 336:60, 1990.
2. Asano Y, et al: *Lancet* 335:862, 1990.

Presentation of Human Minor Histocompatibility Antigens by HLA-B35 and HLA-B38 Molecules
Yamamoto J, Kariyone A, Akiyama N, Kano K, Takiguchi M (University of Tokyo, Japan)
Proc Natl Acad Sci USA 87:2583–2587, 1990   24–4

Introduction.—Graft rejection and graft-vs.-host reaction in bone marrow transplantation between HLA-identical siblings may be the result of disparity of human minor histocompatibility antigens (hmHAs). Establishment of hmHA-specific cytotoxic T lymphocyte (CTL) clones and delineation of their specificities and restriction elements is crucial for the study of hmHA.

Methods.—Clones of hmHA-specific CTL with respectable and reproducible lytic activities were generated from a patient who had multiple renal grafts from his mother and 2 HLA-identical sisters.

Results.—Studies of the lytic activities of 8 CTL clones against target cells from family members demonstrated recognition of 3 distinct hmHA specificities and killing patterns. Five amino acid substitutions on the α_1 domain between HLA-B35 and HLA-Bw53 had a critical role in the relationship of hmHA-1 to HLA-B35 molecules. It was also found that 8 amino acid substitutions on the α_2 domain can affect the recognition of hmHA-1 by the HLA-B35–restricted CTL clones.

▶ This report adds additional data demonstrating that immune T cells are capable of recognizing certain polymorphic non-HLA minor histocompatibility antigens, and these reactions appear to be the in vitro corollary to the alloimmune response to transplanted tissue. T cell recognition, however, depends on the presentation of peptide fragments by class I and class II HLA molecules. Specific peptides appear to be presented by only certain HLA molecules; thus, the response of an individual may be determined not only by the repertoire of the T cell-receptor gene but also by the HLA alleles present on grafted tissue. The practical significance of this is unclear and depends on the number of cellular proteins that can function as minor histocompatibility antigens and the extent of their polymorphism. There is almost no information concerning the potential number of minor histocompatibility antigens. It may be possible to type for these only when the human genome has been fully defined and oligonucleotide probes for identifying functionally relevant polymorphisms are available. Ultimately, matching may not be feasible for logistic reasons, or new methods for inducing tolerance may abrogate the necessity of matching for minor histocompatibility antigens. Nevertheless, studies such as this are very important for elucidating the basic elements of the alloimmune response.—J.A. Hansen, M.D.

Immunomodulatory and Antimicrobial Efficacy of Intravenous Immuno-globulin in Bone Marrow Transplantation
Sullivan KM, Kopecky KJ, Jacom J, Fisher L, Buckner CD, Meyers JD, Counts GW, Bowden RA, Petersen FB, Witherspoon RP, Budinger MD, Schwartz RS, Appelbaum FR, Clift RA, Hansen JA, Sanders JE, Thomas ED, Storb R (Fred Hutchinson Cancer Research Ctr, Seattle; Univ of Washington, Seattle; Miles Inc, Berkeley, Calif)
N Engl J Med 323:705–712, 1990   24–5

Background.—Two major complications of allogeneic bone marrow transplantation are graft-vs.-host disease (GVHD) and infection. Because intravenous immunoglobulin has been shown to be beneficial in several immunodeficiency and autoimmune disorders, its antimicrobial and immunomodulatory roles after marrow transplantation were studied.

Methods.—Three hundred eighty-two patients were enrolled in the randomized trial. Transplant recipients given immunoglobulin were compared with control subjects who were not.

Findings.—Control patients who were seronegative for cytomegalovirus and received seronegative blood products remained seronegative. However, seronegative patients who received immunoglobulin and screened blood had a passive transfer of cytomegalovirus antibody. None of the 61 evaluable seronegative patients contracted interstitial pneumonia. Among the 308 seropositive patients evaluated, 22% of control subjects and 13% of immunoglobulin recipients had this complication (p = .021). Control patients had an increased risk of gram-negative septicemia and local infection (rr = 2.65; p = .0039). They received 51 more units of platelets than did the immunoglobulin recipients. Immunoglobulin did not change survival or the risk of relapse. Patients aged 20 years and older, however, had a reduction in the incidence of acute GVHD and in deaths from transplant-related causes after transplantation of HLA-identical marrow.

Conclusions.—Passive immunotherapy with intravenous immunoglobulin can reduce the risk of acute GVHD, gram-negative septicemia and interstitial pneumonia in CMV seropositive patients after bone marrow transplantation. However, survival and risk of relapse was not affected by immunoglobulin therapy in this study.

▶ The results of this randomized study of intravenous immunoglobulin therapy supports the importance and usefulness of adoptive immunotherapy in marrow transplant patients and suggests that diminished B cell function may contribute to the increased risk of bacterial and viral infection observed during the first 100 days after transplantation. The mechanism by which immunoglobulin therapy may ameliorate GVHD, however, is not clear. The observation that control patients had a higher incidence of clinically significant GVHD compared to treated patients is consistent with the hypothesis that infection may potentiate GVHD by inducing cytokines that nonspecifically activate the immune system and mediate inflammation. Although the findings in this study were significant, the degree of improvement overall may be minimal. Optimal cost effectiveness will require more careful definition of patients and clinical situations where the relative advantage of immunoglobulin therapy will be greatest.—J.A. Hansen, M.D.

Cyclosporine-Associated Seizures in Bone Marrow Transplant Recipients Given Busulfan and Cyclophosphamide Preparative Therapy
Ghany AM, Tutschka PJ, McGhee RB Jr, Avalos BR, Cunningham I, Kapoor N, Copelan EA (Ohio State Univ, Columbus)
Transplantation 52:310–315, 1991   24–6

Introduction.—Cyclosporine A (CsA) is effective in preventing acute graft-vs.-host disease (GVHD) but neurologic side effects, including seizures, have been reported with its use. Contributing factors implicated in CsA-associated seizures include high CsA blood levels, hypomagnesemia, concurrent treatment with high-dose corticosteroids, hemolytic-uremic syndrome, hypertension, hypocholesterolemia and total-body irradiation. Seizures developed in 5 of 182 recipients of allogeneic bone marrow transplants while receiving CsA after a radiation-free preparative regimen consisting of busulfan and cyclosphosphamide.

Patients.—Seizures developed in 2 patients who received HLA-mismatched allografts and 3 who received marrow from HLA-identical sibling donors while receiving standard doses of CsA and methylprednisolone to prevent acute GVHD. Preparative therapy for all patients was a radiation-free regimen of busulfan and cyclophosphamide.

Results.—Cranial MRI and CT showed bilateral abnormalities primarily in the posterior temporal, occipital, and parietal lobes. Sequential MRI scans in 2 patients revealed these abnormalities as transient. Both seizures and radiologic abnormalities resolved when CsA was stopped and 2 patients who resumed CsA at lower doses have no recurrences.

Conclusion.—The cause of CsA-associated seizures is multifactorial. The findings in these patients demonstrated CsA-associated seizures with radiation-free as well as radiation-containing preparative regimens. Treatment with CsA should be withheld and antiseizure medications should be started at the onset of seizures. Resumption of CsA during MRI examination is recommended.

▶ Seizures and significant central nervous system pathology occur in marrow transplant patients for a number of reasons. The differential diagnosis and likely mechanisms of cyclosporine-associated seizures are thoroughly discussed by Ghany et al. The manifestation of cyclosporine toxicity is highly variable, especially as it affects the central nervous system. Renal and hepatic dysfunction, and alternations in drug metabolism can have profound metabolic effects on the central nervous system further complicating the identification of the primary and contributing agents responsible. Nevertheless, it is clear from this and similar reports that cyclosporine has to be considered whenever these complications occur.—J.A. Hansen, M.D.

Chronic Cyclosporine-Associated Nephrotoxicity in Bone Marrow Transplant Patients

Dieterle A, Gratwohl A, Nizze H, Huser B, Mihatsch MJ, Thiel G, Tichelli A, Signer E, Nissen C, Speck B (Children's Hospital, Basel, Switzerland; Wilhelm Pick University, Rostock, Germany)
Transplantation 49:1093–1100, 1990   24–7

Introduction.—Cyclosporine (CsA) is gaining acceptance as an immunosuppressive agent in organ transplantation although it can cause severe nephrotoxicity and other side effects. The prevalence and degree of chronic cyclosporine associated nephropathy and accompanying risk factors were investigated in renal histology samples from 169 bone marrow transplantation (BMT) patients.

Methods.—Patients who received a BMT between July 13, 1979, and the end of 1987 were included in the study. A total of 51 renal histology specimens were obtained from 49 patients (25 female, 24 male) by biopsy (12 samples) or autopsy (39 samples). Group A patients included those with impaired renal function or lethal outcome. In group B the patients were considered long-term survivors without histology samples being available, and this group included 72 patients who survived for more than 1 year after BMT. Eight of the 72 had 1 biopsy and were included in group A. Thirty-five of the remaining 64 patients (30 female, 34 male) (55%) took CsA for more than 12 months. At the end of the study period, 59 of these patients (92%) had not taken CsA for a median of 32 months.

Findings.—Overall, the mean CsA dose was 6.5 mg/kg/day at 3 months and 5 mg/kg/day at 6 months. The serum level of creatinine was within normal limits before receipt of CsA in all patients. After 90 days of CsA therapy mean serum level of creatinine declined, and it stabilized after 6 months. Thirty-seven patients had creatinine values above the normal limit. No correlation was found between serum cholesterol levels and histopathologic lesions in the samples. Slight or moderate glomerular changes were observed in 9 patients, but severe tubular atrophy and fibrosis were never found. The degree of CsA arteriolopathy, striped interstitial fibrosis, tubular atrophy, and glomerular obsolescence increased over time in a significant manner. Patients with histologic changes of CsA nephrotoxicity at 3 months demonstrated a significantly higher serum level of creatinine at day 14 than patients without these changes. The mean CsA dose at day 14 was significantly lower in persons with histologic changes. Despite similar doses of CsA in groups A and B, increases in serum level of creatinine were significantly higher in group A.

Conclusions.—Irreversible CsA-associated alterations in renal tissue do occur in many patients with BMT. The major risk factor for this nephropathy is the duration of CsA therapy, followed by additional sources of kidney damage, such as irradiation. Because CsA-associated renal changes increase over time, patients with BMT should be continuously monitored for renal function even if they have normal serum levels of creatinine.

▶ This study demonstrates that significant irreversible lesions in renal tissue occur in some marrow transplant patients receiving cyclosporine. The major risk factor appeared to be the duration of cyclosporine therapy; however, the authors reported that in their patient population prior radiation therapy may have predisposed to renal damage. It remains unclear, however, that cyclosporine is the primary cause of these renal lesions or whether other variables such as persistent graft-vs.-host disease and infection may contribute. Nevertheless, this study illustrates the need for improved methods for assessing renal function and it reinforces the importance of developing better methods for GVHD prophylaxis and treatment, thereby sparing patients from prolonged cyclosporine therapy.—J.A. Hansen, M.D.

Evidence that Oral Pentoxifylline Reverses Acute Renal Dysfunction in Bone Marrow Transplant Recipients Receiving Amphotericin B and Cyclosporine: Results of a Pilot Study

Bianco JA, Almgren J, Kern DL, Ballard B, Roark K, Andrews F, Nemunaitis J, Shields T, Singer JW (VA Med Ctr; Fred Hutchinson Cancer Research Ctr; Univ of Washington, Seattle)

Transplantation 51:925–927, 1991   24–8

Introduction.—Renal functional impairment is a significant complication of bone marrow transplantation, with 24% of all patients requiring dialysis during the early posttransplant period. The use of amphotericin B is a most significant risk, and combined with cyclosporine A therapy, incidences of acute renal toxicity as high as 80% have been demonstrated. The use of pentoxifylline to reverse nephrotoxicity in marrow transplant recipients was evaluated.

Methods.—Renal insufficiency developed in 5 allograft recipients while receiving amphotericin B and cyclosporine A. Pentoxifylline was administered orally for 2 weeks or longer after discontinuing treatment with amphotericin B. The control group consisted of 10 consecutive disease-, regimen-, and age-matched patients who were not required to have renal insufficiency to be included in the group. Within 4–5 days of starting amphotericin B therapy, renal dysfunction developed in 90% of the control patients. These patients received the standard supportive therapy for renal insufficiency without pentoxifylline.

Results.—Renal insufficiency resolved significantly sooner in patients treated with pentoxifylline than in the control patients. Additionally, no dose reductions for cyclosporine A were required in the treated group, whereas cyclosporine A had to be significantly reduced because of renal dysfunction in the control group.

Conclusion.—Posttransplant patients must receive adequate immunosuppression, such as that achieved with adequate doses of cyclosporine A. The use of pentoxifylline allows the continued use of cyclosporine A in recommended dosages, thus protecting the allograft patient from graft-vs.-host disease. Future studies may indicate successful prophylactic use of pentoxifylline for preserving renal function in these patients and preventing other posttransplant complications.

▶ These are exciting preliminary results and, if confirmed, could represent substantial potential benefit not only to marrow transplant patients, but to other transplant patients receiving potentially nephrotoxic drugs and to cancer patients receiving chemotherapy. The mechanisms by which pentoxifylline may protect renal function is not fully known, but it has been reported to increase production of vasodilator prostaglandins (1) and block the synthesis of tumor necrosis factor alpha (TNFα) (2), a cytokine that mediates expression of adhesion molecules on leukocytes and endothelial cells, and local inflammatory reactions.—J.A. Hansen, M.D.

References

1. Fahr A, Langer R, Ziegoleit S: *Biomed Bioclin Acta* 14:29, 1988.
2. Streiter RM et al: *Biochem Biophys Res Commun* 155:1230, 1988.

Variation in Blood Component Irradiation Practice: Implications for Prevention of Transfusion-Associated Graft-Versus-Host Disease
Anderson KC, Goodnough LT, Sayers M, Pisciotto PT, Kurtz SR, Lane TA, Anderson CS, Silberstein LE (Harvard Med School, Boston; Case Western Reserve Univ, Cleveland; Univ of Washington, Seattle; Univ of Connecticut, Hartford; Lahey Clinic, Burlington, Mass)
Blood 77:2096–2102, 1991   24–9

Introduction.—Transfusion-associated graft-vs.-host disease (TA-GVHD) is a serious yet rarely reported, complication of transfusion. A national survey of transfusion in medical practice was undertaken to identify patients at risk for TA-GVHD and to evaluate methods for its prevention.

Methods.—A survey completed by 2,250 blood centers, hospital blood banks, and transfusion services provided data regarding the number of blood components transfused and the number of blood components irradiated in 1989. Questions also addressed the dose of irradiation used and the patient groups receiving irradiated products.

Results.—Only 10.1% of blood components transfused in 1989 were irradiated. Doses of gamma irradiation ranged from 15 to 50 Gy. Cellular products alone were irradiated by 80.8% of the institutions performing irradiation; 19.2% irradiated both cellular and acellular products. Most institutions provided irradiated components for recipients of allogeneic bone marrow transplants (BMT) (88%), recipients of autologous BMT (81.4%), and patients with congenital immunodeficiency syndromes (68.4%). Although a majority (88.9%) of institutions irradiate directed donations from first degree family members, most (90%) do not irradiate directed donations from nonblood relatives. Documented cases of TA-GVHD reported by the institutions were most common in patients with Hodgkin's disease (11 cases) and after allogeneic BMT (12 cases).

Conclusion.—Patients with profound congenital or acquired immune dysfunction that predisposes them to GVHD should receive only irradiated blood components, but this practice is not universally followed. Neither term newborns nor all patients with hematologic malignancies or tumors of solid organs routinely require irradiation. Because the cost of irradiation facilities is high, a regional approach to this service is recommended.

▶ The transfusion of blood and blood products containing immunocompetent T cells can lead to fatal GVHD in immunodeficient patients. Despite multiple case reports clearly demonstrating evidence of engraftment and the severe tragic consequences of transfusion-associated GVHD, the radiation of blood products for transfusion recipients at risk of GVHD is not universally practiced.—J.A. Hansen, M.D.

25 Immune Reconstitution and Long-Term Follow-Up

Reconstitution of Antibody Response After Allogeneic Bone Marrow Transplantation: Effect of Lymphocyte Depletion by Counterflow Centrifugal Elutriation on the Expression of Hemagglutinins
Bär BMAM, Santos GW, Donnenberg AD (Johns Hopkins School of Medicine)
Blood 76:1410–1418, 1990   25–1

Background.—Counterflow centrifugal elutriation (CCE) is an efficient and safe means of removing lymphocytes from bone marrow allografts and thereby preventing acute graft-vs.-host disease. Studies of how hemagglutinins are expressed in recipients of CCE and non-CCE–processed marrow are a simple and biologically meaningful way of prospectively assessing the development of T- and B-lymphocyte–dependent immunity.

Study Plan.—Generation of ABO hemagglutinins was examined in 29 recipients of elutriated HLA-matched marrow allografts, and in 40 other patients given non-elutriated allografts. A major ABO mismatch was present in 11 of the former recipients and in 16 of the latter.

Findings.—Removal of graft lymphocytes by CCE did not prolong the presence of host-derived hemagglutinins in recipients of major ABO-mismatched grafts. In recipients of minor ABO-mismatched grafts, however, counterflow centrifugal elutriation totally abrogated the adoptive transfer of donor-derived antibody. The recipients nevertheless had hemagglutinin levels comparable to those in patients given nonelutriated grafts within 6 months of transplantation.

Interpretation.—Recipients of nonelutriated grafts received adoptively transferred memory B cells capable of secreting donor-derived hemagglutinin. Recipients of elutriated grafts, in contrast, do not have donor-derived antibody early after transplantation, but their responses are generated de novo. The transfer and later loss of donor antirecipient antibody in patients given unaltered grafts strongly suggests the induction of tolerance.

▶ An unmodified marrow graft contains both stem cells and mature lymphocytes capable of transferring specific antibody-secreting donor B cells. As these passively transferred cells go through senescence, and tolerance to host devel-

311

ops, antibodies reactive with the host are lost. Elutriation (CCE) removes mature lymphoid cells and thereby prevents the passive transfer of immune cells. In the case of a minor ABO mismatch, CCE grafts do not contain the cells capable of secreting antihost hemagglutinins, and these "autoimmune" responses do not occur de novo when stem cells have undergone B cell differentiation, selection, and maturation within the host.—J.A. Hansen, M.D.

B-Cell Differentiation Following Autologous, Conventional, or T-Cell Depleted Bone Marrow Transplantation: A Recapitulation of Normal B-Cell Ontogeny

Small TN, Keever CA, Weiner-Fedus S, Heller G, O'Reilly RJ, Flomenberg N (Mem Sloan Kettering Cancer Ctr, New York)
Blood 76:1647–1656, 1990

25–2

Background.—Humoral immune deficiency after bone marrow transplant (BMT) is thought to be caused by T cell suppression and an intrinsic B cell defect. The condition is exacerbated by graft-vs.-host disease (GVHD). Recently an increase has been reported in circulating CD1c (M241), CD38 (OKT10), CD5 (Leu-1), CD23 (PL13) positive B cells in untreated children who have severe combined immunodeficiency disease (SCID), in cord blood, and even in healthy young children. After undergoing T cell depleted bone marrow transplantation (BMT), sIg positive cells of consecutive patients were analyzed serially for surface antigen expression and function and compared with those seen in normal children.

Methods.—Study patients included 88 children who had had autologous, conventional, or T cell-depleted BMT. Twenty-nine patients with a median age of 12.3 years received a conventional transplant for acute lymphoblastic (ALL) or acute myelogenous leukemia (AML). Forty-four patients with a median age of 24.3 years received a T cell depleted transplant for chronic myelogenous leukemia (CML) or ALL or AML. Eight patients with a median age of 4 years underwent an autologous transplant for neuroblastoma, and 7 patients with a median age of 11.5 years had the same procedure for AML.

Results.—Serial phenotype analyses of the circulating lymphocytes in the 88 patients demonstrated that after transplantation the number of CD20$^+$ B cells increased quickly 3 months posttransplant. After 3 months most patients (except those with chronic GVHD) had the normal or higher number of circulating B cells. Some 85% of the patients with chronic GVHD who had less than normal circulating B cells had had conventional transplantations. The circulating CD20$^+$ cells expressed HLA-DR, CD19 (B4), CD21, (B2), sig, TQ1, Leu-8, but not CD10 (CALLA) after BMT. Most of the circulating B cells were CD1c, CD38, and CD23 positive during the first 6–12 months after transplantation, but the expression of these antigens decreased during the second year. Older normal children (at least age 2 years) and healthy adults also exhibit similar antigen expression. Significant IgG production did not begin until the second year after transplantation.

Implications.—The B cells in the early posttransplant months share a number of phenotypic and functional characteristics with B cells found in cord blood. The CD1c, CD5, CD38, and CD23 positive B cells evolve into minor subsets of cells as a patient acquired humoral immune competence.

▶ The entire immune system including B lymphocytes will be reconstituted with cells and immunoglobulins of donor origin after marrow ablative chemoradiotherapy and transplantation of allogeneic hematopoietic stem cells (1). Small et al. demonstrate that B-cell reconstitution after transplantation requires approximately 1 year to normalize. Cell surface phenotype and switching from IgM to IgG secretion appears to follow a course of differentiation similar to that seen in newborns. This recapitulation of B cell ontogeny suggests that posttransplant recovery depends on a clonal evolution that presumably is driven by specific antigens. B-cell recovery is further delayed in patients with chronic GVHD. These results provide further rationale for immunoglobulin replacement therapy, especially in patients with chronic GVHD. Furthermore, the immature B cell phenotype and deficiency of IgG secretion in vitro provides a means for identifying patients at increased risk of infection.—J.A. Hansen, M.D.

Reference

1. Witherspoon RP, et al: *Transplantation* 26:407, 1978.

Development of IgA Deficiency After Bone Marrow Transplantation: The Influence of Acute and Chronic Graft-Versus-Host Disease
Abedi MR, Hammarström L, Ringdén O, Smith CIE (Karolinska Institute, Huddinge; Stockholm University, Sweden)
Transplantation 50:415–421, 1990   25–3

Introduction.—Bone marrow transplantation (BMT) has become an acceptable therapy for immunodeficiency disorders, hematologic malignancies, and aplastic anemia. Depression of humoral function and of the immune system in patients undergoing BMT, however, appears to correlate with the severity of potential graft-vs.-host disease (GVHD). The temporal course of serum IgA levels during the initial 2 years after BMT was examined in 134 patients given T-cell–depleted bone marrow.

Methods.—The series included 131 allogeneic and 3 syngeneic BMT recipients (49 females and 85 males) who had survived for more than 6 months after transplantation. Bone marrow donors were 122 HLA-identical, mixed lymphocyte culture-nonreactive sibling donors and 9 HLA partially compatible family members, whose median age was 22 years. Patients received varying doses of cyclophosphamide before BMT. Prophylaxis for GVHD included methotrexate (43 patients), cyclosporine A (31 patients), both drugs (41 patients), and T-cell–depleted bone marrow with anti-CD8 and anti-CD12 antibodies (14 patients).

Findings.—When all 134 patients were considered, the mean serum IgA level at 3 months after the BMT was low and equal to that obtained

6 months after surgery. The mean serum IgA level was significantly increased at 1 year when compared to the levels observed at 3 months and 6 months after BMT. A small but significant difference in serum levels was found when comparing patients younger than 15 years and 15 years of age or older. Patients receiving either methotrexate or cyclosporine A had significantly lower IgA concentrations during the first 2 years after BMT compared to patients receiving a combination of both drugs. Those given T-cell–depleted bone marrow had significantly higher IgA levels up to 1 year after BMT. Low serum IgA concentrations were linked to the severity of acute GVHD, whereas patients with chronic GVHD had significantly lower mean IgA levels at 1 year and 2 years posttransplantation. Of 21 patients (16% of the total) whose IgA levels were no more than .1 g/L 1 year or more after BMT, 16 had acute GVHD of grades I to III, and in 14 patients chronic GVHD developed. Four of 5 patients with no GVHD had cytomegalovirus infection after transplantation.

Conclusions.—Acute GVHD emerged as the most important factor for the development of IgA deficiency after BMT in this study. Monitoring serum IgA concentrations may be a sensitive means of detecting impairment of the immune system in patients who have undergone BMT.

▶ Immunodeficiency is a constant feature of the postmarrow transplant convalescence in both autografts and allografts (1–3). This presumably occurs because the high-dose marrow ablative chemotherapy or chemoradiotherapy administered before transplantation destroys the mature lymphoid system, and a significant amount of time is required to regenerate a normal T and B cell clonal repertoire and to fully reconstitute specific primary and secondary immune responses. Posttransplant immune deficiency is greater in allografts, and the severity and duration of immune deficiency correlates with the severity of acute and chronic GVHD. The current study shows that serum IgA levels remained low the first 6 months, but did not completely normalize for 1–2 years. The most important risk factor was severe acute GVHD followed by persistent chronic GVHD. Cytomegalovirus infection was also a significant but independent risk factor.—J.A. Hansen, M.D.

References

1. Halterman RH, et al: *Transplantation* 14:689, 1972.
2. Fass L, et al: *Transplantation* 16:630, 1973.
3. Witherspoon RP, Lum Storb R: *Semin Hematol* 21:2, 1984.

Response to Immunization Against Polio After Allogeneic Marrow Transplantation
Ljungman P, Duraj V, Magnius L (Huddinge Hospital, Huddinge, Sweden; National Bacteriological Laboratory, Stockholm)
Bone Marrow Transplant 7:89–93, 1991

25–4

Background.—The immune system reconstitutes gradually after bone marrow transplantation (BMT). A high proportion of allogeneic BMT recipients apparently lose their preexisting immunity to measles, mumps, and rubella.

Study Design.—The long-term immunity of BMT recipients to polioviruses and the immunization response to inactivated poliovirus vaccine (IPV) were investigated in 55 patients. Neutralization assays were used to determine antibodies. The patients were examined before BMT, 12 months after BMT, and 12 months after immunization.

Findings.—At 12 months after BMT, 37 patients were seropositive to all poliovirus types. Between BMT and 12 months later there was at least a fourfold reduction in antibody level in 55% of the patients to poliovirus type 1, in 41% to type 2, and in 45% to type 3. One dose of trivalent IPV was used to immunize 19 patients. Response with at least a fourfold antibody titer increase to poliovirus type 1, 2, and 3 occurred in 42%, 36%, and 21% of these immunized patients, respectively. Among 29 patients primarily immunized with 3 IPV doses, the response rates were 52%, 48%, and 48% of poliovirus types 1, 2, and 3, respectively. Patients who did or did not have chronic graft vs. host disease had similar responses to immunization.

Conclusions.—A poliovirus reimmunization program is needed for long-term survivors of allogeneic BMT. Three doses of IPV are necessary to obtain protective immunity in most BMT recipients.

▶ As described by Bär et al. (Abstract 25–1), a significant passive transfer of donor-derived humoral immunity occurs after marrow transplantation. The data presented by Ljungman et al., however, emphasizes the marginal nature and limited duration of transferred immunity. The majority of the patients included in this study (49 of 55) received an unmodified marrow graft (non-T cell–depleted) from an HLA-matched donor. Three doses of IPV were required to achieve an adequate immunization response; however, 4 patients failed to respond at all to the 3 immunizations. As T cell-depletion of donor marrow and especially purified stem cell grafts become more prevalent, the number of mature donor-derived immune cells passively transferred during transplantation will decrease. Lacking this passive immunity, the duration of immune deficiency and risk of infection may be prolonged. Active immunizations as proposed here, and administered as soon as they are safe and effective, will be very important.—J.A. Hansen, M.D.

Reconstitution of T-Cell Function After CD6-Depleted Allogeneic Bone Marrow Transplantation
Soiffer RJ, Bosserman L, Murray C, Cochran K, Daley J, Ritz J (Dana-Farber Cancer Inst, Boston; Harvard Med School)
Blood 75:2076–2084, 1990   25–5

Introduction.—Patients with chronic myelogenous leukemia (CML) and other infections after bone marrow transplantation (BMT) appear to have a greater chance for BMT failure. Previous in vitro research indicates that T-cell abnormalities may occur after engraftment in BMT patients, and lymphocyte subsets may recur over time after transplantation. A proliferation assay analysis of intracellular calcium levels and surface expression of the interleukin-2 (IL-2) receptor was done in a series of BMT patients who received HLA-compatible sibling marrow grafts after removal of T cells with anti-CD6 monoclonal antibody and complement.

Methods.—Forty patients aged 18 to 55 were included in the study: 15 had acute myelogenous leukemia (AML), 8 had acute lymphocytic leukemia (ALL), 13 had CML, and 4 had other hematologic malignancies. Before infusion, the donor bone marrow underwent treatment with T12 monoclonal antibody (CD6) and rabbit complement. Analyses included phenotypic testing, proliferation studies, IL-2 receptor expression measurement, and intracellular calcium flux measurement.

Findings.—The number of T lymphocytes steadily increased so that these cells predominated 5 to 6 weeks after BMT. By 10 weeks post-BMT, T-cell levels were nearly normal. Overall T-cell composition, however, was abnormal for more than 2 years. For example, the T4:T8 ratio was found to be well under 1.0 for the first 24 months and was continuously inverted in half the patients. Late, CD3$^+$ and CD5$^+$ T cells began to predominate. A significant portion of the CD3$^+$ T cells do not coexpress CD6 after 2 years. The ability of unstimulated peripheral blood mononuclear cells to respond to recombinant IL-2 remained. The induction of IL-2 receptor (p55) in vitro recovered by 6 months after BMT. Stimulation with CD2 did not affect calcium flux in T cells right after engraftment. Yet, anti-CD3 antibody stimulation of T cells caused these cells not to develop intracellular calcium flux as compared to control cells.

Conclusions.—Although T lymphocytes recover to normal levels early after engraftment of CD6-depleted bone marrow, these T cells demonstrate several physiologic and functional problems that persist for various periods after BMT.

▶ Although successful T cell-depletion of donor marrow for transplantation from HLA-identical siblings spares the recipient the need for posttransplant immunosuppressive therapy and prevents clinically severe acute and chronic GVHD; T cell function remains abnormal for 12 to 18 months or longer. The defects described are relatively subtle, however, they underscore the complex nature of posttransplant immune reconstitution. Given the known risk of late infections, the importance of the GVL effect and the occurrence of secondary malignancies, posttransplant immune function remains a critical area of investigation.—J.A. Hansen, M.D.

Clonal Analysis of T-Cell Deficiencies in Autotransplant Recipients
Miller RA, Daley J, Ghalie R, Kaizer H (Boston Univ; Rush Univ, Chicago)
Blood 77:1845–1850, 1991   25–6

Introduction.—Poor immune function after bone marrow transplantation may be partially attributable to graft-vs.-host disease.

Methods.—Limiting dilution culture methods were used to determine the frequency of mitogen-responsive T cells in peripheral blood of patients after bone marrow autotransplantation, and their responses were compared with those of allotransplant recipients and normal controls. The 26 autologous transplant patients received cryopreserved marrow, and the 20 allogeneic recipients were given marrow from sibling donors.

Results.—Clone counting limiting dilution assays showed autotransplant patients to be more severely retarded than allorecipients in recovery of functional T cells. Autotransplant patients had lower responder-cell frequencies in tests for lymphokine-secreting helper function and for interleukin-2-dependent proliferator and cytotoxic function. Multiple regression analysis showed function to be lower in autotransplant patients than in allorecipients and lower in male patients for all 3 functional assays. Graft vs. host disease was associated with lower T-cell function only in the allotransplant group.

Conclusion.—More severe deficits of T-cell regeneration were observed in autotransplant patients than in allorecipients. Cellular immunodeficiency after bone marrow transplantation may reflect limitations in thymic-dependent repopulation rather than an effect of genetic disparity between host and donor.

▶ The findings that T cell precursor frequencies as measured by limiting dilution assays (LDA) were more severely impaired in marrow autotransplant patients compared to allotransplant patients was remarkable and unexpected. These investigators have previously used LDA to analyze immunodeficiency in marrow allograft recipients (1). They have also shown that increasing the number of donor T cells administered to marrow-allografted mice increased the severity of GVHD, and that the latter correlated with a decrease in the precursor frequencies of helper and cytotoxic T cells (2). Clearly GVHD does not contribute to the immune deficiency observed in autotransplants. Thus, there must be at least 2 or more distinct causes of posttransplant immunodeficiency. One is GVHD, which occurs only in allografts, and there must be host factors contributing to the prolonged immunodeficiency, including the patient's age or injury to host tissues (especially the thymus) induced by chemotherapy or radiation. Another factor is the intrinsic time dependency of T cell-immune reconstitution. The more marked severity seen in autografts may also suggest that the stem cells present in autografts may not have the same functional capacity as stem cells from normal donors.—J.A. Hansen, M.D.

318 / Transplantation

References

1. Rozans MK, et al: *J Immunol* 136:4040, 1986.
2. Ferrara JLM, et al: *J Immunol* 138:3598, 1987.

Chronic Graft-Versus-Host Disease and Other Late Complications of Bone Marrow Transplantation
Sullivan KM, Agura E, Anasetti F, Appelbaum F, Badger C, Bearman S, Erickson K, Flowers M, Hansen J, Loughran T, Martin P, Matthews D, Petersdorf E, Radich J, Riddell S, Rovira D, Sanders J, Schuening F, Siadak M, Storb R, Witherspoon RP (Fred Hutchinson Cancer Research Ctr; Univ of Washington, Seattle)
Semin Hematol 28:250–259, 1991   25–7

Introduction.—Complications after allogeneic bone marrow transplantation were reviewed.

Results.—Chronic graft-vs.-host disease (GVHD) is the major cause of late allogeneic bone marrow transplant-related morbidity (Fig 25–1). The incidence of chronic GVHD is significantly higher in patients who receive HLA-nonidentical marrow than in patients who receive HLA-identical marrow (Fig 25–2). Chronic GVHD also has a more rapid onset in the mismatched recipients. The probability of chronic GVHD increases with age (Fig 25–3). In patients with limited disease, the prognosis is favorable without therapy, but in those with multiorgan disease, chronic GVHD should be treated by immunosuppression. Resolution of dermal activity, as monitored by skin biopsy, correlates with a favorable outcome. Chronic GVHD has been associated with an antileukemic effect, which can contribute to disease-free survival. Impaired immunologic functioning is common for the first few months after allogeneic marrow transplantation. Infections are common. Secondary malignancies can also occur after transplantation.

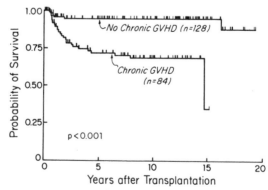

Fig 25–1.—Probability of survival in 212 patients with severe aplastic anemia who underwent transplant through August 1990 and survived at least 150 days after marrow transplantation from HLA-identical siblings. Patients were prepared for transplant with cyclophosphamide and were analyzed in relation to the presence or absence of clinical extensive chronic GVHD. In this and subsequent figures, probability estimates are determined by the Kaplan-Meier method, and significance tests are given as log rank *P* values. (Courtesy of Sullivan KM, Agura E, Anasetti F, et al: *Semin Hematol* 28:250–259, 1991.)

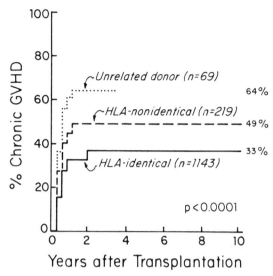

Fig 25–2.—Probability of developing clinical extensive chronic GVHD in patients with hematologic malignancies who underwent transplant through December, 1989 and survived at least 150 days after marrow transplantation from HLA-identical siblings, HLA-nonidentical family members, and unrelated marrow donors. HLA-nonidentical donor recipients significantly differed from HLA-identical (*P* < .0001) and unrelated marrow recipients (*P* = .0401). (Courtesy of Sullivan KM, Agura E, Anasetti F, et al: *Semin Hematol* 28:250–259, 1991.)

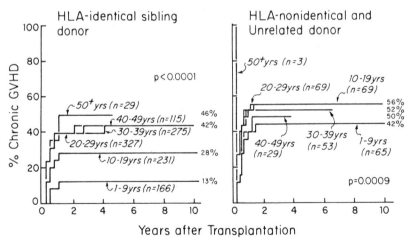

Fig 25–3.—Probability of developing clinical extensive chronic GVHD in patients with hematologic malignancies who underwent transplant through December, 1989 and survived at least 150 days after marrow transplantation from HLA-identical siblings *(left panel)* and HLA-nonidentical family members or unrelated donors *(right panel)*. Results are displayed in relation to patient age at the time of transplantation. (Courtesy of Sullivan KM, Agura E, Anasetti F, et al: *Semin Hematol* 28:250–259, 1991.)

Conclusion.—Chronic GVHD is the major determinant of late alloge-neic marrow transplant-related morbidity and mortality. Early diagnosis and treatment are important in preventing disability. For those transplant patients who are free of GVHD, a return to normal life is possible.

▶ This is a comprehensive but concise review of the late complications occurring in patients who have received marrow allografts from HLA-identical siblings, HLA partially matched relative, and HLA matched unrelated donors. Major emphasis is focused on the risk, diagnosis, treatment, and complications associated with chronic GVHD, but late complications of total body irradiation including neurological and endocrine abnormalities, secondary malignancies, and quality of life are also discussed. These are important issues that will receive increasing attention as larger numbers of patients become long-term marrow allograft survivors.—J.A. Hansen, M.D.

Health, Functional Status, and Employment of Adult Survivors of Bone Marrow Transplantation
Wingard JR, Curbow B, Baker F, Piantadosi S (Johns Hopkins Univ, Baltimore)
Ann Intern Med 114:113–118, 1991   25–8

Background.—Marrow transplantation is increasingly used to treat patients with bone marrow failure and lymphohematopoietic malignancies. The long-term outcome was assessed in 135 patients aged 18 or older at the time of marrow transplantation. The patients were followed for at least 6 months (mean, 47 months). The mean patient age was 31 years. The most frequent indications for transplantation were acute and chronic myelogenous leukemia, aplastic anemia, and acute lymphoblastic leukemia.

Outcome.—More than 90% of the patients were able to carry out normal activities without major physical problems. In general, perceived health and physical and social functioning were good to excellent. Some patients, however, were substantially impaired. One third had clinically significant illness, usually chronic graft-vs.-host disease. Half of the patients were working full-time at the time of evaluation, and another 14% were working part-time. Illness had in some way affected the work plans of 65% of the patients, and 10% reported substantial discrimination with regard to jobs.

Conclusions.—Most patients who survive bone marrow transplantation have generally good health and functional capacity. A large proportion of the patients in the present series were working or enrolled in school.

▶ As pointed out by these authors, more than 2,000 allogeneic and 1,500 autologous marrow transplants were being performed annually by 1988, and a total of more than 15,000 marrow transplants had been performed by the end of 1988. Thus there should be substantial impetus for evaluating the general health and quality of life of long-term marrow transplant survivors. One of the problems in doing so has been the cost and inconvenience of maintaining contact and performing adequate interviews, physical examination, and laboratory studies. Part of this problem can be addressed by using self-reports of health and functional ability as described above by Wingard et al. Fortunately, the results of these preliminary studies indicate that eventual rehabilitation after this intensive therapy is comparable to survivors given conventional less intensive cancer chemotherapy.—J.A. Hansen, M.D.

Increased Incidence of Solid Malignant Tumors After Bone Marrow Transplantation for Severe Aplastic Anemia
Socié G, Henry-Amar M, Cosset JM, Devergie A, Girinsky T, Gluckman E (Hôpital Saint-Louis, Paris; Institut Gustave Roussy, Villejuif, France)
Blood 78:277–279, 1991   25–9

Background.—Allogeneic marrow transplantation is increasingly practiced in patients with hematologic malignancy and nonmalignant hematologic disease. Because secondary neoplasia has been described after chemoradiotherapy, and tumors can develop after solid organ transplantation, human marrow recipients who receive high-dose chemotherapy and/or radiotherapy as well as postgraft immunosuppression may be at high risk for the development of a secondary malignancy.

Findings.—Marrow transplantation was performed after conditioning with cyclophosphamide and thoracoabdominal irradiation in 107 patients with nonconstitutional severe aplastic anemia and 40 with Fanconi's anemia. During a mean follow-up of about 5 years, a solid malignancy developed within the field of radiation in 4 patients. The median interval from marrow transplantation to tumor development was 7 years. No clinical correlates of tumor development were identified. The cumulative 8-year incidence rate was 22%.

Conclusion.—The possibility of a solid malignancy should be considered when following patients after marrow transplantation for severe anemia.

▶ Studies in canine radiation chimeras have demonstrated an increased incidence of tumors (1), and secondary malignancies have been reported in patients undergoing allogeneic marrow transplantation for the treatment of leukemia, severe aplastic anemia, or Fanconi's anemia (2–4). Major risk factors appear to be chronic GVHD, intensive immunosuppressive therapy, and systemic irradiation. The current study and one by Storb et al. (4) report a cumulative incidence of tumors in transplanted aplastic anemia patients of 22% and 6%, respectively. Together these data reveal a problem of great potential concern. Careful prospective surveillance of long-term marrow allograft survivors will be required to assess more accurately the occurrence of tumors and relevant risk factors.—J.A. Hansen, M.D.

References

1. Deeg HJ, et al: *Blood* 55:233, 1980.
2. Witherspoon RP, et al: *N Engl J Med* 321:784, 1989.
3. Lishner M, et al: *Cancer* 64:473, 1990.
4. Storb R, et al: Allogeneic marrow transplantation for aplastic anemia: Major issues, in Gale RP, Champlin RE (eds): *New Strategies in Bone Marrow Transplantation* New York, Wiley-Liss, 1991, p 73.

26 Marrow Transplantation for Patients With Nonmalignant and Genetic Diseases

▶ ↓ The overall results of these HLA-identical transplants for children with severe aplastic anemia (24 to 26 surviving between 21 months and nearly 10 years; median survival, 5¾ years) are very encouraging. A major factor in this success was the ability of methotrexate and cyclosporine to provide safe and effective GVHD prophylaxis.—J.A. Hansen, M.D.

Graft-Versus-Host Disease Prophylaxis With Methotrexate/Cyclosporine in Children With Severe Aplastic Anemia Treated With Cyclophosphamide and HLA-Identical Marrow Grafts
Storb R, Sanders JE, Pepe M, Anasetti C, Appelbaum FR, Buckner CD, Deeg HJ, Doney K, Hansen J, Martin P, Stewart P, Sullivan KM, Thomas ED, Witherspoon RP (Fred Hutchinson Cancer Research Ctr; Univ of Washington, Seattle)
Blood 78:1144–1149, 1991   26–1

Introduction.—In 26 children with aplastic anemia, marrow transplantation was performed with a regimen of methotrexate and cyclosporine (MTX/CSP) administered for graft-vs.-host disease (GVHD) prophylaxis. Before transplantation, all patients were conditioned with cyclophosphamide. In 22 patients there were genotypically HLA-identical sibling grafts and in 4 there were phenotypically HLA-identical parental grafts.

Methods.—Patients were administered MTX intravenously on days 1, 3, 6, and 11. Cyclosporine was administered on the day before grafting and was continued until day 50, when the dose was decreased and continued until 6 months after transplant.

Results.—The week after transplantation, 1 patient died, and 25 patients engrafted. Significant acute GVHD developed in 3 patients and chronic GVHD developed in 8. Seven patients rejected their grafts from days 51 to 408 after transplant, but 6 of the 7 were successfully retransplanted after conditioning with cyclophosphamide and antithymocyte globulin. Of 26 patients, 24 were still alive with successful grafts between 21 months and nearly 10 years later.

Conclusion.—The MTX/CSP regimen has been effective in preventing serious acute GVHD and has improved survival in pediatric marrow transplantation patients conditioned with cyclosporine. A conditioning program of cyclosporine and antithymocyte, which has been effective in conditioning patients for a second transplant, may be tried to prevent graft rejection.

Successful Allogeneic Bone Marrow Transplantation in a 6.5-Year-Old Male for Severe Aplastic Anemia Complicating Orthotopic Liver Transplantation for Fulminant Non-A–Non-B Hepatitis
Kawahara K, Storb R, Sanders J, Petersen FB (Fred Hutchinson Cancer Research Ctr, Seattle)
Blood 78:1140–1143, 1991   26–2

Introduction.—Non-A–non-B (NANB) hepatitis may occasionally result in fulminant hepatic necrosis. Cadaveric hepatic transplantation is the accepted treatment for fulminant hepatitis, but aplastic anemia has occurred in up to 28% of patients in some studies. Transplantation of HLA-identical marrow for severe aplastic anemia has produced survival rates of 75% to 90% in children and adults.

Case Report.—Boy, 6.5 years had a short history of abdominal pain and malaise. Hepatic coma developed rapidly and he received a cadaveric ABO incompatible orthoptic liver transplant. The coma subsided, but he was left with persistent cognitive deficits and a mental age of 24 months. The severe aplastic anemia that developed was treated with transfusions for 2 years. At that time, he was referred for marrow transplantation with his genotypically HLA-identical sister after conditioning with cyclophosphamide and antithymocyte. Occlusive disease of the liver or graft-vs.-host disease (GVHD) did not develop. Almost 2 years after marrow transplantation, the patient was alive without chronic active hepatitis or need for blood product therapy.

Conclusion.—In this patient, allogeneic marrow transplantation was well tolerated in a child with a cadaveric liver allograft. The patient experienced no organ rejection, GVHD, or regimen-related hepatotoxicity. After conditioning with cyclophosphamide, the use of multiple organ allografts from different donors appears feasible.

▶ Absence of acute or chronic GVHD and absence of hepatic dysfunction in this child marrow grafted from an HLA-identical sibling for treatment of severe aplastic anemia after orthotopic liver transplantation for fulminant non-A–non-B hepatitis suggests that immunologic tolerance of marrow donor-derived cells to both the recipient and cadaveric liver was established without any significant reactivity to host or the HLA-incompatible liver. The success of this case should encourage consideration of marrow transplantation for other similar patients who can be saved from hepatitis-induced liver failure by cadaveric liver transplantation but who subsequently develop severe aplastic anemia.—J.A. Hansen, M.D.

Bone Marrow Transplantation in Canine GM1 Gangliosidosis

O'Brien JS, Storb R, Raff RF, Harding J, Appelbaum F, Morimoto S, Kishimoto Y, Graham T, Ahern-Rindell A, O'Brien SL (Univ of California, San Diego; Fred Hutchinson Cancer Ctr, Seattle; Cutwater Kennels, Darien, Conn)

Clin Genet 38:274–280, 1990   26–3

Introduction.—The lysosomal storage disease GM1 gangliosidosis is transmitted as an autosomal trait and is caused by a deficiency of acid β-galactosidase in dogs, cats, cattle, and human beings. Bone marrow transplantation (BMT) has been suggested as treatment for human lysosomal-storage disease, but results in 1 study showed no benefit of BMT performed on a 3-month-old patient. Therapeutic early BMT with full engraftment was tested in canine GM1 gangliosidosis diagnosed at birth.

Methods.—Allogeneic BMT using a DLA-identical sibling as donor was performed on an 81-day-old Portuguese water dog with GM1 gangliosidosis. There was complete successful donor marrow engraftment. Beta-galactosidase activity in leukocytes of the transplanted dog was similar to that of the donor.

Results.—The transplanted dog showed neurologic deterioration similar to untreated dogs with GM1 gangliosidosis during the 2.5-month observation period. Examination after death showed cerebral ganglioside GM1 concentrations were not diminished and cerebral β-galactosidase activity was negligible.

Conclusion.—Early allogeneic BMT in canine GM1 gangliosidosis was ineffective in increasing brain acid β-galactosidase activity or slowing the neurologic deterioration.

▶ The use of hematopoietic stem cell containing marrow transplants from normal donors is being considered potential therapy for an increasing number of genetic deficiency diseases. This study illustrates the value of an experimental animal model in determining the potential use of marrow transplantation for reversing the effects of a specific lysosomal storage disease resulting from an abnormality of acid β-galactosidase. In this case, donor and recipient were major histocompatibility complex identical but sex mismatched; thus, it was possible to prove that sustained engraftment of hematopoietic stem cells of donor origin was achieved. Activity of β-galactosidase in posttransplant leukocytes and in the liver normalized. Ganglioside GM1 concentrations diminished in the liver but not in cerebral tissue, and the recipient suffered progressive neurologic disease. There were no data presented, however, to show whether or nor marrow-derived cells of donor origin had repopulated the central nervous system. The latter may be necessary to efficiently process ganglioside GM1. Studies in humans and experimental animals have documented that dendritic cells in the skin, Kupffer cells in the liver, and pulmonary macrophages are eventually replaced by cells of donor origin, but the kinetics of repopulation can be variable.—J.A. Hansen, M.D.

27 Marrow Transplantation for Patients With Malignant Disease

---

Interphase Cytogenetic Analysis Detects Minimal Residual Disease in a Case of Acute Lymphoblastic Leukemia and Resolves the Question of Origin of Relapse After Allogeneic Bone Marrow Transplantation
Anastasi J, Thangavelu M, Vardiman JW, Hooberman AL, Bian ML, Larson RA, Le Beau MM (Univ of Chicago)
Blood 77:1087–1091, 1991   27–1

Introduction.—Recent advances in methodology have allowed the detection of numerical chromosomal abnormalities in interphase nuclei. Interphase cytogenetic testing was used in a patient with acute lymphoblastic leukemia (ALL) with a hyperdiploid karyotype and trisomy X. The information was used to determine the origin of relapse after a sex-mismatched bone marrow transplant (BMT).

Case Report.—Man, 23, had ALL and an abnormal hyperdiploid male karyotype (60 chromosomes) based on conventional cytogenetic testing of unstimulated BM and peripheral blood (PB) cells. He received standard systemic and intrathecal chemotherapy for the ALL and entered remission after 3 months. The remission BM cells demonstrated no evidence of leukemia. A routine BM biopsy showed relapse 6 months later, and the patient had a BMT with his sister as donor. Three months after BMT, all marrow metaphase cells were female. Relapse occurred again about 9 months later. All 40 metaphase cells examined in a BM biopsy specimen were of normal female karyotype, leading to speculation that the relapse occurred in the donor cells.

Methods.—The BM cells underwent routine cytogenetic analysis after air drying on glass slides and hybridization with a probe to the α-satellite region of the X chromosome. Four control BM samples were obtained from male patients undergoing BMT for nonhematopoietic malignancies.
Findings.—More than 80% of the patient's BM and PB cells showed 3 hybridization signals, indicating trisomy for the X chromosome. Interphase testing of the remission cells obtained 6 months before BMT showed that most nuclei had a single hybridization signal, indicating the normal complement of 1 X chromosome in a male. Yet, 16 of 1,000 nu-

clei showed 3 signals, which was a highly significant indication of trisomy X. The remission specimens taken after BMT contained no cells with 3 signals.

Conclusions.—Interphase testing may prove useful as an adjunct to conventional cytogenetic analysis for minimal disease after BMT. Previous reports of leukemia relapses in donor cells may have been inaccurate if they were verified by cytogenetic testing alone.

▶ This case report convincingly demonstrates how in situ hybridization with an informative probe to interphase cells from marrow and peripheral blood can add to the findings of conventional cytogenetic analysis, which is informative only for metaphase cells. Relying only on the latter, posttransplant relapse in this patient might have been attributed to a leukemic transformation in cells from the normal donor. Interphase hybridization with an X chromosome-specific probe, however, demonstrated the presence of nonmetaphase residual host cells bearing 3 X chromosomes. The original leukemia was known to have a hyperdiploid karyotype and trisomy X. Interphase analysis with informative probes will greatly improve the detection of minimal residual malignant disease and improve the sensitivity of testing for split chimerism.—J.A. Hansen, M.D.

Chemotherapy Compared With Bone Marrow Transplantation for Adults With Acute Lymphoblastic Leukemia in First Remission
Horowitz MM, Messerer D, Hoelzer D, Gale RP, Neiss A, Atkinson K, Barrett AJ, Büchner T, Freund M, Heil G, Hiddemann W, Kolb H-J, Löffler H, Marmont AM, Maschmeyer G, Rimm AA, Rozman C, Sobocinski KA, Speck B, Thiel E, Weisdorf DJ, Zwaan FE, Bortin MM (Med College of Wisconsin, Milwaukee; Biometric Center for Therapeutic Studies, Munich; Johann Wolfgang Goethe University, Frankfurt; Univ of California, Los Angeles; Universitat Innsbruck, Austria, et al)
Ann Intern Med 115:13–18, 1991   27–2

Introduction.—Chemotherapy and allogeneic or autologous bone marrow transplants are primary treatments for patients with acute lymphoblastic leukemia (ALL). To compare the efficacy of intensive postremission chemotherapy with allogeneic bone marrow transplantation in adults with ALL in first remission, data on 2 patient cohorts were retrospectively reviewed.

Methods.—Intensive postremission chemotherapy was administered to 484 patients and HLA-identical sibling bone marrow transplantation was performed in 251 patients. All patients were treated between 1980 and 1987. The chemotherapy cohort included all patients entered prospectively into 2 German multicenter trials, and the transplant cohort included data reported to the International Bone Marrow Transplant Registry (IBMTR) by 98 transplant teams.

Results.—The 5-year survival rates for both the transplant and chemotherapy groups were similar. The leukemia-free survival probability at 5 years was 38% for chemotherapy patients and 44% for transplant recipients. For both treatments, similar prognostic factors predicted treatment failures. There was no benefit of 1 treatment group over the other for any prognostic factor.

Conclusion.—There was no significant 5-year survival differences in either chemotherapy or bone marrow transplant patients in first remission ALL. Relapse rates were lower in the transplant group, but the 5-year survival rates for both groups were still similar.

▶ Lacking randomized trials to compare the ultimate benefit of consolidation and maintenance chemotherapy vs. autologous marrow transplants or allogeneic marrow transplants in first remission, there are no data available to directly compare comparable patient groups. Partial selection and time to treatment variables can bias the analysis in unpredictable ways. What is clear is that relapse rates are lower in patients who have received allogeneic marrow transplants, but nonleukemic causes of death are higher in these patients, and overall leukemia-free survival is not significantly different.—J.A. Hansen, M.D.

Treatment of Adult Acute Lymphoblastic Leukemia With Allogeneic Bone Marrow Transplantation. Multivariate Analysis of Factors Affecting Acute Graft-Versus-Host Disease, Relapse, and Relapse-Free Survival
Doney K, Fisher LD, Appelbaum FR, Buckner CD, Storb R, Singer J, Fefer A, Anasetti C, Beatty P, Bensinger W, Clift R, Hansen J, Hill R, Loughran TP Jr, Martin P, Petersen FB, Sanders J, Sullivan KM, Stewart P, Weiden P, Witherspoon R, Thomas ED (Fred Hutchinson Cancer Research Ctr; Univ of Washington, Seattle)
Bone Marrow Transplant 7:453–459, 1991   27–3

Background.—Acute lymphoblastic leukemia (ALL) has been treated with allogeneic marrow transplantation since 1972 at 4 institutions. Most of the patients have been children. A review of the results of marrow grafts in adults with ALL included a multivariate analysis to identify factors associated with acute graft-vs.-host disease (GVHD) or relapse and with increased relapse-free survival.

Patients.—During a 15.8-year period, 192 patients age 18 years or more with ALL were treated with genotypically HLA-identical marrow transplantation. Median age was 23 years. Eighty-nine patients were treated during a remission, the first remission in 41 cases and a second or subsequent remission in 46 cases. One hundred three patients were treated in marrow relapse, 37 in their first relapse and 50 in their second or later relapse. All patients received preparative treatment depending on their clinical state—3 received chemotherapy alone; the rest also received 9.2 to 17.5 Gy of total body irradiation. Methotrexate, cyclosporine, or both were given as prophylaxis against GVHD.

Findings.—Grade II to IV acute GVHD developed in 79 patients. Chronic GVHD developed in 28 of 122 patients who survived at least

100 days. For patients treated in their first remission, 5-year relapse-free survival was 21%, compared with 15% for those treated in a second or greater remission and 12% for those treated in relapse. On multivariate analysis, risk of developing acute GVHD was increased with increasing donor age. Transplantation during a first remission, younger patient age, and freedom from interstitial pneumonia were significantly associated with both increased survival and relapse-free survival. Patients treated during their first remission, male gender, and grades II to IV acute GVHD were associated with decreased probability of relapse.

Conclusions.—Adult patients with ALL treated early in the course of their disease and younger patients have improved relapse-free survival. Interstitial pneumonia has been the most significant factor affecting long-term survival. Improved control of GVHD and decrease in relapse rates are the major challenges for this group of patients.

▶ Relapse and, until recently, cytomegalovirus pneumonia have been the major causes of treatment failure for patients undergoing allogeneic marrow transplantation for ALL. Cure rates have been modest, as described by Doney et al., and results are improved when transplants have been performed in first remission as compared to relapse or subsequent remissions. It is assumed that ALL evolves into a more resistant disease when relapse occurs after intensive chemotherapy, but patient selection may also contribute to the better outcome of first remission transplants. Although there are prognostic factors that predict for high risk of relapse, some of these patients may have been already cured of ALL before transplantation. A prospective study in which patients are first stratified for relapse risk and then assigned to treatment arms at the time of initial diagnosis is needed to directly and critically address this important question. Eligibility for the transplant arm might be based on risk of relapse and availability of an HLA-identical sibling marrow donor.—J.A. Hansen, M.D.

▶ ↓ The following 2 studies (Abstracts 27–4 and 27–5) report results of randomized trials comparing 2 different dose schedules of total body irradiation (TBI) in combination with cyclophosphamide as preparative marrow ablative therapy for patients receiving HLA-identical marrow transplants for treatment of chronic myeloid leukemia (CML) and acute myeloid leukemia (AML). The overall results were remarkably similar for both studies. Probability of post-transplant relapse was lower in the higher dose TBI group (15.75 Gy over 7 days), but the probability of graft-vs.-host disease (GVHD) and transplant-related mortality was lower in the lower dose TBI group (12.0 Gy over 6 days). Overall disease-free survival, however, was equivalent in the 2 groups. The important finding here is that both AML and CML are radiation sensitive, and 15.75 Gy is a very effective antitumor dose. However, the toxicity of 15.75 Gy is significantly greater than 12.0 Gy. In addition, patients receiving 15.75 Gy were not as likely to complete the prescribed doses of methotrexate and cyclosporine administered for GVHD prophylaxis, and patients receiving incomplete GVHD prophylaxis were more likely to develop clinically significant GVHD. Relapsing leukemia is still a major problem in both CML and AML, thus efforts to deliver more intensive treatment safely, and better strategies for reducing regimen-related toxicity must be pursued.—J.A. Hansen, M.D.

Allogeneic Marrow Transplantation in Patients With Chronic Myeloid Leukemia in the Chronic Phase: A Randomized Trial of Two Irradiation Regimens
Clift RA, Buckner CD, Appelbaum FR, Bryant E, Bearman SI, Petersen FB, Fisher LD, Anasetti C, Beatty P, Bensinger WI, Doney K, Hill RS, McDonald GB, Martin P, Meyers J, Sanders J, Singer J, Stewart P, Sullivan KM, Witherspoon R, Storb R, Hansen JA, Thomas ED (Fred Hutchinson Cancer Research Ctr, Seattle; VA Med Ctr, Seattle; Univ of Washington, Seattle)
Blood 77:1660–1665, 1991   27–4

Introduction.—Total body irradiation (TBI) has been used to improve survival of patients undergoing allogeneic bone marrow transplantation during the chronic phase of chronic myeloid leukemia (CML). Previous trials in patients with advanced leukemia suggested that 15.75 Gy TBI given in 2.25 Gy daily fractions was the maximum tolerable exposure after 120 mg/kg cyclophosphamide followed by an allograft. In this randomized trial, 12.0 Gy and 15.75 Gy TBI regimens were compared in patients with CML in chronic phase receiving graft-vs.-host disease (GVHD) prophylaxis with cyclosporine and methotrexate.

Methods.—During the study period (May 1985 to September 1988) 57 patients were randomized to receive 12.0 Gy over 6 days and 59 were randomized to receive 15.75 Gy over 7 days. Marrow from HLA-identical siblings was infused within 24 hours of the last TBI exposure.

Results.— One patient died 13 days posttransplant of *Pseudomonas* septicemia without achieving engraftment. The remaining patients achieved engraftment as evidenced by recovery of peripheral granulocyte and platelet counts. Veno-occlusive disease of the liver (VOD) caused 2 deaths, both in the 15.75-Gy group. Twenty-eight of 32 transplant-related deaths occurred during the first year after transplantation. Probabilities of relapse at 4 years were 0.25 for the 12.0 group and 0 for the 15.75 group, but the lower relapse rate associated with higher doses of TBI did not improve survival because of higher mortality rates from causes other than relapse.

Conclusion.—The benefit of a low relapse rate with the 15.75-Gy regimen was offset by this regimen's increased transplant-related mortality. An improvement in overall outcome might be achieved by an intermediate dose of TBI, improved methods of delivering GVHD prophylaxis, effective measures to prevent or treat severe VOD, and the posttransplant administration of interferon.

Allogeneic Marrow Transplantation in Patients With Acute Myeloid Leukemia in First Remission: A Randomized Trial of Two Irradiation Regimens

Clift RA, Buckner CD, Appelbaum FR, Bearman SI, Petersen FB, Fisher LD, Anasetti C, Beatty P, Bensinger WI, Doney K, Hill RS, McDonald GB, Martin P, Sanders J, Singer J, Stewart P, Sullivan KM, Witherspoon R, Storb R, Hansen JA, Thomas ED (Fred Hutchinson Cancer Research Ctr, Seattle; Univ of Washington, Seattle)

Blood 76:1867–1871, 1990   27–5

Background.—Outcome in a group of 19 patients treated between 1976 and 1978 by the Seattle Marrow Transplant Team established the efficacy of allogeneic marrow transplantation as early consolidation therapy for acute myeloid leukemia (AML) in first remission. Since that time, a series of randomized trials evaluated approaches for improving survival in such patients. The results of 2 regimens of total body irradiation (TBI) in patients with AML in first remission receiving graft-vs.-host disease (GVHD) prophylaxis with cyclosporine (CSP) and methotrexate (MTX) were reported.

Patients.—Thirty-four patients were randomized to receive 12.0 Gy of TBI over 6 days and 37 were randomized to receive 15.75 Gy over 7 days after preparation with 120 mg/kg cyclophosphamide. Marrow from HLA-identical siblings was infused within 24 hours of the last TBI exposure.

Results.—Seventy patients had successful engraftment, as evidenced by recovery of peripheral granulocyte and platelet counts. The 3-year probability of transplant-related mortality was greater (Fig 27–1) for the 15.75-Gy group (0.32) than for the 12.0-Gy group (0.12). The probability of relapse was greater (Fig 27–2) in the 12.0-Gy group (0.35) than in the 15–75-Gy group (0.12). The 3-year actuarial probabilities for re-

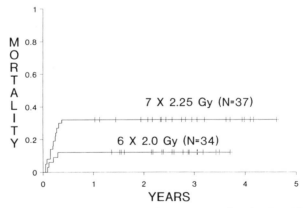

Fig 27–1.—Mortality in patients not relapsing after marrow transplantation ($P = .04$). Patients who relapsed were censored at the time of relapse. (Courtesy of Clift RA, Buckner CD, Appelbaum FR, et al: *Blood* 76:1867–1871, 1990.)

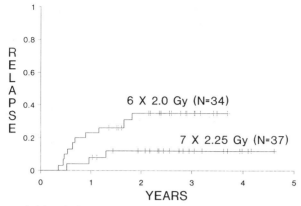

Fig 27–2.—Probability of relapse (P = .06). (Courtesy of Clift RA, Buckner CD, Appelbaum FR, et al: *Blood* 76:1867–1871, 1990.)

lapse-free survival were similar (Fig 27–3) for the 2 groups (0.58 with 12.0 Gy and 0.59 with 15.75 Gy) The incidence of moderate-to-severe GVHD was higher with the increased dose of TBI.

Conclusion.—Although the larger dose of TBI significantly reduced the probability of relapse, survival was not thereby improved because of increased mortality from other causes. In most cases, this increased mortality resulted from obstruction of the GVHD prophylaxis by radiation-induced tissue damage. An intermediate dose of TBI may permit the effective delivery of CSP and MTX.

Treatment for Acute Myelocytic Leukemia With Allogeneic Bone Marrow Transplantation Following Preparation With BuCy2

Copelan EA, Biggs JC, Thompson JM, Crilley P, Szer J, Klein JP, Kapoor N, Avalos BR, Cunningham I, Atkinson K, Downs K, Harmon GS, Daly MB, Brodsky I, Bulova SI, Tutschka PJ (Ohio State Univ, Columbus; St Vincent's Hospital, Sydney, Australia; Wilford Hall USAF Med Ctr, San Antonio; Hahnemann Univ, Philadelphia; Alfred Hospital, Melbourne)
Blood 78:838–843, 1991   27–6

Objective.—Allogeneic bone marrow transplantation (BMT) following high-dose chemotherapy and total body irradiation (TBI) can cure 45% to 50% of patients with acute myelocytic leukemia (AML). The combination of cyclophosphamide and TBI is a standard conditioning regimen for BMT, but a radiation-free regimen of oral busulfan and intravenous cyclophosphamide has been investigated. Results were assessed in 127 individuals with AML who underwent allogeneic marrow transplantation after receiving busulfan and cyclophosphamide.

Methods.—Patients with AML were given a radiation-free regimen of busulfan, 4 mg/kg, on each of 4 days plus cyclophosphamide, 60 mg/kg,

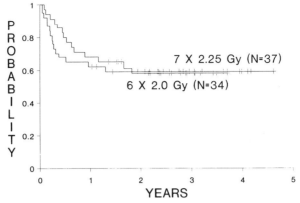

Fig 27–3.—Probability of surviving relapse-free after transplantation. (Courtesy of Clift RA, Buckner CD, Appelbaum FR, et al: *Blood* 76:1867–1871, 1990.)

on each of 2 days (BuCy2). Allogeneic bone marrow transplantation from an HLA-identical or 1-antigen-disparate sibling was performed.

Results.—The combined drugs produced a comparatively brief period of neutropenia and hospitalization compared to the regimen of cyclophosphamide plus TBI. The 3-year leukemia-free survival rate among 71 patients in first remission was 63.1%; it was 32.6% in the 23 patients in second complete remission or complete relapse, and 24.2% in 33 patients with primary refractory disease, second or subsequent relapse, or a preceding hematologic disorder. Relapse and decreased leukemia-free survival were associated with an advanced disease phase and with an M4/M5 French-American-British classification.

Conclusions.—The radiation-free preparative regimen of busulfan plus cyclophosphamide before allogeneic transplantation in patients with AML was as effective as a regimen including TBI. Prognostic factors for relapse and leukemia-free survival were similar for the 2 regimens described. Therapy with busulfan plus cyclophosphamide resulted in a low incidence of transplant-related deaths.

▶ This paper reports results of an alternate approach to achieving marrow ablation in patients with AML before allogeneic marrow transplantation. Clift et al. (Abstract 27–5) reported on the use of 2 TBI-containing regimens (cyclophosphamide, 120 mg/kg and TBI, 12.0 Gy or 15.75 Gy) and Copelan et al. (Abstract 27–6) describe results for a chemotherapy only regimen (busulfan, 16 mg/kg; and cyclophosphamide, 12.0 mg/kg): Overall probability of disease-free survival was not significantly different for the Bu/Cy vs. Cy/TBI regimens. Potential long-term complications were not addressed by either study. A more critical comparison of the 2 regimens would require a randomized trial. This endeavor has been initiated by the European Group for Bone Marrow Transplantation (1).—J.A. Hansen, M.D.

Reference

1. Blaise D, et al: *J Cell Biochem* 14A:282, 1990.

Bone Marrow Transplantation in Multiple Myeloma

Barlogie B, Gahrton G (Univ of Arkansas, Little Rock; Huddinge University Hospital, Huddinge, Sweden)
Bone Marrow Transplant 7:71–79, 1991   27–7

Background.—Because they are generally older and debilitated, patients with multiple myeloma have traditionally not been considered good candidates for high-dose treatment or marrow-ablative therapy requiring autologous or allogeneic stem cell grafting. However, some investigators are beginning to explore high-dose cytotoxic treatment for such patients.

Discussion.—The prognosis of patients with multiple myeloma has not improved with modifications of standard treatment. High doses of intravenously administered melphalan have yielded encouraging results and prompted interest in marrow-ablative treatment with hematopoietic stem cell support. Experience with about 400 patients given alkylating agents, occasionally with total body irradiation added, showed partial remissions in virtually all of those with advanced and refractory myeloma. Complete remissions, however, occurred in less than half of the patients, even when transplants were done for responsive disease with a low tumor burden.

Conclusions.—Hematopoietic stem cell grafting should be considered as part of an overall treatment strategy for patients with multiple myeloma to avoid irreversible normal hematopoietic stem cell damage from nitrosoureas and radiation to marrow-containing bones. Allogeneic bone marrow transplantation should be reserved for patients younger than 50 years, among whom transplant-related mortality usually does not exceed 30%. Forty percent will achieve complete remission, with a 3-year relapse-free survival expectation of 70%. Also, with autologous transplantation, a death rate of less than 10% and marked treatment benefits seem attainable if transplantation is performed when the tumor bulk is low and standard doses of treatment are still effective.

▶ As explained by Barlogie and Gahrton, multiple myeloma has not been a disease where high-dose cytotoxic therapy or marrow transplantation have played a significant role. However, as also explained by these investigators, the indications and expectations for aggressive therapy are becoming more apparent, and the likelihood of achieving complete remission as well as cure, especially for younger patients, argues strongly for a more determined approach to the treatment of this disease.—J.A. Hansen, M.D.

Treatment of Hemophagocytic Lymphohistiocytosis With Chemotherapy and Bone Marrow Transplantation: A Single-Center Study of 22 Cases

Blanche S, Caniglia M, Girault D, Landman J, Griscelli C, Fischer A (Hôpital des Enfants-Malades, Paris; Institut Gustave Roussy, Villejuif, France)
Blood 78:51–54, 1991   27–8

Background.—Familial hemophagocytic lymphohistiocytosis (FHL) is a rare and fatal disease characterized by onset before 18 months of age, high fever, hepatosplenomegaly, neurological symptoms, low fibrinogen levels, hypertriglyceridemia and pancytopenia with lymphocytes and histiocytes infiltrating the bone marrow, liver, and central nervous system. Phagocytosis of blood cells is a distinctive feature of this disease. The cause is unknown. Long-term remission has been reported with the cytotoxic drug epipodophylotoxin (VP16), but most patients eventually relapse. The long-term outcome of patients treated with chemotherapy is compared with that of patients who underwent marrow transplantation from a normal donor.

Methods.—Twenty-two children with FHL were treated with a regimen of VP16, corticosteroids, and intrathecal methotrexate. Nine patients received allogeneic BMT after treatment with VP16, busulfan, and cyclophosphamide.

Results.—Of the 22 children treated with chemotherapy alone, a sustained complete remission was obtained in 15 patients with a partial remission in 1 child. Ten of these children received maintenance chemotherapy alone leading to long-term remission in 2 children and a relapse in 8 children after cessation of therapy. Relapses were less sensitive to subsequent therapy, and death occurred within .5 to 6 months. Nine patients underwent BMT, 6 in remission and 3 in relapse. Four of the 6 children transplanted in remission are disease-free 1 to 6 years after transplant.

Conclusions.—Treatment of FHL with chemotherapy alone does not achieve cure, but marrow transplantation from an identical HLA match was successful in most cases in maintaining a prolonged remission without therapy. The relatively poor results of chemotherapy alone may justify studies of new chemotherapy protocols and HLA-mismatched or unrelated HLA-matched BMT.

▶ Although epidemiologic data suggest that FHL may be an autosomal-recessive disease, there is known genetic marker, and the disease often appears to be triggered by a viral illness (1, 2). Hyperactivation of monocytes and histocytes is the predominate pathologic feature of this disease. The underlying abnormality in these phagocytic cells may be genetic or acquired, possibly secondary to chronic activation or transformation of B cells or macrophages. The transplantation of hematopoietic stem cells after marrow-ablative high-dose cytotoxic therapy provides the opportunity for replacing the defective cells with normal donor-derived cells. Regardless of the mechanism responsible for FHL, the data presented here indicate that the pathogenesis of this disease is reversible after successful marrow transplantation.—J.A. Hansen, M.D.

References

1. Janka GE: *Eur J Pediatr* 140:221, 1983.
2. Nezelof C: *Pediatr Hematol Oncol* 6:207, 1989.

Subject Index

A

Acalculous
  cholecystitis after marrow transplant in
    acute leukemia, 298
Adhesion molecules
  ICAM-1 expression on epidermal
    keratinocytes in cutaneous
    graft-vs.-host disease, 271
  vessel-associated, in graft-vs.-host
    disease, 272
Age
  donor, influence on outcome, 113
  graft-vs.-host disease and, 254
Alloantigen
  induction of specific nonresponsiveness
    in T cells by, 179
Allogeneic
  lymphocyte proliferation in mixed
    lymphocyte kidney cell culture,
    failure of nephron components to
    induce (in rat), 204
Allograft (see Transplantation)
Alloreactivity
  regulation in vivo by IL-4 and soluble
    IL-4 receptor (in mice), 195
Allorecognition
  class II-restricted, impairment due to
    mutations affecting antigen
    processing, 209
Alveolar
  macrophages after lung transplantation,
    78
Amphotericin
  B nephrotoxicity after marrow
    transplant, effect of pentoxifylline
    on, 308
Anemia
  aplastic, marrow transplantation in
    graft-vs.-host disease prophylaxis in,
      in children, 323
    after liver transplant, in children,
      324
    solid malignant tumors after, 321
  Fanconi's, anti-LFA-1 CD11a and
    marrow transplant in, in children,
    241
Angiocardiography
  exercise radionuclide, before renal
    transplantation, 22
Anti-allo-class I H-2
  immune responses, heterogeneity of
    CD4$^+$ cells in (in mice), 210
Anti-asialo
  GM1 antiserum before marrow
    transplantation (in mice), 239

Anti-B-cell monoclonal antibodies
  for B-cell lymphoproliferative syndrome
    after marrow and organ
    transplantation, 131
Antibody(ies)
  anti-HLA
    adsorption with HLA class I
      immunosorbent beads, 8
    extracorporeal removal in transplant
      candidates, 7
    in heart transplantation, 72
  antiidiotypic
    production of (in rat), 73
    renal transplant outcome and, 139
  anti-OKT3, effect of cyclosporine on, 187
  to cytomegalovirus related to antibodies
    to T cell receptor/CD3 complex, 124
  mediated cardiac xenograft rejection,
    deoxyspergualin in (in rat), 170
  monoclonal
    anti-B-cell, for lymphoproliferative
      syndrome after marrow and organ
      transplantation, 131
    anti-CD3 (see Anti-CD3 antibody)
    anti-CD4, in heart transplantation (in
      rat), 137
    anticytomegalovirus, in marrow
      transplantation, 295
    anti-LFA-1 (see Anti-LFA-1 CD11a)
    anti-Tac (see Anti-Tac monoclonal
      antibody)
    anti-Tac-H, in heart transplantation
      (in monkey), 188
    ART-18, in heart and kidney
      transplantation (in rat), 12
    BWH-4, effect on accelerated
      rejection (in rat), 184
    in graft-vs.-host disease treatment,
      264, 265
    OKT3 (see OKT3)
  response after marrow transplantation,
    reconstitution of, 311
  to T cell receptor/CD3 complex,
    relation to antibodies to
    cytomegalovirus, 124
  to tumor necrosis factor, effects on
    allograft survival (in rat), 193
  2A3 in prevention of graft-vs.-host
    disease, 262
  xenoreactive, natural, ELISA assay for,
    199
Anti-CD3 antibody
  in hypersensitivity, delayed-type (in
    mice), 183
  induction of specific nonresponsiveness
    in T cells by, 179
  in islet transplantation (in mice), 183

337

lymphoproliferative syndrome after
transplantation, anti-B-cell
monoclonal antibodies for, 131
production in bone marrow, effect of
graft-vs.-host reaction on (in mice),
128
stimulation after transplantation and
interleukin-6 expression, 132
Beta-blockers
discontinuance before thallium stress
testing in renal transplant
candidates, 24
Biliary
cirrhosis, primary, symptom
development and prognosis in, 48
lipid metabolism after liver
transplantation, 50
Binephrectomy
before transplantation in autosomal
dominant polycystic kidney disease,
29
Biohybrid artificial pancreas
(in dog), 95, 96
Biopsy
aspiration, fine needle, differentiating
cytomegalovirus infection from
acute rejection in renal transplant,
122
CT-guided, of pancreas transplant, 89
cytoscopically directed needle, of
pancreatoduodenal allograft
dysfunction, 89
endoscopic, in intestinal graft-vs.-host
disease, 275
liver, donor, before transplantation, 49
percutaneous, of pancreas transplant,
87
Bleeding
complications of ventricular assist
device, 65
Blood
cells
red, CMV-seronegative, for
prevention of CMV infection after
marrow transplant, 288
white (*see* Leukocyte)
dendritic cells in, mature host, failure to
migrate into cardiac or skin
allografts (in mice), 206
peripheral, stem cells in (*see under* Stem
cells)
products
marrow donor, gamma irradiation of
(in dog), 301
radiation of, in prevention of
transfusion-associated graft-vs.-host
disease, 309

screening for prevention of CMV
infection after marrow
transplantation, 287
transfusion (*see* Transfusion)
B lymphocyte (*see* B cell)
BMT (*see* Bone marrow transplantation)
Bone marrow
B lymphocyte production in, effect of
graft-vs.-host reaction on (in mice),
128
interleukin-2-activated, adoptive
transfer of anti-cytomegalovirus
effect of (in mice), 290
stem cells transplanted to, IV, molecular
basis of homing to (in mice), 227
stromal cells transformed with simian
virus 40, regulation of cytokine and
growth factor gene expression in,
251
Bone marrow transplantation
allogeneic
GM-CSF after, 250
after irradiation, total body (in mice),
235
in anemia, aplastic (*see* Anemia,
aplastic, marrow transplantation
in)
anti-asialo GM1 antiserum before (in
mice), 239
antibody response after, reconstitution
of, 311
anticytomegalovirus monoclonal
antibody in, 295
anti-LFA-1 CD11a in (*see* Anti-LFA-1
CD11a)
autologous
in cancer patients, estimation of
circulating hematopoietic
progenitors for, 231
4-hydroxyperoxycyclophosphamide-
purged, hematologic recovery after,
243
stem cells after, peripheral blood, 229
T cell deficiencies after, clonal
analysis of, 317
B-cell differentiation after, 312
in breast cancer, CD34$^+$ cells in, 231
busulfan/cyclophosphamide
conditioning for (*see* Busulfan,
/cyclophosphamide)
CD6-depleted, reconstitution of T cell
function after, 315
chimerism after (*see* Chimerism)
colony-stimulating factor after,
granulocyte (in mice), 245
complications of, late, 318
cross-species, 143

C

hepatitis (*see* Hepatitis)
herpesvirus-6 infection, human, and interstitial pneumonitis after marrow transplant, 303
immunodeficiency, human, infection, and organ transplantation, 116
infectious, and graft-vs.-host reactions (in mice), 268
simian virus 40-transformed marrow stromal cells, regulation of cytokine and growth factor gene expression in, 251
vaccine, Towne live, effect on cytomegalovirus infection after renal transplant, 119

W

White blood cell (*see* Leukocyte)

X

Xenogeneic
stromal environment, stem cell engraftment in, 143

Xenoreactive
antibodies, natural, ELISA assay for, 199
Xenotransplantation
bone marrow, 143
cardiac
anti-Tac antibody in, yttrium-90-labeled (in monkey), 190
deoxyspergualin in (in rat), 170
induction of long-term survival (in rat), 197
ELISA assay for natural xenoreactive antibodies in, 199
islet
rejection prevention by masking donor HLA class I antigens (in mice), 198
survival and local release of mouse and rat antilymphocyte sera at transplant site, 200

Y

Yttrium-90
-labeled anti-Tac antibody in xenotransplantation (in monkey), 190

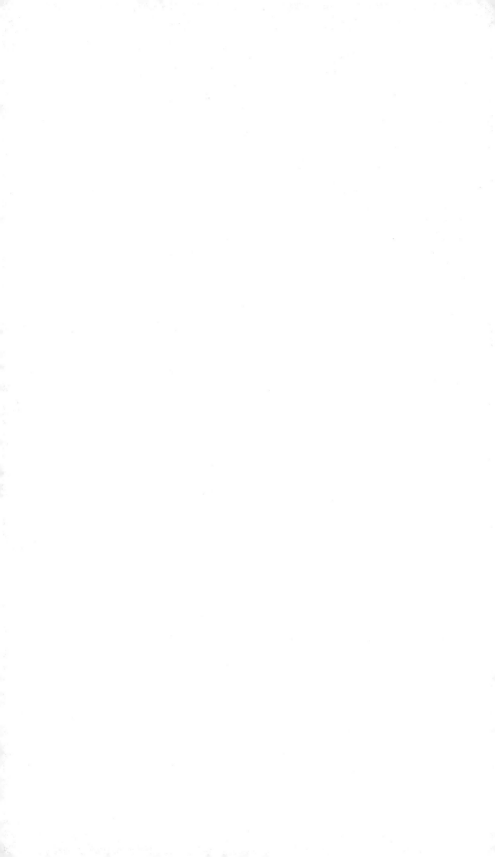

Author Index

A

Abe F, 274
Abedi MR, 313
Abramowicz D, 268
Adams DH, 59, 62
Adams RJ, 16
Aebischer P, 200
Agah R, 290
Agura E, 318
Ahern-Rindell A, 325
Akiyama N, 304
Alard P, 9
Alberti A, 300
Alessiani M, 151
Alexander JW, 113
Alexander SR, 109
Alfrey EJ, 182
Allen RDM, 87
Allison AC, 172
Almawi WY, 176
Almgren J, 308
Al-Muzairai IA, 139
Al-Saffar N, 270, 272
Alvord WG, 239
Ambinder RF, 283
Anasetti C, 179, 224, 261,
    262, 263, 323, 329, 331,
    332
Anasetti F, 318
Anastasi J, 327
Andersen J, 246
Anderson CB, 94, 142
Anderson CS, 309
Anderson J, 248
Anderson KC, 237, 309
Andrews DF III, 251
Andrews F, 308
Andrews RG, 231
Angelin B, 50
Angrisani L, 53
Appelbaum FR, 224, 247,
    250, 261, 262, 263, 265,
    301, 305, 318, 323, 325,
    329, 331, 332
Aragona E, 102
Arce CA, 246
Armbrust MJ, 15, 56
Armitage JM, 70
Armitage JO, 232, 248
Aroldi A, 158
Arthur M, 97
Arthur RS, 23
Arulnaden J-L, 51
Aschan J, 256, 259, 299
Aschendorff C, 31
Ascher NL, 46
Ash RC, 223, 295, 303
Aspinall R, 197
Asplund MW, 182
Atasoylu AA, 236, 281
Atkinson K, 249, 255, 328,
    333

Atluru D, 175
Atluru S, 175
Auchincloss H Jr, 86
Ault KA, 16
Austyn JM, 206
Avalos BR, 306, 333
Ayukawa K, 148
Azuma T, 210

B

Bach FH, 199
Bach J-F, 19, 186
Bacigalupo A, 258, 267, 300
Badger C, 318
Baker F, 320
Bakker A, 222
Bakris GL, 39
Balfour HH Jr, 116, 287
Ballard B, 308
Baltzan BL, 3
Baltzan MA, 3
Baltzan RB, 3
Banchereau J, 230
Banfi G, 32
Bär BMAM, 311
Barba L, 122
Barbier F, 101
Barker C, 119
Barker CF, 149, 182
Barker H, 206
Barlogie B, 335
Barr D, 89
Barrett AJ, 328
Bartucci MR, 156
Båryd I, 256
Bassett D, 91
Bastos MG, 183
Batchelor JR, 217
Bean MA, 301
Bearman SI, 224, 318, 331,
    332
Beatty PG, 224, 261, 262,
    263, 329, 331, 332
Beaumont P, 122
Beckmann MP, 195
Bélanger R, 221
Bell PRF, 91
Belli N, 231
Belzer FO, 15, 49, 56, 71,
    125
Benacerraf B, 209
Benhamou J-P, 37, 51
Benjamin WR, 188
Bensinger W, 231, 261, 329,
    331, 332
Berden JHM, 32
Berenson RJ, 231
Bernardino M, 89
Bernstein ID, 231
Bétuel H, 101
Bian ML, 327

Bianco J, 250, 308
Bickel U, 132
Bierman PJ, 248
Biggs J, 249
Biggs JC, 333
Bignon JD, 218
Billingham ME, 137
Bilo HJG, 160
Bismuth A, 51
Bismuth H, 51
Blakeman BM, 66
Blanche S, 131, 241, 335
Blazar B, 254, 276
Boehm DH, 169
Boggs SS, 143
Bohman S-O, 17, 18
Boland GJ, 121
Bolman RM III, 199
Bonadonna G, 231
Boon AP, 62
Bordigoni P, 131
Borland K, 95, 96
Bortin MM, 223, 255, 328
Bosserman L, 237, 315
Bowden RA, 288, 305
Bowman R, 287
Boxall JA, 21
Boyle PJ, 94
Brando B, 231
Brayman K, 119
Brechbiel MW, 190
Brechot C, 51
Breggia AC, 16
Bregni M, 231
Brehm G, 285
Brenner CA, 177
Bretan PN, 122
Breur-Vriesendorp BS, 215
Brezina M, 97
Bridge J, 217
Brinker KR, 155
Brochu S, 221
Brockmöller J, 132
Brodehl J, 31
Brodsky I, 333
Broelsch CE, 45
Bromberg JS, 182
Bronsther OL, 110
Brookes PA, 217
Brown PS Jr, 188
Brunner FP, 81
Bryant E, 331
Brynger H, 81
Bryson JS, 278
Büchner T, 328
Buckels JAC, 53, 62
Buckner CD, 224, 231, 247,
    250, 261, 305, 323, 329,
    331, 332
Budinger MD, 305
Bukowski MA, 188
Bulova SI, 333
Bunzendahl H, 61
Burakoff SJ, 240

363

A SIMPLE, ONCE-A-YEAR DOSE!

Review the partial list of titles below. And then request your own FREE 30-day preview. When you subscribe to a Year Book, we'll also send you an automatic notice of future volumes about two months before they publish.

This system was designed for your convenience and to take up as little of your time as possible. If you do not want the Year Book, the advance notice makes it easy for you to let us know. And if you elect to receive the new Year Book, you need do nothing. We will send it on publication.

No worry. No wasted motion. And, of course, every Year Book is yours to examine FREE of charge for thirty days.

Year Book of **Anesthesia**® (22141)
Year Book of **Cardiology**® (22640)
Year Book of **Critical Care Medicine**® (22639)
Year Book of **Dermatology**® (22645)
Year Book of **Dermatologic Surgery**® (21171)
Year Book of **Diagnostic Radiology**® (22613)
Year Book of **Digestive Diseases**® (22625)
Year Book of **Drug Therapy**® (22630)
Year Book of **Emergency Medicine**® (22080)
Year Book of **Endocrinology**® (21174)
Year Book of **Family Practice**® (22124)
Year Book of **Geriatrics and Gerontology** (22611)
Year Book of **Hand Surgery**® (22618)
Year Book of **Hematology**® (22646)
Year Book of **Health Care Management**® (21177)
Year Book of **Infectious Diseases**® (22650)
Year Book of **Infertility** (22637)
Year Book of **Medicine**® (22638)
Year Book of **Neonatal-Perinatal Medicine** (22629)
Year Book of **Nephrology** (21175)
Year Book of **Neurology and Neurosurgery**® (22616)
Year Book of **Neuroradiology**® (21849)
Year Book of **Nuclear Medicine**® (22627)
Year Book of **Obstetrics and Gynecology**® (22636)
Year Book of **Occupational and Environmental Medicine** (22619)
Year Book of **Oncology** (22651)
Year Book of **Ophthalmology**® (22133)
Year Book of **Orthopedics**® (22644)
Year Book of **Otolaryngology – Head and Neck Surgery**® (22609)
Year Book of **Pathology and Clinical Pathology**® (21176)
Year Book of **Pediatrics**® (22130)
Year Book of **Plastic and Reconstructive Surgery**® (22635)
Year Book of **Psychiatry and Applied Mental Health**® (22649)
Year Book of **Pulmonary Disease**® (22624)
Year Book of **Sports Medicine**® (22111)
Year Book of **Surgery**® (22641)
Year Book of **Transplantation**® (21854)
Year Book of **Ultrasound** (21169)
Year Book of **Urology**® (22621)
Year Book of **Vascular Surgery**® (22612)

Mosby-Year Book, Inc. • 11830 Westline Industrial Drive • St. Louis, MO 63146